RN
Expert
Guides

Neurologic Care

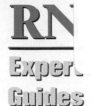

Wolters Kluwer | Lippincott Williams & Wilkins
Health
Philadelphia • Baltimore • New York • London
Buenos Aires • Hong Kong • Sydney • Tokyo

STAFF

EXECUTIVE PUBLISHER
Judith A. Schilling McCann, RN, MSN

EDITORIAL DIRECTOR
H. Nancy Holmes

CLINICAL DIRECTOR
Joan M. Robinson, RN, MSN

ART DIRECTOR
Elaine Kasmer

EDITORS
Jennifer A. Kowalak, Julie Munden

CLINICAL PROJECT MANAGER
Kate Stout, RN, MSN, CCRN

COPY EDITORS
Kimberly Bilotta (supervisor),
Heather Ditch, Jeannine Fielding,
Amy Furman, Dona Perkins,
Pamela Wingrod

DESIGNER
Debra Moloshok

DIGITAL COMPOSITION SERVICES
Diane Paluba (manager),
Joyce Rossi Biletz, Donna S. Morris

MANUFACTURING
Beth J. Welsh

EDITORIAL ASSISTANTS
Megan L. Aldinger, Karen J. Kirk,
Jeri O'Shea, Linda K. Ruhf

INDEXER
Patricia Perrier

RNEGN010707

**Library of Congress
Cataloging-in-Publication Data**

RN expert guides. Neurologic care.
    p. ; cm.
    Includes bibliographical references and index.
    1. Neurological nursing—Handbooks, manuals, etc. I. Lippincott Williams & Wilkins.
    [DNLM: 1. Nervous System Diseases—nursing. 2. Nursing Care—methods. WY 160.5 R627 2008]
    RC350.5.R54 2008
    616.8'04231—dc22
ISBN-13: 978-1-58255-706-9 (alk. paper)
ISBN-10: 1-58255-706-3 (alk. paper)
               2007012521

Contents

───────○───────

Contributors and consultants

Laura M. Criddle, RN, PhD(c), CCRN, CEN, CNRN
Clinical Nurse Specialist
Premier Jets/Lifeguard Air Ambulance
Hilsboro, Ore.

Diana Everley, RN, BSN, CNRN, BC
Staff Development Specialist
Deaconess Hospital
Evansville, Ind.

Ellie Franges, APRN-BC, MSN, CNRN
Nurse Practitioner—Neurosurgery
St. Luke's Hospital and Health Network
Bethlehem, Pa.

Fiona S. Johnson, RN, MSN, CCRN
Clinical Education Specialist
CCU/CVICU RN
Memorial Health University Medical Center
Savannah, Ga.

Debi Murphy, RN, MSN, CRNP
Stroke Program Coordinator
Abington (Pa.) Memorial Hospital

Angela Starkweather, PhD, ACNP, CCRN, CNRN
Assistant Professor
Washington State University
Intercollegiate College of Nursing
Spokane

Patricia Ann Zrelak, RN, PhD, CNAA-BC, CNRN
Administrative Nurse Researcher
Center for Health Services Research in Primary Care
University of California, Davis
Adjunct Professor of Nursing
Samuel Merritt College
Sacramento

Anatomy and physiology

The nervous system serves as the body's communication network. It processes information from the outside world, through the sensory portion, and coordinates and organizes the functions of all other body systems. Its far-reaching effects can be seen when patients, who suffer from diseases of other body systems, develop neurologic impairments related to the disease. For example, the patient who has heart surgery could suffer a stroke.

The neurologic system is divided into the central nervous system (CNS), the peripheral nervous system, and the autonomic nervous system (ANS). Through complex and coordinated interactions, these three systems integrate all physical, intellectual, and emotional activities. Understanding how each works is essential to conducting an accurate neurologic assessment.

NERVOUS SYSTEM CELLS

Two major cell types, neurons and neuroglia, compose the nervous system. The neuron is the fundamental unit of the nervous system. It's a highly specialized conductor cell that transmits and receives electrochemical nerve impulses. Delicate, threadlike nerve fibers extend from the central cell body to transmit impulses—axons carry these impulses away from the cell body, whereas dendrites carry impulses to it. Most

STRUCTURE OF THE NEURON

The basic structure of the neuron is composed of the cell body, axon, and dendrites, as depicted below.

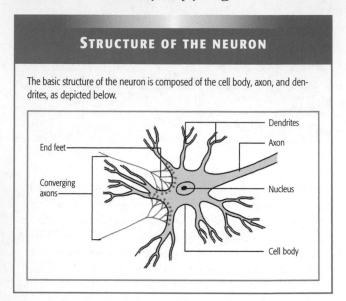

neurons have multiple dendrites but only one axon. (See *Structure of the neuron.*)

Sensory (afferent) neurons transmit impulses from special receptors to regulate activity in the brain and spinal cord. Motor (efferent) neurons transmit impulses from the CNS to regulate activity in muscles or glands, whereas interneurons (connecting or association neurons) shuttle signals through complex pathways between sensory and motor neurons. Interneurons account for 99% of all the neurons in the nervous system and include most of the neurons in the brain itself.

Neuroglial cells, or *glial cells* (derived from the Greek word for glue because they hold the neurons together), serve as the supportive cells of the CNS and form roughly 40% of the brain's bulk. The four types of neuroglial cells include:

■ *Astroglia,* or astrocytes, exist throughout the nervous system and form part of the blood-brain barrier. They supply nutrients to the neurons and help maintain their electrical potential.

- *Ependymal cells* line the brain's four ventricles and the choroid plexus and help produce cerebrospinal fluid (CSF).
- *Microglia* phagocytize waste products from injured neurons and are deployed throughout the nervous system.
- *Oligodendroglia* support and electrically insulate CNS axons by forming protective myelin sheaths.

CENTRAL NERVOUS SYSTEM

The CNS includes the brain and the spinal cord. These two major structures collect and interpret voluntary and involuntary motor and sensory stimuli. (See *Major structures of the central nervous system,* page 4.)

The brain and spinal cord engage in an intricate network of interlocking receptors and transmitters, ultimately forming a dynamic control system — a "living computer" — that oversees and regulates every mental and physical function. Indeed, from birth to death, the CNS efficiently organizes the body's affairs — controlling the smallest action, thought, or feeling; monitoring communication and the instinct for survival; and allowing introspection, wonder, and abstract thought.

The brain, the center of the CNS, is a large, soft mass of nervous tissue that's housed within the cranium and supported by the meninges. The brain and spinal cord are protected by bone (the skull and vertebrae), which cushions CSF, and three membranes:

- *dura mater,* or outer sheath, made of tough, white fibrous tissue
- *arachnoid membrane,* the delicate, lacelike middle layer
- *pia mater,* the inner meningeal layer, consisting of fine blood vessels held together by connective tissue. (This membrane is thin and transparent and clings to the brain and spinal cord surfaces, carrying branches of the cerebral arteries deep into the brain's fissures and sulci.)

Between the dura matter and the arachnoid membrane is the subdural space; between the arachnoid membrane and the

MAJOR STRUCTURES OF THE CENTRAL NERVOUS SYSTEM

This illustration shows a cross section of the major structures of the central nervous system – the brain and spinal cord. The brain joins the spinal cord at the base of the skull and ends between the first and second lumbar vertebrae. Note the H-shaped mass of gray matter in the spinal cord.

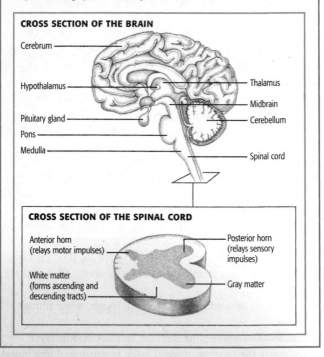

CROSS SECTION OF THE BRAIN

Cerebrum

Hypothalamus

Pituitary gland

Pons

Medulla

Thalamus

Midbrain

Cerebellum

Spinal cord

CROSS SECTION OF THE SPINAL CORD

Anterior horn
(relays motor impulses)

White matter
(forms ascending and
descending tracts)

Posterior horn
(relays sensory
impulses)

Gray matter

pia mater is the subarachnoid space. Within the subarachnoid space and the brain's four ventricles is the aforementioned CSF — a substance comprised of water and traces of organic materials (especially protein), glucose, and minerals. CSF is formed from blood in capillary networks called *choroid plexi*, which are located primarily in the brain's lateral ventricles.

CSF is eventually reabsorbed into the venous blood through the arachnoid villi, in dural sinuses on the brain's surface.

Brain

The brain consists of the cerebrum, or cerebral cortex, the brain stem, the cerebellum, the limbic system, and the reticular activating system (RAS). It collects, integrates, and interprets all stimuli and initiates and monitors voluntary and involuntary motor activity.

CEREBRUM

The cerebrum, the largest portion of the brain, houses the nerve center that controls motor and sensory functions and intelligence. It's encased by the skull and enclosed by three membrane layers called *meninges*. If blood or fluid accumulates between these layers, pressure builds inside the skull and compromises brain function. The surface layer of the cerebrum is the cerebral cortex, which is composed of unmyelinated cell bodies called *gray matter.* Additionally, the cerebrum has a rolling surface made up of convolutions, called *gyri,* and creases or fissures, called *sulci.*

The cerebrum consists of a left and right hemisphere, joined by the corpus callosum — a mass of nerve fibers that allows for communication between the hemispheres and for sharing learning and intellect. However, these two hemispheres don't share equally; one always dominates, giving one side control over the other. Because motor impulses descending from the brain through the pyramidal tract intersect in the medulla, the right hemisphere controls the left side of the body, whereas the left hemisphere controls the right side of the body.

Several fissures divide the cerebrum into lobes, each of which is associated with specific functions. To that end, each hemisphere is divided into four lobes, based on anatomic landmarks and functional differences. The lobes are named for the cranial bones that lie over them: the frontal, temporal, parietal, and occipital.

- The *frontal lobe* influences personality, judgment, abstract reasoning, social behavior, language expression, and movement.
- The *temporal lobe* controls hearing, language comprehension, and the storage and recall of memories, although some memories are stored throughout the brain.
- The *parietal lobe* interprets and integrates sensations, including pain, temperature, and touch. It also interprets size, shape, distance, and texture. The parietal lobe of the non-dominant hemisphere, usually the right, is especially important for awareness of body schema or shape.
- The *occipital lobe* functions primarily in interpreting visual stimuli.

In addition, cranial nerves (CNs) I and II originate in the cerebrum. The cerebrum is considered the area involving upper motor neuron function. (See *The cerebrum and its functions*.)

The diencephalon, a division of the cerebrum, contains the thalamus and hypothalamus. The thalamus is a relay station for sensory impulses as they ascend to the cerebral cortex. Its functions include primitive awareness of pain, screening of incoming stimuli, and focusing of attention and emotional response. The *hypothalamus* lies beneath the thalamus and is an autonomic center that has connections with the brain, spinal cord, ANS, and pituitary gland. It regulates temperature, appetite, blood pressure, breathing, sleep patterns, and peripheral nerve discharges that occur with behavioral and emotional expression. It also partially controls pituitary gland secretion and stress reaction.

BRAIN STEM

The brain stem lies below the diencephalon and is divided into the midbrain, pons, and medulla. These three parts provide two-way conduction between the spinal cord and brain.

The brain stem relays messages between the parts of the nerous system. It has three main functions that include producing the rigid autonomic behaviors necessary for survival,

THE CEREBRUM AND ITS FUNCTIONS

The cerebrum is divided into four lobes, based on anatomic landmarks and functional differences. The lobes – parietal, occipital, temporal, and frontal – are named for the cranial bones that lie over them.

This illustration shows the locations of the cerebral lobes and explains their functions. It also shows the location of the cerebellum.

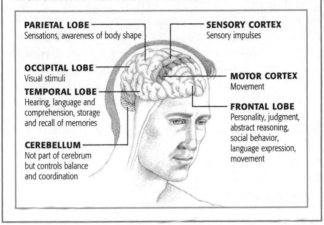

PARIETAL LOBE
Sensations, awareness of body shape

OCCIPITAL LOBE
Visual stimuli

TEMPORAL LOBE
Hearing, language and comprehension, storage and recall of memories

CEREBELLUM
Not part of cerebrum but controls balance and coordination

SENSORY CORTEX
Sensory impulses

MOTOR CORTEX
Movement

FRONTAL LOBE
Personality, judgment, abstract reasoning, social behavior, language expression, movement

such as increasing the heart rate and stimulating the adrenal medulla to produce epinephrine; providing the pathways for nerve fibers between higher and lower neural centers; and serving as the origin for 10 of the 12 pairs of cranial nerves.

The midbrain is the origination site for CNs III and IV and the corticospinal tract, which is the main motor pathway from the cerebrum. The midbrain mediates the auditory and visual reflexes.

The pons is the origination site for CNs V, VI, and VII and it contains one of the respiratory centers. The pons connects the cerebellum to the cerebrum and the midbrain to the medulla. The pons mediates such actions as chewing, taste, saliva secretion, hearing, and equilibrium.

The medulla is the origination site for CNs VIII to XII. It joins the spinal cord at the level of the foramen magnum — an opening in the occipital portion of the skull. The medulla regulates respiratory, vasomotor, and cardiac function. It's the center that controls vomiting, coughing, and hiccupping reflexes. Areas below the cerebrum are considered the areas involving lower motor neuron function.

CEREBELLUM

The cerebellum, the most posterior part of the brain lying behind and below the cerebrum, is the brain's second largest region. It contains the major motor and sensory pathways. It facilitates smooth, coordinated muscle movement and helps to maintain equilibrium.

LIMBIC SYSTEM

The limbic system is a primitive brain area deep within the temporal lobe. In addition to initiating basic drives, such as hunger, aggression, and emotional and sexual arousal, the limbic system screens all sensory messages traveling to the cerebral cortex.

RETICULAR ACTIVATING SYSTEM

The RAS is a diffuse network of hyperexcitable neurons. It fans out from the brain stem through the cerebral cortex. After screening all incoming sensory information, the RAS channels it to appropriate areas of the brain for interpretation. It functions as the arousal, or alerting, system for the cerebral cortex, and its functioning is crucial for maintaining consciousness.

VASCULAR SUPPLY

Four major arteries — two vertebral and two carotid — supply the brain with oxygenated blood. The two vertebral arteries, which are branches of the subclavians, converge to become the basilar artery. The basilar artery supplies oxygen to the posterior brain.

The two carotid arteries branch into the two internal carotids, which divide further to supply oxygen to the anterior brain and the middle brain. These arteries interconnect through the circle of Willis—an anastomosis at the base of the brain. The circle of Willis ensures that oxygen is continuously circulated to the brain despite interruption of any of the brain's major vessels.

Spinal cord

The spinal cord is the primary pathway for messages traveling between the body's peripheral areas and the brain. It extends from the upper border of the first cervical vertebrae to the lower border of the first lumbar vertebrae. The spinal cord is encased in the spinal column by the uninterrupted meningeal linings and spinal fluid that protect the brain. The spinal cord is further protected by the bony vertebrae and the intervertebral disks. At the spinal cord's inferior end, nerve roots cluster in the cauda equina.

A cross section of the spinal cord reveals a central H-shaped mass of gray matter divided into dorsal (posterior) and ventral (anterior) horns. These horns are primarily made up of neuron cell bodies. Cell bodies in the two dorsal horns relay sensory, or afferent, impulses; those in the two ventral horns relay motor, or efferent, impulses, thus playing a part in voluntary and reflex motor activity. White matter surrounds the horns and consists of myelinated axons of sensory and motor nerve fibers grouped in vertical columns, or tracts, which form the ascending and descending tracts. (See *Cross section of the spinal cord,* page 10.)

SENSORY PATHWAYS

Sensory impulses travel via the afferent, also called *sensory* or *ascending,* neural pathways to the sensory cortex in the brain's parietal lobe. Here, the impulses are interpreted using two major pathways: the dorsal horn and the ganglia.

Pain and temperature sensations enter the spinal cord through the dorsal horn. After immediately crossing over to

CROSS SECTION OF THE SPINAL CORD

The cross section of the spinal cord below shows the anterior and posterior segments.

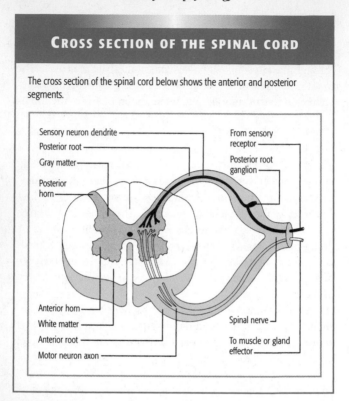

Sensory neuron dendrite
Posterior root
Gray matter
Posterior horn
Anterior horn
White matter
Anterior root
Motor neuron axon

From sensory receptor
Posterior root ganglion
Spinal nerve
To muscle or gland effector

the opposite side of the spinal cord, these impulses then travel to the thalamus via the spinothalamic tract.

Touch, pressure, and vibration sensations enter the spinal cord via relay stations called *ganglia*. Ganglia are knotlike masses of nerve cell bodies on the dorsal roots of spinal nerves. Impulses travel up the spinal cord in the dorsal column to the medulla, where they cross to the opposite side and enter the thalamus. The thalamus relays all incoming sensory impulses, except olfactory impulses, to the sensory cortex for interpretation.

MOTOR PATHWAYS

Motor impulses travel from the brain to the muscles via the efferent, also known as the *motor* or *descending,* neural pathways. Motor impulses originate in the motor cortex of the frontal lobe and reach the lower motor neurons of the peripheral nervous system via upper motor neurons.

Upper motor neurons originate in the brain and form two major systems that include the pyramidal system and extrapyramidal system.

The pyramidal system, or corticospinal tract, is responsible for the fine, skilled movements of skeletal muscle. Impulses in this system travel from the motor cortex through the internal capsule to the medulla. At the medulla they cross to the opposite side and continue down the spinal cord.

The extrapyramidal system, or extracorticospinal tract, controls gross motor movements. Impulses originate in the premotor area of the frontal lobes and travel to the pons. At the pons the impulses cross to the opposite side, then travel down the spinal cord to the anterior horns, where they're relayed to the lower motor neurons. These neurons, in turn, carry the impulses to the muscles. (See *How neurotransmission occurs,* page 12.)

REFLEXES

The spinal cord mediates the sensory-to-motor transmission path known as the *reflex arc.* Because the reflex arc enters and exits the spinal cord at the same level, reflex pathways don't need to travel up and down as other stimuli. Reflex responses occur automatically, without brain involvement, to protect the body. For example, if the brain can't send a message to a patient's leg after a severe spinal cord injury, a stimulus can still cause a knee jerk, or patellar, reflex as long as the spinal cord remains intact at the level of the reflex. (See *Functioning of the reflex arc,* page 13.)

Spinal nerves, which have sensory and motor portions, mediate deep tendon reflexes (DTRs; involuntary contractions

How neurotransmission occurs

Neurotransmission occurs when sensory and motor impulses travel through different pathways to the brain for interpretation. Typically, these impulses trigger sensations, such as touch, pressure, and vibration as well as muscle movement.

Sensory pathways

Sensory impulses travel through two major sensory (afferent or ascending) pathways to the sensory cortex in the cerebrum.

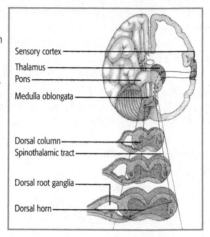

Sensory cortex
Thalamus
Pons
Medulla oblongata

Dorsal column
Spinothalamic tract

Dorsal root ganglia

Dorsal horn

Motor pathways

Motor impulses travel from the motor cortex in the cerebrum to the muscles via motor (efferent, or descending) pathways.

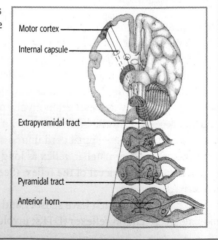

Motor cortex
Internal capsule

Extrapyramidal tract

Pyramidal tract
Anterior horn

FUNCTIONING OF THE REFLEX ARC

Spinal nerves, which have sensory and motor portions, control deep tendon and superficial reflexes. A simple reflex arc requires a sensory, or afferent, neuron and a motor, or efferent, neuron. The knee jerk, or patellar, reflex illustrates the sequence of events in a normal reflex arc.

First, a sensory receptor detects the mechanical stimulus produced by the reflex hammer striking the patellar tendon. Then, the sensory neuron carries the impulse along its axon by way of the spinal nerve to the dorsal root, where it enters the posterior horn of the spinal cord.

Next, in the anterior horn of the spinal cord, as illustrated here, the sensory neuron joins with a motor neuron, which carries the impulse along its axon by way of a spinal nerve to the muscle. The motor neuron transmits the impulse to the muscle fibers through stimulation of the motor end plate. This triggers the muscle to contract and the leg to extend.

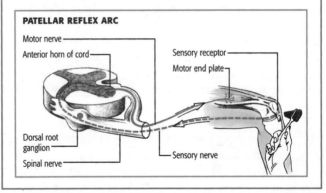

PATELLAR REFLEX ARC

Motor nerve
Anterior horn of cord
Sensory receptor
Motor end plate
Dorsal root ganglion
Sensory nerve
Spinal nerve

of a muscle after brief stretching caused by tendon percussion), superficial reflexes (withdrawal reflexes elicited by noxious or tactile stimulation of the skin, cornea, or mucous membranes) and, in infants, primitive reflexes.

DTRs include reflex responses of the biceps, triceps, brachioradialis, patellar, and Achilles tendons. The biceps reflex contracts the biceps muscle and forces flexion of the forearm, whereas the triceps reflex contracts the triceps muscle and forces extension of the forearm. The brachioradialis reflex causes supination of the hand and flexion of the forearm at the elbow. The patellar reflex forces contraction of the quadriceps muscle in the thigh with extension of the leg. Last, the Achilles reflex forces plantar flexion of the foot at the ankle.

Superficial reflexes are reflexes of the skin and mucous membranes. Successive attempts to stimulate these reflexes provoke increasingly limited responses. Superficial reflexes include plantar flexion of the toes, the cremasteric reflex, and the abdominal reflex. Plantar flexion of the toes occurs when the lateral sole of an adult's foot is stroked from heel to great toe with a tongue blade. Babinski's reflex causes upward movement of the great toe and fanning of the little toes in children younger than age 2 in response to stimulation of the outer margin of the sole of the foot. In men, the cremasteric reflex is stimulated by stroking the inner thigh. This forces the contraction of the cremaster muscle and elevation of the testicle on the side of the stimulus. The abdominal reflex is induced by stroking the sides of the abdomen above and below the umbilicus, moving from the periphery toward the midline. Movement of the umbilicus toward the stimulus is normal.

AGE AWARE Primitive reflexes are abnormal in an adult but normal in an infant, whose CNS is immature. As the nervous system matures, these reflexes disappear. Primitive reflexes include grasping, sucking, and glabella. Grasping involves the application of gentle pressure to an infant's palm, which results in grasping. The infantile sucking reflex to ingest milk is a primitive response to oral stimuli. The glabella reflex is elicited by repeatedly tapping the bridge of the infant's nose, with a normal response being persistent blinking.

DERMATOMES

For the purpose of documenting sensory function, the body is divided into dermatomes. Each dermatome represents an area supplied with afferent, or sensory, nerve fibers from an individual spinal root — cervical, thoracic, lumbar, or sacral. This body "map" is used when testing sensation and trying to identify the source of a lesion. (See *Identifying dermatomes.*)

IDENTIFYING DERMATOMES

Knowledge of dermatomes is useful to localize neurologic lesions. These illustrations demonstrate the patterns of dermatomes on the body.

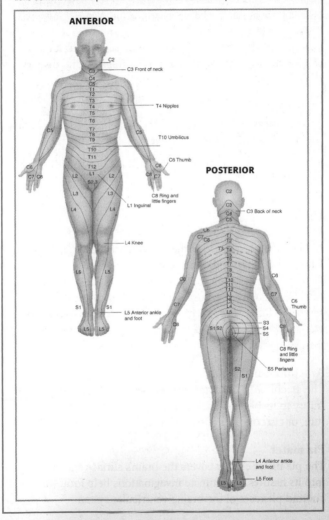

Protective structures

Bone, meninges, and CSF protect the brain and the spinal cord from shock and infection.

BONE

Formed of cranial bones, the skull completely surrounds the brain and opens at the base, called the *foramen magnum,* where the spinal cord exits.

The vertebral column protects the spinal cord. It consists of 30 vertebrae, each separated by an intervertebral disk that allows flexibility.

MENINGES

The meninges cover and protect the cerebral cortex and spinal column. They consist of three layers of connective tissue that include the dura mater, the arachnoid membrane, and the pia mater. (See *Protecting the central nervous system.*)

Dura mater

The dura mater lines the skull and forms folds, called *reflections,* that descend into the brain's fissures and provide stability. The dural folds include the falx cerebri, which lies in the longitudinal fissure and separates the cerebrum's hemispheres; the tentorium cerebelli, which separates the cerebrum from the cerebellum; and the falx cerebelli, which separates the two cerebellar lobes. The arachnoid villi, projections of the dura mater into the superior sagittal and transverse sinuses, serve as the exit points for CSF drainage into venous circulation.

Arachnoid membrane

The arachnoid membrane lies between the dura and pia mater. Injury to its blood vessels during head trauma, lumbar puncture, or cisternal puncture may cause hemorrhage.

Pia mater

The pia mater closely covers the brain's surface and extends into its fissures. Its intimate invaginations help form the choroid plexuses of the brain's ventricular system.

PROTECTING THE CENTRAL NERVOUS SYSTEM

Three primary membranes, or meninges, help protect the central nervous system: the dura mater, the arachnoid membrane, and the pia mater.

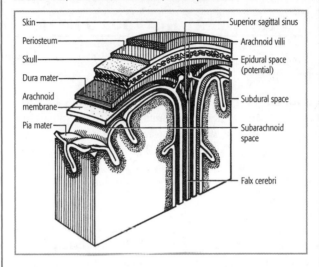

Additional layers

Three layers of space further cushion the brain and spinal cord against injury. The epidural space (a potential space) lies over the dura mater. The subdural space lies between the dura mater and the arachnoid membrane and is commonly the site of hemorrhage after head trauma. The subarachnoid space, which is filled with CSF, lies between the arachnoid membrane and the pia mater.

CEREBROSPINAL FLUID

CSF nourishes cells, transports metabolic waste, and cushions the brain. This colorless fluid circulates through the ventricular system, into the subarachnoid space of the brain and spinal cord, and back to the venous sinuses on top of the brain where it's reabsorbed. The ependymal cells that cover the surface of the choroid plexus, which is a tangled mass of tiny blood vessels lining the ventricles, constantly produce CSF at a rate of about 150 ml per day.

PERIPHERAL NERVOUS SYSTEM

The peripheral nervous system consists of the peripheral and cranial nerves.

Peripheral nerves

Peripheral sensory nerves transmit stimuli to the spinal cord's dorsal horn from sensory receptors located in the skin, muscles, sensory organs, and viscera. The upper motor neurons of the brain and the lower motor neurons of the cell bodies in the spinal cord's ventral horn carry impulses that affect movement.

Cranial nerves

The 12 pairs of cranial nerves transmit motor or sensory messages, or both, primarily between the brain or brain stem and the head and neck. All cranial nerves, except the olfactory and optic nerves, exit from the midbrain, pons, or medulla oblongata of the brain stem. (See *Functions of the cranial nerves.*)

AUTONOMIC NERVOUS SYSTEM

The vast autonomic nervous system (ANS) enervates all internal organs. Also known as the *visceral efferent nerves,* the nerves of the ANS carry messages to the viscera from the brain stem and neuroendocrine system. The ANS has two major divisions: the sympathetic and the parasympathetic nervous systems.

FUNCTIONS OF THE CRANIAL NERVES

The 12 pairs of cranial nerves (CNs) transmit motor or sensory messages, or both, primarily between the brain or brain stem and the head and neck. All cranial nerves, except for the olfactory and optic nerves, exit from the midbrain, pons, or medulla of the brain stem.

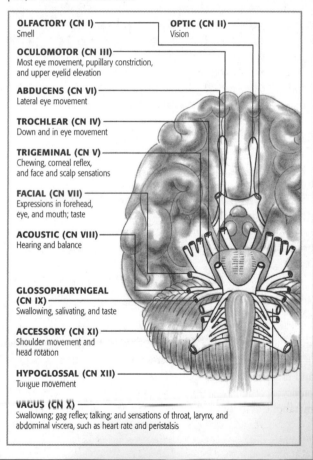

OLFACTORY (CN I)
Smell

OPTIC (CN II)
Vision

OCULOMOTOR (CN III)
Most eye movement, pupillary constriction, and upper eyelid elevation

ABDUCENS (CN VI)
Lateral eye movement

TROCHLEAR (CN IV)
Down and in eye movement

TRIGEMINAL (CN V)
Chewing, corneal reflex, and face and scalp sensations

FACIAL (CN VII)
Expressions in forehead, eye, and mouth; taste

ACOUSTIC (CN VIII)
Hearing and balance

GLOSSOPHARYNGEAL (CN IX)
Swallowing, salivating, and taste

ACCESSORY (CN XI)
Shoulder movement and head rotation

HYPOGLOSSAL (CN XII)
Tongue movement

VAGUS (CN X)
Swallowing; gag reflex; talking; and sensations of throat, larynx, and abdominal viscera, such as heart rate and peristalsis

Sympathetic nervous system

Sympathetic nerves, called *preganglionic neurons,* exit the spinal cord between T1 and L2. After these nerves leave the spinal cord, they enter small relay stations, the ganglia, near the spinal cord. The ganglia form a chain that disseminates the impulse to postganglionic neurons. These neurons reach many organs and glands and can produce widespread, generalized responses.

The physiologic effects of sympathetic activity include vasoconstriction; elevated blood pressure; enhanced blood flow to skeletal muscles; increased heart rate and contractility; heightened respiratory rate; smooth-muscle relaxation of the bronchioles, GI tract, and urinary tract; sphincter contraction; pupillary dilation and ciliary muscle relaxation; increased sweat gland secretion; and reduced pancreatic secretion.

Parasympathetic nervous system

The fibers of the parasympathetic nervous system leave the CNS via the cranial nerves from the midbrain and medulla and from the spinal nerves between S2 and S4.

After leaving the CNS, the long preganglionic fiber of each parasympathetic nerve travels to a ganglion near a particular organ or gland; the short postganglionic fiber enters the organ or gland. This creates a more specific response involving only one organ or gland.

The physiologic effects of parasympathetic system activity include reduced heart rate, contractility, and conduction velocity; bronchial smooth-muscle constriction; increased GI tract tone and peristalsis with sphincter relaxation; urinary system sphincter relaxation and increased bladder tone; vasodilation of external genitalia, causing erection; pupillary constriction; and increased pancreatic, salivary, and lacrimal secretions. The parasympathetic system has a minimal effect on mental or metabolic activity.

Assessment

Because the neurologic system is so complex and intricate, evaluating it may seem daunting. However, routine tests for assessing neurologic status, although extensive, are basic and straightforward. In fact, you may include some of these tests in your daily practice.

Just talking with a patient helps assess his orientation, level of consciousness, and ability to formulate and produce speech. Having him perform a simple task such as walking allows you to evaluate motor ability. Further, knowledge of neurologic anatomy, physiology, and assessment will enhance patient care and may save a patient from irreversible neurologic damage. If possible, you should start with taking a thorough health history and then proceed with performing a complete physical assessment.

HEALTH HISTORY

Begin the health history by asking about the patient's chief complaint. Then gather details about his current illness, past illnesses, family history, drug history, and psychosocial history. Also perform a body systems review.

If possible, include the patient's family members or close friends when taking the history. Don't assume that the patient remembers accurately; corroborate the details with others to get a clearer picture.

AGE AWARE When obtaining a child's health history, ask questions about the child's development, including a prenatal history up to the present. Also evaluate the child's achievement of developmental milestones, such as sitting up, walking, and talking at the appropriate age.

Chief complaint

The most common complaints about the neurologic system include headache, dizziness, disturbances in balance and gait, and changes in mental status or level of consciousness (LOC).

When documenting the patient's chief complaint, record the information in the patient's own words. Ask him about the problem's onset and frequency, what precipitates or exacerbates it, and what alleviates it. Also ask whether other symptoms accompany the problem.

Current health history

Ask the patient to elaborate on his chief complaint, using questions to focus the interview. Determine if he's experiencing problems with his activities of daily living (ADLs) due to the complaint. Also question the patient about measures used to treat the problem and if he experienced any adverse effects from those treatments.

Make sure you ask about other aspects of his current health. Help the patient describe problems by asking pertinent focused questions.

AGE AWARE Keep in mind that some neurologic changes, such as decreased reflexes, hearing, and vision, are a normal part of aging. Additionally, because neurons undergo various degenerative changes, aging can lead to diminished reflexes; decreased hearing, vision, taste, and smell; slowed reaction time; decreased agility; decreased vibratory sense in the ankles; and the development of muscle tremors, such as in the head and hands. Remember that not all neurologic changes in elderly patients are caused by aging and that certain drugs can cause changes as well. Find out if the changes are symmetric, indicating a condition, or if other abnormalities need further investigation.

HEADACHE

Ask the patient whether he has headaches. If so, ask him how often they occur and what seems to provoke them. Find out if light bothers his eyes during a headache. Also find out what other symptoms occur with the headache.

AGE AWARE In children older than age 3, headache is the most common symptom of a brain tumor. In a school-age child, ask the parents about recent scholastic performance and about any problems at home that may produce a tension headache. Twice as many young boys have migraine headaches than girls.

Attempt to gather additional information about the headache to aid in ascertaining the possible cause. First, ask the patient where the pain is located, such as across his forehead, on one side of his head, or at the back of his head and neck. Pain that emanates from specific areas of the head characterizes certain types of headaches. For example, tension headaches are usually located in the occipital area, and migraine pain tends to be unilateral.

Ask the patient if the pain is tight, bandlike, boring, throbbing, steady, or dull. Headaches can be identified by the quality of pain they produce. A dull, steady pain may indicate a tension, or muscle, headache; severe or throbbing pain may indicate a vascular problem such as a migraine headache.

Find out from the patient if the pain's onset is sudden or gradual. Migraine headaches may develop suddenly, with no warning, but are usually preceded by a prodromal disturbance. Headaches associated with hemorrhage typically occur suddenly and with increasing severity.

Ask the patient how long the pain usually lasts and if it's continuous or recurrent. Tension and migraine headaches may last from several hours to several days. Cluster headaches last about an hour. Also, find out if the headaches are occurring more frequently because a change in headache pattern may signal a developing condition.

Next, find out when the headaches occur, such as in the evening or if they wake him during the night. Although tension headaches usually occur in the evening, a patient may awaken in the morning with such a headache. A patient who suffers from headaches caused by hypertension, inflammation, or tumors may awaken anytime with the pain. Cluster headaches typically awaken the patient a few hours after he has fallen asleep.

Ask the patient if he sees flashing lights or shining spots or feels tingling, weakness, or numbness immediately before the headache occurs. These are common characteristics of the prodromal (premonitory) neurologic disturbance that commonly precedes a migraine headache.

Ask the patient if the pain worsens when he coughs, sneezes, or bends over. Valsalva's maneuver may exacerbate a headache caused by an intracranial lesion such as a subarachnoid hemorrhage. Find out if he becomes nauseated or vomits during the headache. Such GI distress may accompany a migraine headache, a brain tumor, or hemorrhage.

Headaches that occur daily for a prolonged period may be related to stress or depression. Ask the patient if he's been experiencing these difficult feelings.

Find out about any measures, such as medication, he takes for the headache and whether it's effective. Ask about other therapeutic approaches, such as lying down, applying heat, or sleeping, and if they relieve the headache.

Finally, have your patient describe the last headache he experienced by rating it on a scale of 1 to 10 with 1 being no pain and 10 being the worst headache he has ever had. How a particular headache differs from headaches a patient typically experiences can provide valuable clues to the possible cause.

DIZZINESS

Ask the patient about complaints of feeling dizzy. Find out if he has dizziness, numbness, tingling, seizures, tremors, weakness, or paralysis. Ask how often it occurs and how long each episode lasts. Find out if the dizziness abates spontaneously or if it leads to loss of consciousness. Ask him if the dizziness is triggered by sitting or standing up suddenly or stooping over.

Find out if being in a crowd makes the patient feel dizzy. Ask about emotional stress. Find out if the patient has been irritable or anxious lately. Ask him if he has insomnia or difficulty concentrating. Look for fidgeting and eyelid twitching. Observe the patient to see if he startles easily. Also, ask about palpitations, chest pain, diaphoresis, shortness of breath, and chronic cough.

BALANCE AND GAIT DISTURBANCES

Find out if the patient has problems with walking and keeping his balance. Then ask him when his balance or gait impairment first developed and whether it has worsened recently. Find out if the problem occurred gradually over time or developed suddenly. If he has difficulty remembering, attempt to gain information from family members or friends. Find out if the problem has remained constant or if it's getting progressively worse. Ask about environmental changes such as hot weather, or other conditions, such as fatigue or warm baths or showers that could make his problem worse. Such exacerbation typically is associated with multiple sclerosis. Also, find out if anyone in his family has experienced a similar type of problem.

MENTAL STATUS OR LOC CHANGES

Ask the patient how he would rate his memory and ability to concentrate. Ask him if he ever has trouble speaking or understanding people. Find out if he has difficulty reading or writing. If so, find out how much the problems interfere with his ADLs.

If the patient complains of problems with mental status, such as confusion, ask him how long he has felt confused and how quickly it occurred. Depending on the patient's degree of change, family members may need to be questioned to determine the true nature of the problem. Find out if the change occurred gradually or developed suddenly. An acute onset of confusion can indicate metabolic encephalopathy or delirium; gradual onset usually indicates a degenerative disorder. Ask if the confusion fluctuates. This question can help distinguish between an extracerebral disorder, such as metabolic encephalopathy, and a subdural hematoma caused by intracerebral impairment, such as arteriosclerosis or senile dementia.

If the patient was found unconscious, note where he was found. This answer may provide clues to the cause of the unconsciousness such as a possible reaction to drugs or alcohol. Ask him if unconsciousness occurred abruptly or gradually. Find out if his LOC has fluctuated. Abrupt change in LOC may indicate a stroke. Gradual onset could result from metabolic, extracerebral, toxic, or systemic causes.

A fluctuating LOC may indicate that systemic hypotension is affecting the brain. Find out from the patient what may have served as a trigger to exacerbate an existing condition, resulting in unconsciousness. For example, an infection or a break in treatment of an existing condition can result in unconsciousness.

Drug history

Obtain a thorough drug history, including medication type and dosage. Ask the patient if he has been taking over-the-counter medications, herbal supplements, vitamin supplements, or illegal substances. Find out if the patient has been taking the medication as prescribed. Ask him if any medications are newly prescribed and how they make him feel. Also find out about alcohol intake, frequency, and amount, and type of alcohol ingested.

Past health history

Explore all of the patient's previous major illnesses, recurrent minor illnesses, accidents or injuries, surgical procedures, mental illness, and allergies. Establish when his last physical examination occurred and if any routine examinations, such as an eye examination, took place. Ask about dietary habits and restrictions. Find out if he exercises daily. Ask him if he currently smokes or uses tobacco products or has smoked in the past. Calculate a pack-per-year history. Find out if the patient has ever attempted to stop smoking or using tobacco.

Family history

Information about the patient's family may help uncover hereditary disorders. Ask him if anyone in his family has had diabetes, cardiac or renal disease, high blood pressure, cancer, bleeding disorders, mental disorders, or a stroke.

Some genetic diseases are degenerative; others cause muscle weakness. For example, seizures are more common in patients whose family history shows idiopathic epilepsy, and more than 50% of patients with migraine headaches have a family history of the disorder.

Psychosocial history

Always consider the patient's cultural and social background when planning his care. Note his ethnic background and if it's a factor in his daily living. Find out what religion he practices and if he actively practices his beliefs. Also note the patient's education level and occupation. Find out if he has a stable or erratic employment history. Find out if his employment involves possible exposure to toxic substances, such as heavy metals or carbon monoxide. Ask him if he lives alone or with someone and what type of dwelling he lives in, and find out if he has a support system. Find out what his hobbies are. Ask him how he views his illness. Ask if the patient needs assistance with financial matters. Assess the patient's self-image while gathering this information.

PHYSICAL ASSESSMENT

A complete neurologic examination can be time-consuming and detailed, making it difficult to perform one in its entirety. However, if the initial screening examination suggests a neurologic problem, you may want to perform a more detailed neurologic assessment.

Always examine the patient's neurologic system in an orderly fashion.

Vital signs

The central nervous system (CNS), primarily by way of the brain stem and the autonomic nervous system (ANS), controls the body's vital functions, including body temperature; heart rate and rhythm; blood pressure; and respiratory rate, depth, and pattern. However, because these vital control centers lie deep within the cerebral hemispheres and in the brain stem, changes in these vital signs aren't usually early indicators of CNS deterioration. When evaluating the significance of vital sign changes, consider each sign individually as well as in relation to the others.

TEMPERATURE

Normal body temperature ranges from 96.7° F to 100.5° F (35.9° C to 38.1° C), depending upon the route used for measurement. Damage to the hypothalamus or upper brain stem can impair the body's ability to maintain a constant temperature, resulting in profound hypothermia (temperature below 94° F [34.4° C]) or hyperthermia (temperature above 106° F [41.1° C]). Such damage can result from petechial hemorrhages in the hypothalamus or brain stem; trauma, causing pressure, twisting, or traction; or destructive lesions.

HEART RATE

Because the ANS controls heart rate and rhythm, pressure on the brain stem and cranial nerves slows the heart rate by stimulating the vagus nerve. Bradycardia occurs in patients in the later stages of increasing intracranial pressure (ICP) and with cervical spinal cord injuries; it's usually accompanied by rising systolic blood pressure, widening pulse pressure, and bounding pulse. Tachycardia occurs in patients with acutely increased ICP or a brain injury; it signals decompensation, a condition in which the body has exhausted its compensatory measures for managing ICP, which rapidly leads to death.

BLOOD PRESSURE

Pressor receptors in the medulla continuously monitor blood pressure.

RED FLAG In a patient with no history of hypertension, rising systolic blood pressure may signal rising ICP. If ICP continues to rise, the patient's pulse pressure widens as his systolic pressure climbs and diastolic pressure remains stable or falls. In the late stages of acutely elevated ICP, blood pressure plummets as cerebral perfusion fails, resulting in the patient's death.

Hypotension accompanying a brain injury is also an ominous sign. In addition, cervical spinal cord injuries may interrupt sympathetic nervous system pathways, causing peripheral vasodilation and hypotension.

RESPIRATION

Respiratory centers in the medulla and pons control the rate, depth, and pattern of respiration. Neurologic dysfunction, particularly when it involves the brain stem or both cerebral hemispheres, commonly alters respirations. Assessment of respiration provides valuable information about a CNS lesion's site and severity. (See *Respiratory patterns associated with neurologic impairment,* page 30.)

Mental status assessment

The mental status assessment begins when interviewing the patient during the health history. How he responds to your questions gives clues to his orientation and memory and guides the physical assessment as well as the mental assessment. For example, if he complains about confusion or memory problems, you'll want to concentrate on the mental status part of the examination.

Ask the patient questions that require more than yes-or-no answers. Otherwise, confusion or disorientation might not be immediately apparent. If you have doubts about a patient's mental status, perform a more detailed screening examination. (See *Screening mental status,* page 31.)

RESPIRATORY PATTERNS ASSOCIATED WITH NEUROLOGIC IMPAIRMENT

Several patterns displaying impaired respiration due to neurologic dysfunction include:

● *Cheyne-Stokes respirations* – a waxing and waning period of hyperpnea that alternates with a shorter period of apnea, which usually indicates increased intracranial pressure from a deep cerebral or brain stem lesion, or a metabolic disturbance in the brain.

● *Central neurogenic hyperventilation* – a type of hyperpnea that indicates damage to the lower midbrain or upper pons, which may occur as a result of severe head injury.

● *Apneustic respirations* – an irregular breathing pattern characterized by prolonged, gasping inspiration, with a pause at full inspiration followed by expiration; there may also be a pause after expiration, which is an important localizing sign of severe brain stem damage.

● *Biot's respirations* – late signs of neurologic deterioration, which are rare and may appear abruptly; characterized by irregular and unpredictable rate, rhythm, and depth of respiration, they may reflect increased pressure on the medulla coinciding with brain stem compression.

● *Respiration impairment* – varying degrees can occur due to spinal cord damage above C7, which could weaken or paralyze the respiratory muscles.

The mental status examination consists of checking level of consciousness (LOC), orientation, appearance, behavior, communication, cognitive function, and constructional ability.

LEVEL OF CONSCIOUSNESS

In performing an initial assessment, first evaluate the patient's LOC.

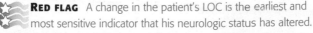 **RED FLAG** A change in the patient's LOC is the earliest and most sensitive indicator that his neurologic status has altered.

If the patient's behavior is threatening while performing this initial assessment, he may not be in immediate danger, but as the health care provider, you may be at risk. Therefore, you may need to change the order of the assessment. Always consider the environment and physical condition of the patient. For example, an elderly patient admitted to the health care fa-

SCREENING MENTAL STATUS

To screen patients for disordered thought processes, ask the questions presented here. An incorrect answer to any question may indicate the need for a complete mental status examination.

QUESTION	FUNCTION SCREENED
What's your name?	Orientation to person
What's your mother's name?	Orientation to other people
What year is it?	Orientation to time
Where are you now?	Orientation to place
How old are you?	Memory
Where were you born?	Remote memory
What did you have for breakfast?	Recent memory
Who's the U.S. president?	General knowledge
Can you count backward from 20 to 1?	Attention span and calculation skills

cility for several days may not be oriented to time, especially if he's bedridden. Also, consider the patient's vital signs and need for immediate lifesaving care.

Speak the patient's name in a normal tone of voice and note the response to an auditory stimulus. If he doesn't respond, use a tactile stimulus, such as touching him gently, squeezing his hand, or shaking his shoulder.

A fully awake patient is alert, open-eyed, and attentive to environmental stimuli. A less-awake patient appears drowsy, has reduced motor activity, and seems less attentive to environmental stimuli. Decreased arousal commonly precedes disorientation.

Use painful stimuli only to assess a patient who's unconscious or who has a markedly decreased LOC and doesn't respond to other stimuli. To test response to pain, apply firm pressure over the patient's nail bed with a blunt, hard object such as a pen. Other acceptable methods include squeezing the trapezius muscle, applying supraorbital pressure, applying mandibular pressure, and performing a sternal rub.

Next, note the type and intensity of stimulus required to elicit a response. Observe if the response is verbally appropriate, if it consists of unintelligible mumbling, body movement or eye opening, or if the patient exhibits no response at all. After you remove the stimulus, observe his level of alertness—for example, if he's wide awake, drowsy, or drifting to sleep.

After assessing the patient's level of alertness, compare the findings with results of previous assessments. Note trends, for example, if he's lethargic more often than usual. Consider factors that could affect patient responsiveness. For example, a normally alert patient may become drowsy after administration of such CNS depressant medications as sedatives and opioids.

Describe a patient's responsiveness objectively. For example, describe a lethargic patient's responses this way: "awakened when called loudly, then immediately fell asleep."

Many terms are used to describe LOC, but their definitions may differ slightly among health care providers. To avoid confusion, clearly describe the patient's response to various stimuli using these guidelines:

- *alert*— follows commands and responds completely and appropriately to stimuli
- *lethargic* — is drowsy; has delayed responses to verbal stimuli; may drift off to sleep during examination
- *stuporous* — requires vigorous stimulation for a response
- *comatose* — doesn't respond appropriately to verbal or painful stimuli; can't follow commands or communicate verbally.

RED FLAG If the patient has sustained a skull fracture, but appears lucid, and later has a decreased LOC, this could indicate an arterial epidural bleed that requires immediate surgery.

To minimize the subjectivity of LOC assessment and to establish a greater degree of reliability, use the Glasgow Coma Scale. This scale evaluates the patient's LOC according to three objective behaviors: eye opening, verbal responsiveness (which includes orientation), and motor response. (See *Using the Glasgow Coma Scale,* pages 34 and 35.)

Several disorders can affect the cerebral hemisphere of the brain stem, and a patient's LOC may be impaired by any one of them. Such disorders include toxic encephalopathy; hemorrhage; extensive, generalized cortical atrophy; and a tumor or intracranial hemorrhage. Rapid deterioration of LOC, from minutes to hours, usually indicates an acute neurologic disorder requiring immediate intervention. A gradually decreasing LOC, from weeks to months, may reflect a progressive or degenerative neurologic disorder.

ORIENTATION

The orientation portion of the mental status assessment measures the ability of the cerebral cortex to receive and accurately interpret sensory stimuli. It includes three aspects: orientation to person, place, and time. Always ask questions that require the patient to provide more than just a yes-or-no answer. First, find out if the patient is oriented to person by asking his name, and note the response. If the patient is disoriented to person, he may look baffled and may stammer or produce an unintelligible or inaccurate answer. Self-identity usually remains intact until late in decreasing LOC, making disorientation to person an ominous sign.

Next, ask the patient about place. Find out if he can correctly state his location. For example, when looking around the room, note if he concludes that he's in a health care facility, or if he thinks he's at home.

A patient in the health care facility disoriented to place most commonly confuses the health care facility's room with home or some other familiar surrounding; a patient who isn't in a health care facility, yet is still disoriented to place, such as a patient with Alzheimer's disease, may fail to recognize famil-

USING THE GLASGOW COMA SCALE

The Glasgow Coma Scale describes a patient's baseline mental status and helps to detect and interpret changes from baseline findings. When using the Glasgow Coma Scale, test the patient's ability to respond to verbal, motor, and sensory stimulation, and grade your findings according to the scale. A score of 15 indicates that the patient is alert, can follow simple commands, and is oriented to time, place, and person. A decreased score in one or more categories may signal an impending neurologic crisis. A score of 7 or less indicates severe neurologic damage.

TEST	SCORE	RESPONSE
EYE OPENING RESPONSE		
Spontaneously	4	Opens eyes spontaneously
To speech	3	Opens eyes when told to
To pain	2	Opens eyes only to painful stimulus
None	1	Doesn't open eyes in response to stimuli
MOTOR RESPONSE		
Obeys	6	Shows two fingers when asked
Localizes	5	Reaches toward painful stimulus and tries to remove it
Withdraws	4	Moves away from painful stimulus

iar home surroundings and may wander off in search of something familiar.

Finally, assess orientation to time by asking the patient to state the year, month, and date. Most people usually answer correctly and can also differentiate day from night if their environment provides enough information; for example, if the room has a window.

 RED FLAG A patient's orientation to time is usually disrupted first and his orientation to person is disrupted last.

TEST	SCORE	RESPONSE
MOTOR RESPONSE (continued)		
Abnormal flexion	3	Assumes a decorticate posture (shown below)
Abnormal extension	2	Assumes a decerebrate posture (shown below)
None	1	No response; just lies flaccid (an ominous sign)
VERBAL RESPONSE (TO QUESTION "WHAT YEAR IS THIS?")		
Oriented	5	Tells correct year
Confused	4	Tells incorrect year
Inappropriate words	3	Replies randomly with incorrect words
Incomprehensible	2	Moans or screams
No response	1	No response
TOTAL SCORE		

If disorientation to time arises from a physiologic problem, the patient is also likely to mistake unfamiliar surroundings or people for familiar ones. For example, he may confuse the health care facility's room with his bedroom or mistake a health care provider for a relative. If the disorientation originates from psychiatric disturbances, such as schizophrenia, he may have an unusually bizarre confusion pattern. Answers, such as 1756 or 2054, may indicate a psychiatric disturbance — or a lack of cooperation.

APPEARANCE

Note how the patient behaves, dresses, and grooms himself. Observe his appearance and if he acts appropriately. Note his personal hygiene. If you observe negative findings, such as disheveled or dirty clothing, discuss them with family members to determine whether this is a change. Even subtle changes can signal a new onset of a chronic disease or a more acute change that involves the frontal lobe.

Look at the patient's color, facial expressions, mobility, deformities, and nutritional state. Observe the patient's gait, posture, and ability to rise from a chair. Note if he needs assistance to walk, rise from a chair, or get undressed. Observe if he can hear and see you when you're talking. Observe him for raccoon eyes. Note if he has otorrhea — cerebrospinal fluid leaking from his ears.

RED FLAG Raccoon eyes could indicate bleeding into the periorbital tissue. Otorrhea could indicate a basilar skull fracture. If the brain stem is lacerated or contused, immediate death can occur. Smaller leakages can resolve in 2 to 10 days.

BEHAVIOR

Assess the patient's thought content by evaluating the clarity and cohesiveness of his ideas. Observe his conversation for smoothness, with logical transitions between ideas. Note if he has hallucinations, which are sensory perceptions that lack appropriate stimuli; or delusions, which are beliefs not supported by reality. Disordered thought patterns may indicate delirium or psychosis.

Test the patient's ability to think abstractly by asking him to interpret a common proverb such as "A stitch in time saves nine." A patient with dementia may interpret a common proverb literally.

Test the patient's judgment by asking him how he would respond to a hypothetical situation. For example, ask him what he would do if he was in a public building and the fire alarm sounded. Evaluate the appropriateness of his answer.

Throughout the interview, assess the patient's emotional status. Note his mood, his emotional stability or lability, and the appropriateness of his emotional responses. Also assess his mood by asking how he feels about himself and his future.

AGE AWARE In elderly patients, symptoms of depression may be atypical — for example, decreased function or increased agitation may occur rather than the usual sad affect.

COMMUNICATION

If the patient's primary language isn't English, he may have difficulty communicating. Engage the assistance of family members when English isn't the patient's primary language. If the family isn't available, attempt to contact an interpreter. Use of body language will also be necessary.

Assess the patient's ability to comprehend speech, writing, numbers, and gestures. Language skills include learning and recalling the parts of the language (such as words), organizing word relationships according to grammatical rules, and structuring message content logically. Speech involves neuromuscular actions of the mouth, tongue, and oropharynx.

Verbal responsiveness

During the interview and physical assessment, observe the patient when you ask a question. If you suspect a decreased LOC, call the patient's name or gently shake his shoulder to try to elicit a verbal response. Note if he speaks in complete sentences, in phrases, or in single words and if he communicates spontaneously or if he rarely speaks.

Assess the quality of the patient's speech, such as if it's unusually loud or soft. Observe the patient for clear articulation, or if his words are difficult to understand. Note the rate and rhythm of his speech.

Note if the patient's verbal responses are appropriate. Observe him for any difficulty finding or articulating his words. Also, note if he uses made-up words, or neologisms.

If communication problems arise, note if the patient is aware of them. If he appears frustrated or angry when communication fails, note if he continues to attempt to talk, unaware that you don't comprehend.

If you suspect a language impairment, show the patient a common object, such as a cup or a book, and ask him to name it. Ask the patient to repeat a word that you say, such as dog or breakfast. If the patient appears to have difficulty understanding spoken language, ask him to follow a simple instruction such as "Touch your nose." If the patient succeeds, then try a two-step command such as "Touch your right knee, then touch your nose." Keep in mind that language performance tends to fluctuate with the time of day and changes in physical condition. A healthy individual may experience language difficulty when ill or fatigued. Increasing language difficulties may indicate deteriorating neurologic status, warranting further evaluation.

Speech impairment or impaired language function can occur from dysphasia, which is the impaired ability to use or understand language, and aphasia, which is the inability to use or understand language, or both, which indicates injury to the cerebral cortex. Several types of aphasia exist, including:

- *expressive or Broca's aphasia* — impaired fluency; difficulty finding words; impairment located in the frontal lobe, the anterior speech area
- *receptive or Wernicke's aphasia* — inability to understand written words or speech; use of made-up words; impairment located in the posterior speech cortex, which involves the temporal and parietal lobes
- *global aphasia* — lack of expressive and receptive language; impairment of both speech areas
- *facial muscle paralysis* — difficulty in articulation and slurred speech
- *dysarthria* — impairment of neuromuscular speech
- *dysphonia* — impairment of voice.

Formal language skills evaluation
The formal language skills evaluation identifies the extent and characteristics of the patient's language deficits. Usually per-

formed by a speech pathologist, it may help pinpoint the site of a CNS lesion. For example, identifying expressive aphasia, when the patient knows what he wants to say but can't speak the words, may help diagnose a frontal lobe lesion.

When evaluating the patient, assess these language skills:

- *Spontaneous speech* — show the patient a picture, and ask him to describe what's going on.
- *Comprehension* — Ask the patient a series of simple yes-or-no questions and evaluate his answers. Use questions with obvious answers. For example: "Does it snow in July?"
- *Naming* — Show the patient various common objects, one at a time, and then ask him to name each one. Typical objects include a comb, ball, cup, and pencil.
- *Repetition* — Ask him to repeat words or phrases such as "no ifs, ands, or buts."
- *Vocabulary* — Ask the patient to explain the meaning of each of a series of words.
- *Reading* — Ask him to read printed words on cards and perform the action described. For example: "Raise your hand."
- *Writing* — Ask the patient to write something such as his name and address.
- *Copying figures* — Show the patient several figures, one at a time, and then ask him to copy them. The figures usually become increasingly complex, starting with a circle, an X, and a square and proceeding to a triangle and a star.

COGNITIVE FUNCTION

Assessing cognitive function involves testing the patient's memory, orientation, attention span, calculation ability, thought content, abstract thinking, judgment, insight, and emotional status.

To test your patient's orientation, memory, and attention span, use the mental status screening questions discussed previously. Always consider the patient's environment and physical condition when assessing orientation. Also, when the person is intubated and can't speak, ask questions that require only a nod, such as "Do you know you're in the hospital?" and

"Are we in Pennsylvania?" The patient with an intact short-term memory can generally repeat five to seven nonconsecutive numbers right away and again 10 minutes later.

 RED FLAG   Short-term memory is commonly affected first in the patient with a neurologic disease.

When testing attention span and calculation skills, keep in mind that lack of mathematical ability and anxiety can affect the patient's performance. If he has difficulty with numeric computation, ask him to spell the word "world" backward. While he's performing these functions, note his ability to pay attention.

CONSTRUCTIONAL ABILITY

The patient's ability to perform simple tasks and use various objects reflects constructional ability. Apraxia and agnosia are two types of constructional disorders.

Apraxia is the inability to perform purposeful movements and make proper use of objects and is commonly associated with parietal lobe dysfunction. It can appear in any of four types. Ideomotor apraxia is the inability to understand the effect of motor activity; the ability to perform simple activities, but without awareness of performing them; and the inability to perform actions on command. Ideational apraxia is the awareness of actions that need to be done accompanied by an inability to perform them. Constructional apraxia is the inability to copy a design, such as a square or the face of a clock. Finally, dressing apraxia is the inability to understand the meaning of various articles of clothing or the sequence of actions required to get dressed.

Agnosia is the inability to identify common objects and may indicate a lesion in the sensory cortex. Agnosia types include visual, which is the inability to identify common objects unless they're touched; auditory, the inability to identify common sounds; and body image, the inability to identify body parts by sight or touch, the inability to localize a stimulus, or denial of existence of half of the body.

Cranial nerve assessment

There are 12 pairs of cranial nerves (CNs). These nerves transmit motor or sensory messages, or both, primarily between the brain and brain stem and the head and neck. Cranial nerve assessment provides valuable information about the condition of the CNS, particularly the brain stem.

OLFACTORY (CN I)

To assess the olfactory nerve, first check the patency of both nostrils, then instruct the patient to close his eyes. Occlude one nostril and hold a familiar, pungent-smelling substance — such as coffee, lemon, soap, or peppermint — under his nose and ask its identity. Repeat this technique with the other nostril.

If the patient reports detecting the smell but can't name it, offer a choice such as "Do you smell lemon, coffee, or peppermint?" The patient should be able to detect and identify the smell correctly. The location of the olfactory nerve makes it especially vulnerable to damage from facial fractures and head injuries.

Damage to CN I may be due to disorders of the base of the frontal lobe, such as tumors or arteriosclerotic changes.

RED FLAG The sense of smell remains intact as long as one of the two olfactory nerves exists; it's permanently lost (anosmia) if both nerves are affected. Anosmia may also result from non-neurologic causes, such as nasal congestion, sinus infection, smoking, and cocaine use. Once anosmia is present, it can also impair the sense of taste. Therefore, a complaint about food taste may signal CN I damage.

OPTIC (CN II) AND OCULOMOTOR (CN III)

To assess the optic nerve, check visual acuity, visual fields, and the retinal structures. To assess the oculomotor nerve, check pupil size, pupil shape, and pupillary response to light.

To test visual acuity and retinal structure quickly and informally, have the patient read a newspaper, starting with large headlines and moving to small print.

DETECTING VISUAL FIELD DEFECTS

Here are some examples of visual field defects. The black areas represent vision loss.

	LEFT	RIGHT
1. Blindness of right eye	○	●
2. Bitemporal hemianopsia, or loss of half the visual field	◐	◑
3. Left homonymous hemianopsia	◐	◐
4. Left homonymous hemianopsia, superior quadrant	◕	◕

Test visual fields with a technique called *confrontation*. To do this, stand 2′ (0.6 m) in front of the patient, and have him cover one eye. Then close one of your eyes and bring your moving fingers into the patient's visual field from the periphery. Ask him to tell you when he sees your hand. Test each quadrant of the patient's visual field, and compare his results with your own. Chart any defects you find. (See *Detecting visual field defects*.)

A visual field defect may signal a stroke, head injury, or brain tumor. The area and extent of the loss depend on the lesion's location.

When assessing pupil size, look for trends. For example, watch for a gradual increase in the size of one pupil or the appearance of unequal pupils in a patient whose pupils were previously equal. The pupils should be equal, round, and reactive to light.

 RED FLAG In a blind patient with a nonfunctional optic nerve, light stimulation will fail to produce either a direct or a consensual pupillary response. However, a legally blind patient may have some optic nerve function, which causes the blind eye to respond to direct light. In a patient who's totally blind in only one eye, the pupil of the eye with the intact optic nerve will react to direct light stimulation, whereas the blind eye, because it receives sensory messages from the functional optic nerve, will respond consensually.

Pupil size can be affected by increased ICP, which causes a change in responsiveness or pupil size on the affected side, resulting in dilation of the pupil ipsilateral to the mass lesion; as ICP rises, the other oculomotor nerve becomes affected, causing both pupils to become oval or react sluggishly to light shortly before dilating. Without treatment, both pupils become fixed and dilated. The hippus phenomenon causes brisk pupil constriction in response to light followed by a pulsating dilation and constriction, which may be normal in some patients but may also reflect early oculomotor nerve compression. Optic and oculomotor nerve damage may also affect pupil size by impairing the pupillary response to light, which indicates neurologic demise. Lastly, anisocoria, or unequal pupils, which are normal in about 20% of people, occurs when pupil size doesn't change with the amount of illumination. (See *Understanding pupillary changes,* page 44.)

OCULOMOTOR (CN III), TROCHLEAR (CN IV), AND ABDUCENS (CN VI)

To test the coordinated function of the oculomotor, trochlear, and abducens nerves, assess them simultaneously by evaluating the patient's extraocular eye movement. (See *Testing extraocular muscles,* page 45.) The patient's eyes should move smoothly and in a coordinated manner through all six directions of eye movement including left superior, left lateral, left inferior, right superior, right lateral, and right inferior.

Observe each eye for rapid oscillation, known as *nystagmus;* movement not in unison with that of the other eye, called *disconjugate movement;* or inability to move in certain directions, known as *ophthalmoplegia.* Also note any complaint of double vision, or diplopia. Nystagmus may indicate a disorder

UNDERSTANDING PUPILLARY CHANGES

Use this chart as a guide when observing your patient for pupillary changes.

PUPILLARY CHANGE	POSSIBLE CAUSES
Unilateral, dilated (4 mm), fixed, and nonreactive 	● Uncal herniation with oculomotor nerve damage ● Brain stem compression ● Increased intracranial pressure ● Tentorial herniation ● Head trauma with subdural or epidural hematoma ● May be normal in some people
Bilateral, dilated (4 mm), fixed, and nonreactive 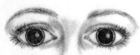	● Severe midbrain damage ● Cardiopulmonary arrest (hypoxia) ● Anticholinergic poisoning
Bilateral, midsize (2 mm), fixed, and nonreactive 	● Midbrain involvement caused by edema, hemorrhage, infarctions, lacerations, contusions
Bilateral, pinpoint (< 1 mm), and usually nonreactive 	● Lesions of pons, usually after hemorrhage
Unilateral, small (1.5 mm), and nonreactive 	● Disruption of sympathetic nerve supply to the head caused by spinal cord lesion above T1

TESTING EXTRAOCULAR MUSCLES

The coordinated action of six muscles controls eyeball movements. To test the function of each muscle and the cranial nerve (CN) that innervates it, ask the patient to look in the direction controlled by that muscle. The six directions you can test make up the cardinal fields of gaze. The patient's inability to turn the eye in the designated direction indicates muscle weakness or paralysis.

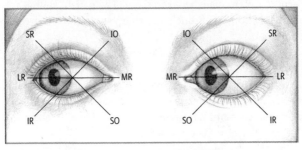

SR–superior rectus (CN III)
LR–lateral rectus (CN VI)
IR–inferior rectus (CN III)

IO–inferior oblique (CN III)
MR–medial rectus (CN III)
SO–superior oblique (CN IV)

of the brain stem, the cerebellum, or the vestibular portion of CN VIII. It may also imply drug toxicity such as from the anticonvulsant, phenytoin.

RED FLAG Increased ICP can put pressure on CN IV, causing impaired extraocular eye movement inferiorly and medially, and CN VI, causing impaired extraocular eye movement laterally.

The oculomotor nerve is also responsible for eyelid elevation and pupillary constriction. Drooping of the patient's eyelid, or ptosis, can result from a defect in the oculomotor nerve. To assess ptosis more accurately, have the patient sit upright.

TRIGEMINAL (CN V)

To assess the sensory portion of the trigeminal nerve, gently touch the right side and the left side of the patient's forehead with a cotton ball while his eyes are closed. Instruct him to state the moment the cotton touches the area. Compare his response on both sides. Repeat the technique on the right and left cheek and on the right and left jaw. Next, repeat the entire procedure using a sharp object. The cap of a disposable ball-point pen can be used to test light touch with the dull end and sharp stimuli with the sharp end. If an abnormality appears, test for temperature sensation by touching the patient's skin with test tubes filled with hot and cold water and asking the patient to differentiate between them. The patient should report feeling both light touch and sharp stimuli in all three tested areas.

Peripheral nerve damage can create a loss of sensation in any or all three regions supplied by the trigeminal nerve. Trigeminal neuralgia causes severe, piercing, or stabbing pain over one or more of the facial dermatomes. A lesion in the cervical spinal cord or brain stem can produce impaired sensory function in each of the three areas.

To assess the motor portion of the trigeminal nerve, ask the patient to clench his jaws. Palpate the temporal and masseter muscles bilaterally, checking for symmetry. Try to open his clenched jaws. Next, watch the patient while he's opening and closing his mouth for asymmetry. The jaws should clench symmetrically and remain closed against resistance.

A lesion in the cervical spinal cord or brain stem can produce impaired motor function in regions supplied by the trigeminal nerve, weakening the patient's jaw muscles, causing the jaw to deviate toward the affected side when chewing, and allowing residual food to collect in the affected cheek.

To assess the patient's corneal reflex, stroke a wisp of cotton lightly across a cornea. The lids of both eyes should close. (See *Eliciting the corneal reflex.*) An absent corneal reflex may result from peripheral nerve or brain stem damage. However, a diminished corneal reflex commonly occurs in patients who wear contact lenses.

ELICITING THE CORNEAL REFLEX

To elicit the corneal reflex, have the patient turn her eyes away from you to avoid involuntary blinking during the procedure. Then approach the patient from the opposite side, out of her line of vision, and brush the cornea lightly with a fine wisp of sterile cotton. Repeat the procedure on the other eye. The lids of both eyes should close.

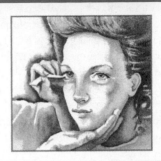

FACIAL (CN VII)

To test the motor portion of the facial nerve, ask the patient to wrinkle his forehead, raise and lower his eyebrows, smile to show his teeth, and puff out his cheeks. Also, with the patient's eyes tightly closed, attempt to open the eyelids. With each of these movements, observe closely for symmetry.

Unilateral facial weakness can reflect an upper motor neuron problem, such as a stroke or a tumor that has damaged neurons in the facial control area of the motor strip in the cerebral cortex. If the weakness originates in the cerebral cortex, the patient will retain the ability to wrinkle his forehead because the forehead receives motor messages from both hemispheres of the brain — which explains why when one side is damaged, such as in a stroke, the other side takes over. However, if CN VII is damaged, the weakness will extend to the forehead, and the eye on the affected side won't close.

To test the sensory portion of the facial nerve, which supplies taste sensation to the anterior two-thirds of the tongue, first prepare four marked, closed containers, with one containing salt; another sugar; a third, vinegar (or lemon); and a fourth, quinine (or bitters). Then, with the patient's eyes closed, place salt on the anterior two-thirds of his tongue using a cotton swab or dropper. Ask him to identify the taste as sweet, salty, sour, or bitter. Rinse his mouth with water. Repeat this procedure, alternating flavors and sides of the tongue, until all four flavors have been tested on both sides. Taste sensations to the posterior third of the tongue are supplied by the glossopharyngeal nerve (CN IX) and are usually tested at the same time. The patient should have symmetrical taste sensations.

An impaired sense of taste can signify damage to the patient's facial or glossopharyngeal nerve, or it may simply reflect a part of the normal aging process. Chemotherapy or head and neck radiation can also alter taste by damaging taste bud receptors.

ACOUSTIC (CN VIII)

To assess the acoustic portion of the acoustic nerve, test the patient's hearing acuity. Ask the patient to cover one ear, and then stand on his opposite side and whisper a few words. See whether he can repeat what you said. Test the other ear the same way.

To assess the vestibular portion of this nerve, observe for nystagmus and disturbed balance and note reports of dizziness or the room spinning.

The patient should be able to hear a whispered voice, rubbing of fingers, or a watch ticking. He should have normal eye movement and balance and no dizziness or vertigo. With sensorial hearing loss, the patient may have trouble hearing high-pitched sounds, or he may have a total hearing loss in the affected ear due to lesions of the cochlear branch of CN VIII. With nystagmus and vertigo, the patient may have a disturbance of the vestibular centers. If caused by a peripheral lesion, vertigo and nystagmus will occur 10 to 20 seconds after the patient changes position, and symptoms will gradually lessen with the repetition of the position change. If the vertigo is of central origin, there's no latent period, and the symptoms don't diminish with repetition.

GLOSSOPHARYNGEAL (CN IX) AND VAGUS (CN X)

To assess the glossopharyngeal and vagus nerves, which have overlapping functions, first listen to the patient's voice for indications of a hoarse or nasal quality. Then watch his soft palate when he says "ah." Next, test the gag reflex by touching the posterior wall of the pharynx with a cotton swab or tongue blade.

The patient's voice should sound strong and clear. The soft palate and the uvula should rise when he says "ah," and the uvula should remain midline. The palatine arches should remain symmetrical during movement and at rest. The gag reflex should be intact. If it diminishes or if the pharynx moves asymmetrically, evaluate each side of the posterior pharyngeal wall to confirm the integrity of both cranial nerves.

Glossopharyngeal neuralgia produces paroxysmal pain, which radiates from the patient's throat to his ear. Damage to CN IX or X impairs swallowing. Furthermore, during swallowing, the palate fails to rise and close off the nasal passageways, allowing nasal regurgitation of fluids.

Because the vagus nerve innervates most viscera through the parasympathetic nervous system, vagal damage can affect involuntary vital functions, producing tachycardia, other cardiac arrhythmias, and dyspnea.

ACCESSORY (CN XI)

To assess the spinal accessory nerve, press down on the patient's shoulders while he attempts to shrug against this resistance. Note shoulder strength and symmetry while inspecting and palpating the trapezius muscle.

Then apply resistance to his turned head while he attempts to return to a midline position. Note neck strength while inspecting and palpating the sternocleidomastoid muscle. Repeat for the opposite side.

RED FLAG If the patient complains of stiffness in the neck, suspect nuchal rigidity, an early sign of meningeal irritation. Passively flex the patient's neck and touch his chin to his chest. Nuchal rigidity is present if the patient experiences pain and muscle

ELICITING KERNIG'S AND BRUDZINSKI'S SIGNS

If, during your spinal accessory nerve assessment (cranial nerve XI), you observe nuchal rigidity, indicating meningeal irritation, test the patient for Kernig's and Brudzinski's signs.

Kernig's sign

To elicit Kernig's sign, place the patient in a supine position. Flex the leg at the hip and knee, as shown. Then try to extend the leg while keeping the hip flexed. If the patient experiences pain and possibly spasm in the hamstring muscle and resists further extension, assume that meningeal irritation has occurred.

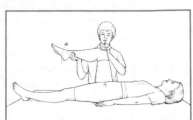

Brudzinski's sign

To test for Brudzinski's sign, place the patient in the supine position with your hands behind the neck and lift the patient's head toward the chest.

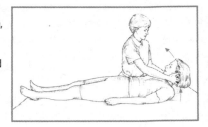

The patient with meningeal irritation will flex the hips and knees in response to passive neck flexion.

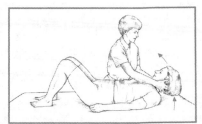

spasms. If positive, check for Kernig's and Brudzinski's signs. (See *Eliciting Kernig's and Brudzinski's signs.*)

Both shoulders should be able to overcome the resistance equally well. The neck should overcome resistance in both directions. Unilateral weakness, atrophy, or paralysis of the muscles innervated by the spinal accessory nerve suggests a peripheral nerve lesion. Signs include a drooping shoulder or a scapula that appears displaced toward the affected side.

HYPOGLOSSAL (CN XII)

To assess the hypoglossal nerve, observe the patient's protruded tongue for any deviation from midline, atrophy, fasciculations, or very fine muscle flickering, which indicates lower motor neuron disease.

Next, instruct the patient to move his tongue rapidly from side to side with the mouth open, to curl his tongue up toward the nose, and to curl his tongue down toward the chin. Then use a tongue blade or folded gauze pad to apply resistance to his protruded tongue and ask him to try to push the tongue blade to one side. Repeat this procedure on the other side and note the patient's tongue strength.

Listen to the patient's speech for the sounds "d," "n," and "t," which require use of the tongue to articulate. If his general speech suggests a problem, have him repeat a phrase or a series of words that contain these sounds such as "round the rugged rock that ragged rascal ran." The tongue should be midline, and the patient should be able to move it right and left equally. He should also be able to move the tongue up and down. Pressure exerted by the tongue on the tongue blade should be equal on either side. Speech should be clear.

A peripheral nerve lesion creates a unilateral flaccid paralysis of the patient's tongue, atrophy of the affected side, and deviation of the tongue. A unilateral spastic paralysis of the tongue produces poorly articulated, difficult speech, or dysarthria, characterized by an explosive production of words. The tongue deviates toward the affected side.

Sensory function assessment

Evaluation of the sensory system involves assessing five areas of sensation: pain, light touch, vibration, position, and discrimination.

PAIN

To test the patient for pain, have him close his eyes; then touch all the major dermatomes, first with the sharp end of a safety pin and then with the dull end. Proceed in this order: fingers, shoulders, toes, thighs, and trunk. Ask him to identify when he feels the sharp stimulus.

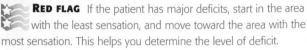 **RED FLAG** If the patient has major deficits, start in the area with the least sensation, and move toward the area with the most sensation. This helps you determine the level of deficit.

LIGHT TOUCH

To test for the sense of light touch, follow the same routine as above, but use a wisp of cotton. Lightly touch the patient's skin — don't swab or sweep the cotton, because you might miss an area of loss. A patient with a peripheral neuropathy might retain his sensation for light touch after he has lost pain sensation.

VIBRATION

To test vibratory sense, apply a tuning fork over certain bony prominences while the patient keeps his eyes closed. Start at the distal interphalangeal joint of the index finger, and move proximally. Test only until the patient feels the vibration, because everything above that level will be intact. (See *Evaluating vibration*.) If vibratory sense is intact, you don't have to check position sense because the same pathway carries both.

POSITION

To assess position sense, have the patient close his eyes. Then grasp the sides of his big toe, move it up and down, and ask him what position it's in. To be tested for position sense, the patient needs intact vestibular and cerebellar function.

EVALUATING VIBRATION

To evaluate the patient's vibratory sense, apply the base of a vibrating tuning fork to the interphalangeal joint of the great toe, as shown.

Ask the patient what he feels. If he feels the sensation, he'll typically report a feeling of buzzing or vibration. If he doesn't feel the sensation at the toe, try the medial malleolus. Then continue moving proximally until he feels the sensation. Note where he feels it, and then repeat the process on the other leg.

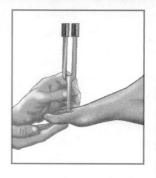

Perform the same test on the patient's upper extremities by grasping the sides of his index finger and moving it back and forth.

DISCRIMINATION

Discrimination testing assesses the ability of the cerebral cortex to interpret and integrate information. Stereognosis is the ability to discriminate an object's shape, size, weight, texture, and form by touching and manipulating it. To test stereognosis, ask the patient to close his eyes and open his hand. Then place a common object, such as a key, in his hand, and ask him to identify it. If he can't identify the key, test graphesthesia next. Have the patient keep his eyes closed and hold out his hand while you draw a large number on his palm. Ask him to identify the number. Both these tests assess the ability of the cortex to integrate sensory input.

To test point localization, have the patient close his eyes; then touch one of his limbs, and ask him where you touched him. Test two-point discrimination by touching the patient simultaneously in two contralateral areas. He should be able to identify both touches. Failure to perceive touch on one side is called *extinction*.

ASSESSMENT FINDINGS

Assessment of the sensory system may reveal several abnormal findings. Reduced sensory acuity is evidenced by a need for repeated, prolonged, or excessive contact to evoke a response. Sensory deficits are indicated by repeated failure to detect tactile stimuli in one body area or a difference in sensory acuity in the same extremity on opposite sides of the body.

Damaged sensory nerve fibers are indicated by a complaint of tingling or dysesthesia in one area, even if the patient can correctly identify the tactile stimulus. A disorder in the posterior tracts and dorsal columns of the spinal cord or a peripheral nerve or root lesion may be evidenced by a loss of the sense of light touch, vibration, and position.

A disorder in the spinothalamic tracts can occur as indicated by impaired pain or temperature sensation. Developing peripheral neuropathy is commonly preceded by loss of the sense of vibration. A bilateral, symmetrical, distal sensory loss also suggests a peripheral neuropathy. A disorder in the dorsal columns or the sensory interpretive regions of the parietal lobe of the cerebral cortex may occur as evidenced by an impaired ability to recognize the distance between two points (discriminative sensation). In addition, lesions of the sensory cortex can occur, indicated by impaired point localization.

Motor function assessment

Assessing the patient's motor system includes inspecting the muscles and testing muscle tone and muscle strength. Cerebellar testing is also performed because the cerebellum plays a role in abnormal smooth-muscle movements, such as tics, tremors, or fasciculations.

MUSCLE TONE

Muscle tone represents muscular resistance to passive stretching. To test arm muscle tone, move the patient's shoulder through passive range-of-motion (ROM) exercises. You should feel a slight resistance. Then let the arm drop to the patient's side. The arm should fall easily.

To test leg muscle tone, guide the hip through passive ROM exercises; then let the leg fall to the bed. If it falls into an externally rotated position, this is an abnormal finding.

Assessment may reveal abnormal muscle movements, including uncontrollable tics that involve sudden, uncontrolled movements of the face, shoulders, and extremities caused by abnormal neural stimuli. They can be normal movements that appear repetitively and inappropriately, such as blinking, shoulder shrugging, and facial twitching. Involuntary tremors may also occur, which involve repetitive, involuntary movements usually seen in the fingers, wrist, eyelids, tongue, and legs. These movements occur when the affected body part is at rest or with voluntary movement. For example, the patient with Parkinson's disease has a characteristic pill-rolling tremor, and the patient with cerebellar disease has an "intention tremor" when reaching for an object. In addition, small-muscle fasciculations — fine twitchings in small muscle groups — may occur, which are most commonly associated with lower motor neuron dysfunction.

MUSCLE STRENGTH
To perform a general examination of muscle strength, observe the patient's gait and motor activities. Assessment may reveal gait abnormalities resulting from disorders of the cerebellum, posterior columns, corticospinal tract, basal ganglia, and lower motor neurons. These abnormalities include hemiparetic, or spastic, gait with characteristics varying according to the amount of upper motor neuron damage. In severe cases, the patient walks with the affected upper extremity abducted and the elbow, wrist, and fingers flexed. The upper body is somewhat stooped, and he tilts slightly to the opposite side. As he walks, he extends his leg and inverts his foot at the ankle with the leg swinging in a circular motion.

RED FLAG During the gait assessment, remain close to an elderly or infirm patient and be ready to help if he should stumble or start to fall.

Ataxic gait may also occur, which is caused by cerebellar damage. The patient has a wide-based and reeling walk, commonly called *drunken gait*. If sensory loss occurs, the patient may not be able to feel where he's placing his foot so he partially flexes his hips and lifts up his legs and then slaps his feet down with each step.

Steppage gait is another abnormality associated with lower motor neuron disease and is commonly accompanied by muscle weakness and atrophy. The patient deliberately lifts up his feet and slaps them down on the floor.

AGE AWARE Aging may cause difficulty in tandem walking. Typically, the elderly person walks with shorter steps and a wider leg stance to achieve better balance and stable weight distribution.

To further evaluate muscle strength, ask the patient to move major muscles and muscle groups against resistance. For instance, to test shoulder girdle strength, have him extend his arms with his palms up and maintain this position for 30 seconds. If he can't maintain this position, test further by pushing down on his outstretched arms. If he lifts both arms equally, look for pronation of the hand and downward drift of the arm on the weaker side. (See *Testing muscle strength,* pages 58 and 59.)

CEREBELLAR FUNCTION

Cerebellar testing looks at the patient's coordination and general balance. Observe the patient to see if he can sit and stand without support. If he can, observe him as he walks across the room, turns, and walks back. Note imbalances or abnormalities.

RED FLAG With cerebellar dysfunction, the patient has a wide-based, unsteady gait. Deviation to one side may indicate a cerebellar lesion on that side.

Ask the patient to walk heel to toe, and observe his balance. Then perform Romberg's test.

Romberg's test
Observe the patient's balance as he stands with his eyes open, feet together, and arms at his sides. Then ask him to close his eyes. Hold your arms out on either side of him to protect him if he sways. If he falls to one side, the result of Romberg's test is positive.

Nose-to-finger test
Test extremity coordination by asking the patient to touch his nose and then touch your outstretched finger as you move it. Have him do this faster and faster. His movements should be accurate and smooth.

Rapid alternating movement tests
Other tests of cerebellar function assess rapid alternating movements.

First, ask the patient to touch the thumb of his right hand to his right index finger and then to each of his remaining fingers. Observe the movements for accuracy and smoothness. Next, ask him to sit with his palms on his thighs. Tell him to turn his palms up and down, gradually increasing his speed.

Finally, have the patient lie in a supine position. Then stand at the foot of the table or bed and hold your palms near the soles of his feet. Ask him to alternately tap the sole of his right foot and the sole of his left foot against your palms. He should increase his speed as you observe his coordination.

Reflex assessment
Evaluating the patient's reflexes involves testing deep tendon and superficial reflexes and observing for primitive reflexes.

DEEP TENDON REFLEXES
Deep tendon reflexes (DTRs), also called *muscle-stretch reflexes,* occur when a sudden stimulus causes the muscle to stretch.

(Text continues on page 61.)

TESTING MUSCLE STRENGTH

Obtain an overall picture of your patient's motor function by testing strength in 10 selected muscle groups in the arms and legs. Ask the patient to attempt normal range-of-motion movements against your resistance. If the muscle group is weak, vary the amount of resistance as required to permit accurate assessment. If necessary, position the patient so his limbs don't have to resist gravity, and repeat the test.

ARM MUSCLES

Biceps. With your hand on the patient's hand, have him flex his forearm against your resistance. Watch for biceps contraction.

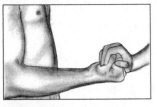

Deltoid. With the patient's arm fully extended, place one hand over his deltoid muscle and the other on his wrist. Ask him to abduct his arm to a horizontal position against your resistance; as he does so, palpate for deltoid contraction.

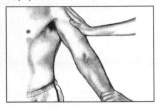

Triceps. Have the patient abduct and hold his arm midway between flexion and extension. Hold and support his arm at the wrist, and ask him to extend it against your resistance. Watch for triceps contraction.

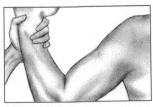

Dorsal interossei. Have the patient extend and spread his fingers, and tell him to try to resist your attempt to squeeze them together.

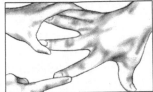

Forearm and hand (grip). Have the patient grasp your middle and index fingers and squeeze as hard as he can. To prevent pain or injury, cross your fingers.

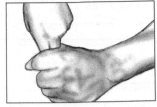

Rate muscle strength on a scale from 0 to 5:
0 = Total paralysis
1 = Visible or palpable contraction, but no movement
2 = Full muscle movement with force of gravity eliminated
3 = Full muscle movement against gravity, but no movement against resistance
4 = Full muscle movement against gravity; partial movement against resistance
5 = Full muscle movement against both gravity and resistance – normal strength

LEG MUSCLES

Anterior tibial. With the patient's leg extended, place your hand on his foot and ask him to dorsiflex his ankle against your resistance. Palpate for anterior tibial contraction.

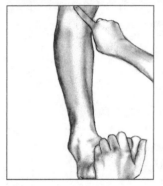

Psoas. While you support his leg, have the patient raise his knee and then flex his hip against your resistance. Watch for psoas contraction.

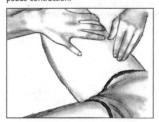

Extensor hallucis longus. With your finger on the patient's great toe, have him dorsiflex the toe against your resistance. Palpate for extensor hallucis contraction.

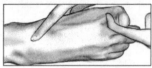

Quadriceps. Have the patient bend his knee slightly while you support his lower leg. Then ask him to extend the knee against your resistance; as he's doing so, palpate for quadriceps contraction.

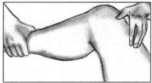

Gastrocnemius. With the patient on his side, support his foot and ask him to plantarflex his ankle against your resistance. Palpate for gastrocnemius contraction.

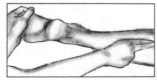

ASSESSING DEEP TENDON REFLEXES

During a neurologic examination, you'll assess the patient's deep tendon reflexes. Test the biceps, triceps, brachioradialis, patellar or quadriceps, and Achilles reflexes.

BICEPS REFLEX

Position the patient's arm so his elbow is flexed at a 45-degree angle and his arm is relaxed. Place your thumb or index finger over the biceps tendon and your remaining fingers loosely over the triceps muscle. Strike your finger with the pointed end of the reflex hammer, and watch and feel for the contraction of the biceps muscle and flexion of the forearm.

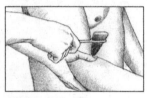

TRICEPS REFLEX

Have the patient adduct his arm and place his forearm across his chest. Strike the triceps tendon about 2" (5 cm) above the olecranon process on the extensor surface of the upper arm. Watch for contraction of the triceps muscle and extension of the forearm.

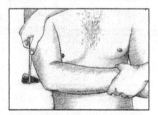

BRACHIORADIALIS REFLEX

Ask the patient to rest the ulnar surface of his hand on his abdomen or lap with the elbow partially flexed. Strike the radius, and watch for supination of the hand and flexion of the forearm at the elbow.

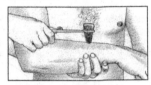

PATELLAR REFLEX

Have the patient sit with his legs dangling freely. If he can't sit up, flex his knee at a 45-degree angle, and place your nondominant hand behind it for support. Strike the patellar tendon just below the patella, and look for contraction of the quadriceps muscle in the thigh with extension of the leg.

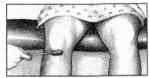

ACHILLES REFLEX

Have the patient flex his foot. Then support the plantar surface. Strike the Achilles tendon, and watch for plantar flexion of the foot at the ankle.

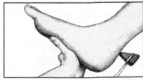

Make sure the patient is relaxed and comfortable during this assessment because tension or anxiety may diminish the reflex. Position the patient comfortably and instruct him to become limp.

If you suspect the patient has depressed reflexes, ask him to perform two isometric muscle contractions. First, to improve leg reflexes, have the patient clench his hands together and tense the arm muscles during the reflex assessment. Second, to improve arm reflexes, have him clench his teeth or squeeze one thigh with the hand not being evaluated.

These maneuvers force the patient to concentrate on something other than the reflexes being tested, which can help to eliminate unintentional inhibition of the reflexes. Hold the reflex hammer loosely, yet securely, between your thumb and fingers so that it can swing freely in a controlled direction. Place the patient's extremities in a neutral position, with the muscle you're testing in a slightly stretched position. Compare reflexes on opposite sides of the body for symmetry of movement and muscle strength. (See *Assessing deep tendon reflexes.*)

Grade DTRs using a 0 for absent impulses; +1 for diminished impulses; +2 for normal impulses; +3 for increased impulses, but may be normal; and +4 for hyperactive impulses. (See *Documenting deep tendon reflexes,* page 62.)

Increased or hyperactive reflexes occur with upper motor neuron disorders, where damaged CNS neurons in the cerebral cortex or corticospinal tracts prevent the brain from inhibiting peripheral reflex activity, thereby allowing a small stimulus to trigger reflexes, which then tend to overrespond. Examples of hyperactive reflexes include spasticity associated with spinal cord injuries or other upper motor neuron disorders such as multiple sclerosis.

Decreased, hypoactive, or absent reflexes indicate a disorder of the lower motor neurons or the anterior horn of the spinal cord, where the peripheral nerve originates. Examples of lower motor neuron disorders characterized by hyporeflexia or areflexia include Guillain-Barré syndrome and amyotrophic lateral sclerosis.

DOCUMENTING DEEP TENDON REFLEXES

Record the patient's deep tendon reflex (DTR) scores by drawing a stick figure and entering the grades on this scale at the proper location. The figure shown here indicates hypoactive DTRs in the legs; other reflexes are normal.

KEY:

    0 = absent
    + = hypoactive (diminished)
  ++ = normal
 +++ = brisk (increased)
++++ = hyperactive (clonus may be present)

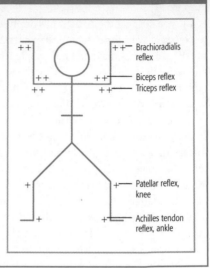

Brachioradialis reflex

Biceps reflex

Triceps reflex

Patellar reflex, knee

Achilles tendon reflex, ankle

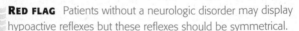

RED FLAG Patients without a neurologic disorder may display hypoactive reflexes but these reflexes should be symmetrical. For example, a compressed spinal nerve root, which can cause a herniated intervertebral disk at L3 or L4, may diminish the patient's knee jerk reflex.

SUPERFICIAL REFLEXES

Stimulating the skin or mucous membranes is a method of testing superficial reflexes. Because these are cutaneous reflexes, the more you try to elicit them in succession, the less of a response you'll get. So observe carefully the first time you stimulate.

Babinski's reflex

Using an applicator stick, tongue blade, or key, slowly stroke the lateral side of the patient's sole from the heel to the great

ELICITING BABINSKI'S REFLEX

To elicit Babinski's reflex, stroke the lateral aspect of the sole of the patient's foot with your thumbnail or another moderately sharp object. Normally, this elicits flexion of all toes — a negative Babinski's reflex — as shown in the left illustration. With a positive Babinski's reflex, the great toe dorsiflexes and the other toes fan out, as shown in the right illustration.

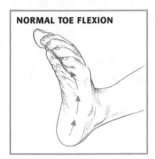

NORMAL TOE FLEXION

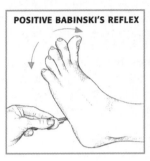

POSITIVE BABINSKI'S REFLEX

toe. The normal response in an adult is plantar flexion of the toes. Upward movement of the great toe and fanning of the little toes — called Babinski's reflex — is abnormal. (See *Eliciting Babinski's reflex*.)

AGE AWARE In normal infants, Babinski's reflex can be elicited, in some cases until age 2. However, plantar flexion of the toes is also seen in more than 90% of normal infants.

Cremasteric reflex

The cremasteric reflex is tested in men by using an applicator stick to stimulate the inner thigh. Normal reaction is contraction of the cremaster muscle and elevation of the testicle on the side of the stimulus.

Abdominal reflex

Test the abdominal reflex with the patient in the supine position with his arms at his sides and his knees slightly flexed.

Briskly stroke both sides of the abdomen above and below the umbilicus, moving from the periphery toward the midline. Movement of the umbilicus toward the stimulus is normal.

PRIMITIVE REFLEXES
The primitive reflexes you'll check for are the grasp, snout, sucking, and glabella reflexes.

AGE AWARE Primitive reflexes are abnormal in an adult but normal in an infant, whose CNS is immature. As the patient's neurologic system matures, these reflexes disappear.

Grasp reflex
Assess the grasp reflex by applying gentle pressure to the patient's palm with your fingers. If the patient grasps your fingers between his thumb and index finger, suspect cortical or premotor cortex damage.

Snout reflex
Assess the snout reflex by lightly tapping on the patient's upper lip. If the patient's lip purses when lightly tapped, suspect frontal lobe damage.

Sucking reflex
Observe the patient while you're feeding him or while he has an oral airway or endotracheal tube in place. A sucking motion while the patient is being fed indicates cortical damage. This reflex is commonly seen in the patient with advanced dementia.

Glabella reflex
Elicit the glabella response by repeatedly tapping the bridge of the patient's nose. If the patient responds with persistent blinking, suspect diffuse cortical dysfunction.

ABNORMAL FINDINGS

A patient may seek care for several signs and symptoms related to the neurologic system. The most significant findings are aphasia; apraxia; Babinski's reflex; Brudzinski's sign; corneal reflex, absent; deep tendon reflexes (DTRs), hyperactive or hypoactive; fasciculations; level of consciousness (LOC), decreased; headache; Kernig's sign; muscle flaccidity; muscle spasticity; paralysis; pupils, nonreactive; Romberg's sign; seizures, generalized tonic-clonic or simple partial; and tremors. The following history, physical assessment, and analysis summaries will help you assess each one quickly and accurately. After obtaining further information, begin to interpret the findings. (See *Neurologic system: Interpreting your findings,* pages 66 to 76.)

Aphasia

Aphasia is the impaired expression or comprehension of written or spoken language. It's indicative of damage to the brain's language centers. Depending on its severity, it may slightly impede communication or may make it virtually impossible.

HISTORY

If the patient doesn't display signs of increased intracranial pressure (ICP), or if aphasia has developed gradually, perform a thorough neurologic examination, starting with the patient history. If necessary, obtain this history from the patient's family because of the patient's impairment. Ask about a history of headaches, hypertension, or seizure disorders and about drug use. Ask about the patient's ability to communicate and to perform routine activities before the aphasia began.

PHYSICAL ASSESSMENT

Check for obvious signs of neurologic deficit, such as ptosis or fluid leakage from the nose and ears. Be aware that assessing the patient's LOC may be difficult because his verbal responses

(Text continues on page 76.)

NEUROLOGIC SYSTEM: INTERPRETING YOUR FINDINGS

After you assess the patient, a group of findings may lead you to suspect a particular neurologic disorder. The chart below shows you some common groups of findings for major signs and symptoms related to the neurologic system, along with their probable causes.

SIGN/SYMPTOM & FINDINGS	PROBABLE CAUSE	SIGN/SYMPTOM & FINDINGS	PROBABLE CAUSE
APHASIA		**APRAXIA**	
● Wernicke's, Broca's, or global aphasia ● Decreased level of consciousness (LOC) ● Right-sided hemiparesis ● Homonymous hemianopsia ● Paresthesia and loss of sensation	Stroke	● Gradual and irreversible motor apraxia ● Amnesia ● Anomia ● Decreased attention span ● Apathy ● Aphasia ● Restlessness, agitation ● Paranoid delusions ● Incontinence ● Social withdrawal ● Ataxia ● Tremors	Alzheimer's disease
● Any type of aphasia occurring suddenly, may be transient or permanent ● Blurred or double vision ● Headache ● Cerebrospinal otorrhea and rhinorrhea ● Disorientation ● Behavioral changes ● Signs of increased intracranial pressure (ICP)	Head trauma	● Occasional apraxia accompanied by headache, fever, drowsiness, decreased mental acuity, aphasia ● Dysarthria ● Hemiparesis ● Hyperreflexia ● Incontinence ● Focal or generalized seizures ● Ocular disturbances such as nystagmus, visual field deficits, unequal pupils	Brain abscess
● Any type of aphasia occurring suddenly and resolving within 24 hours ● Transient hemiparesis ● Paresthesia ● Dizziness, confusion	Transient ischemic attack		

NEUROLOGIC SYSTEM: INTERPRETING YOUR FINDINGS *(continued)*

SIGN/SYMPTOM & FINDINGS	PROBABLE CAUSE
APRAXIA (continued)	
● Progressive apraxia preceded by decreased mental acuity, headache, dizziness, and seizures ● Increased ICP as evidenced by pupillary changes ● Localized signs and symptoms of tumor such as aphasia, dysarthria, visual field deficits, weakness, stiffness, and hyperreflexia	Brain tumor
BABINSKI'S REFLEX	
● Bilateral Babinski's reflex with hyperactive deep tendon reflexes (DTRs) and spasticity ● Fasciculations accompanied by muscle atrophy and weakness ● Incoordination ● Impaired speech ● Difficulty chewing, swallowing, or breathing ● Urinary frequency and urgency ● Occasional choking and drooling	Amyotrophic lateral sclerosis (ALS)
● Unilateral or bilateral Babinski's reflex with hyperreflexia and spasticity ● Weakness and incoordination	Head trauma

SIGN/SYMPTOM & FINDINGS	PROBABLE CAUSE
BABINSKI'S REFLEX (continued)	
● Headache ● Vomiting ● Behavioral changes ● Altered vital signs ● Decreased LOC with abnormal pupil size and response to light	
● Babinski's reflex unilateral, eventually becoming bilateral ● Initially paresthesia, nystagmus, and blurred or double vision ● Scanning speech ● Dysphagia ● Intention tremor ● Weakness, incoordination ● Spasticity ● Gait ataxia ● Seizures ● Paraparesis or paraplegia ● Bladder incontinence ● Occasionally, loss of pain and temperature sensation and proprioception	Multiple sclerosis
● Unilateral Babinski's reflex with hemiplegia or hemiparesis, unilateral hyperactive DTRs, hemianopsia, and aphasia, if stroke involves cerebrum	Stroke

(continued)

NEUROLOGIC SYSTEM: INTERPRETING YOUR FINDINGS *(continued)*

SIGN/SYMPTOM & FINDINGS	PROBABLE CAUSE
BABINSKI'S REFLEX (continued)	
● Bilateral Babinski's reflex with bilateral weakness or paralysis, bilateral hyperreflexia, cranial nerve dysfunction, incoordination and unsteady gait if stroke involves brain stem	
BRUDZINSKI'S SIGN	
● Positive sign occurring within 24 hours of onset of disorder ● Headache ● Positive Kernig's sign ● Nuchal rigidity ● Irritability ● Deep stupor or coma ● Vertigo ● Fever ● Chills, malaise ● Hyperalgesia ● Opisthotonos ● Symmetrical DTRs ● Papilledema ● Ocular and facial palsies ● Nausea and vomiting ● Photophobia, diplopia, and unequal sluggish pupils	Meningitis
● Positive sign within minutes of onset of hemorrhage ● Sudden onset of severe headache	Subarachnoid hemorrhage

SIGN/SYMPTOM & FINDINGS	PROBABLE CAUSE
BRUDZINSKI'S SIGN (continued)	
● Nuchal rigidity ● Altered LOC ● Dizziness ● Photophobia ● Cranial nerve palsies ● Nausea and vomiting ● Fever ● Positive Kernig's sign	
CORNEAL REFLEX, ABSENT	
● Diminished or absent corneal reflex ● Tinnitus ● Unilateral hearing impairment ● Facial palsy and anesthesia ● Palate weakness ● Ataxia, nystagmus if tumor impinging on adjacent cranial nerves	Acoustic neuroma
● Diminished or absent corneal reflex ● Complete hemifacial weakness or paralysis ● Drooling on affected side ● Masklike appearance of affected side ● Constant eye tearing on affected side	Bell's palsy

NEUROLOGIC SYSTEM: INTERPRETING YOUR FINDINGS *(continued)*

SIGN/SYMPTOM & FINDINGS	PROBABLE CAUSE
CORNEAL REFLEX, ABSENT (continued)	
● Diminished or absent corneal reflex with sudden bursts of intense pain or shooting sensation lasting from 1 to 15 minutes, possibly triggered by light touch or exposure to hot or cold temperatures ● Hypersensitivity around mouth and nose	Trigeminal neuralgia
DEEP TENDON REFLEXES, HYPERACTIVE	
● Sudden or gradual onset of hyperactive DTRs with paresthesia, muscle twitching and cramping ● Positive Chvostek's and Trousseau's signs ● Carpopedal spasm and tetany	Hypocalcemia
● Hyperactive DTRs preceded by weakness and paresthesia in one or both arms or legs ● Clonus ● Positive Babinski's reflex ● Tingling sensation down back with passive flexion of neck ● Ataxia ● Diplopia ● Vertigo	Multiple sclerosis

SIGN/SYMPTOM & FINDINGS	PROBABLE CAUSE
DEEP TENDON REFLEXES, HYPERACTIVE (continued)	
● Vomiting ● Urinary retention or incontinence	
● Sudden onset of generalized hyperactive DTRs accompanied by tachycardia, diaphoresis, low-grade fever, and painful involuntary muscle contractions ● Trismus ● Masklike grin	Tetanus
DEEP TENDON REFLEXES, HYPOACTIVE	
● Hypoactive DTRs ● Associated signs and symptoms variable depending on cause and location of dysfunction	Cerebellar dysfunction
● Bilateral hypoactive DTRs progressing rapidly from hypotonia to areflexia ● Muscle weakness beginning in the legs and extending to the arm and possibly trunk and neck muscles ● Cranial nerve palsies ● Pain ● Paresthesia	Guillain-Barré syndrome

(continued)

NEUROLOGIC SYSTEM: INTERPRETING YOUR FINDINGS *(continued)*

SIGN/SYMPTOM & FINDINGS	PROBABLE CAUSE
DEEP TENDON REFLEXES, HYPOACTIVE (continued)	
● Signs of brief autonomic dysfunction such as sinus tachycardia or bradycardia, flushing, fluctuating blood pressure, and anhidrosis	
● Hypoactive DTRs below the level of lesion ● Quadriplegia or paraplegia ● Flaccidity ● Loss of sensation below lesion ● Dry, pale skin ● Urine retention with overflow incontinence ● Hypoactive bowel sounds ● Constipation ● Loss of genital reflex	Spinal cord lesion
FASCICULATIONS	
● Fasciculations of face and tongue early on ● Dysarthria ● Dysphagia ● Hoarseness ● Drooling ● Eventual spreading of weakness to respiratory muscles	Bulbar palsy
● Fasciculations of muscles innervated by compressed nerve roots	Herniated disk

SIGN/SYMPTOM & FINDINGS	PROBABLE CAUSE
FASCICULATIONS (continued)	
● Severe low back pain possibly radiating unilaterally to the leg and exacerbated by coughing, sneezing, bending, and straining ● Muscle weakness, atrophy, and spasms ● Paresthesia ● Footdrop ● Steppage gait ● Hypoactive DTRs in legs	
● Coarse, usually transient, fasciculations accompanied by progressive muscle weakness, spasms, and atrophy ● Decreased DTRs ● Paresthesia ● Coldness and cyanosis in affected limbs ● Bladder paralysis ● Dyspnea ● Elevated blood pressure ● Tachycardia	Poliomyelitis, spinal paralytic
HEADACHE	
● Excruciating headache ● Acute eye pain ● Blurred vision ● Halo vision ● Nausea and vomiting	Acute angle-closure glaucoma

NEUROLOGIC SYSTEM: INTERPRETING YOUR FINDINGS *(continued)*

SIGN/SYMPTOM & FINDINGS	PROBABLE CAUSE
HEADACHE *(continued)*	
● Moderately dilated, fixed pupils	
● Slightly throbbing occipital headache on awakening that decreases in severity during day ● Atrial gallop ● Restlessness ● Blurred vision ● Nausea and vomiting	Hypertension
● Sudden onset of severe generalized or frontal headache ● Stabbing retro-orbital pain ● Weakness, diffuse myalgia ● Fever, chills ● Coughing ● Rhinorrhea	Influenza
KERNIG'S SIGN	
● Positive sign with fever, chills ● Nuchal rigidity ● Hyperreflexia ● Brudzinski's sign ● Opisthotonos ● Headache and vomiting with increasing ICP	Meningitis
● Positive Kernig's sign with positive Brudzinski's sign	Subarachnoid hemorrhage

SIGN/SYMPTOM & FINDINGS	PROBABLE CAUSE
KERNIG'S SIGN *(continued)*	
● Sudden onset of severe headache, initially localized but then spreads ● Pupillary inequality ● Nuchal rigidity ● Decreased LOC	
LEVEL OF CONSCIOUSNESS, DECREASED	
● Slowly decreasing LOC, from lethargy to coma ● Apathy, behavior changes ● Memory loss ● Decreased attention span ● Morning headache ● Sensorimotor disturbances	Brain tumor
● Slowly decreasing LOC, from lethargy to coma ● Malaise ● Tachycardia ● Tachypnea ● Orthostatic hypotension ● Hot skin, flushed, and diaphoretic	Heatstroke

(continued)

NEUROLOGIC SYSTEM: INTERPRETING YOUR FINDINGS (continued)

SIGN/SYMPTOM & FINDINGS	PROBABLE CAUSE

LEVEL OF CONSCIOUSNESS, DECREASED (continued)

- Lethargy, progressing to coma — Shock
- Confusion, anxiety, and restlessness
- Hypotension
- Tachycardia
- Weak pulse with narrowing pulse pressure
- Dyspnea
- Oliguria
- Cool, clammy skin

MUSCLE FLACCIDITY

- Progressive muscle weakness and paralysis accompanied by generalized flaccidity, typically beginning in one hand and spreading to arm, other hand and arm, ultimately spreading to trunk, neck, tongue, larynx, pharynx, and legs — ALS
- Progressive respiratory muscle weakness
- Muscle cramps and coarse fasciculations
- Hyperactive DTRs
- Dysphagia
- Dysarthria
- Excessive drooling
- Depression

- Generalized flaccidity or hypotonia — Cerebellar dysfunction
- Ataxia

SIGN/SYMPTOM & FINDINGS	PROBABLE CAUSE

MUSCLE FLACCIDITY (continued)

- Dysmetria
- Intention tremor
- Slight muscle weakness
- Fatigue
- Dysarthria

- Symmetrical and ascending muscle flaccidity — Guillain-Barré syndrome
- Sensory loss or paresthesia
- Absent DTRs
- Tachycardia, bradycardia
- Fluctuating blood pressure
- Diaphoresis
- Incontinence
- Dysphagia
- Dysarthria
- Hypernasality
- Facial diplegia

MUSCLE SPASTICITY

- Bilateral limb spasticity occurring late — Epidural hemorrhage
- Momentary loss of consciousness after head trauma followed by lucid interval and then rapid deterioration in LOC
- Unilateral hemiparesis or hemiplegia
- Seizures
- Fixed, dilated pupils

NEUROLOGIC SYSTEM: INTERPRETING YOUR FINDINGS *(continued)*

SIGN/SYMPTOM & FINDINGS	PROBABLE CAUSE
MUSCLE SPASTICITY (continued)	
● High fever ● Decreased and bounding pulse ● Widened pulse pressure ● Elevated blood pressure ● Irregular respiratory pattern ● Decerebrate posture ● Positive Babinski's reflex	
● Muscle spasticity, hyperreflexia, and contractures ● Progressive weakness and atrophy ● Diplopia, blurred vision, or loss of vision ● Nystagmus ● Sensory loss or paresthesia ● Dysarthria ● Dysphagia ● Incoordination, ataxic gait ● Intention tremors ● Emotional lability ● Impotence ● Urinary dysfunction	Multiple sclerosis
● Spastic paralysis on affected side following acute stage ● Dysarthria ● Aphasia ● Ataxia	Stroke

SIGN/SYMPTOM & FINDINGS	PROBABLE CAUSE
MUSCLE SPASTICITY (continued)	
● Apraxia ● Agnosia ● Ipsilateral paresthesia or sensory loss ● Vision disturbance ● Altered LOC ● Amnesia ● Personality changes ● Emotional lability ● Bowel and bladder dysfunction	
PARALYSIS	
● Transient, unilateral, facial muscle paralysis with sagging muscles and failure of eyelid closure ● Increased tearing ● Diminished or absent corneal reflex	Bell's palsy
● Transient paralysis that gradually becomes more persistent ● May include weak eye closure, ptosis, diplopia, lack of facial mobility, and dysphagia ● Neck muscle weakness ● Possible respiratory distress	Myasthenia gravis
● Permanent spastic paralysis below the level of back injury	Spinal cord injury

(continued)

NEUROLOGIC SYSTEM: INTERPRETING YOUR FINDINGS *(continued)*

SIGN/SYMPTOM & FINDINGS	PROBABLE CAUSE
PARALYSIS (continued)	
● Absent reflexes may or may not return	
PUPILS, NONREACTIVE OR SLUGGISH	
● Initially sluggish pupils becoming dilated and nonreactive ● Decreased accommodation and cranial nerve palsies ● Decreased LOC ● High fever ● Headache ● Vomiting ● Nuchal rigidity	Encephalitis
● Bilateral midposition nonreactive pupils ● Loss of upward gaze ● Coma ● Central neurogenic hyperventilation ● Bradycardia ● Hemiparesis or hemiplegia ● Decorticate or decerebrate posture	Midbrain lesion
● Dilated nonreactive pupils and loss of accommodation reaction (unilateral or bilateral depending on whether palsy is unilateral or bilateral) ● Diplopia	Oculomotor nerve palsy

SIGN/SYMPTOM & FINDINGS	PROBABLE CAUSE
PUPILS, NONREACTIVE OR SLUGGISH (continued)	
● Ptosis ● Outward deviation of eye	
ROMBERG'S SIGN	
● Positive Romberg's sign with nystagmus, constipation, muscle weakness, and spasticity ● Vision changes, diplopia, and paresthesia early on ● Hyperreflexia ● Dysphagia ● Dysarthria ● Incontinence ● Urinary frequency and urgency ● Impotence ● Emotional instability	Multiple sclerosis
● Positive Romberg's sign with loss of proprioception in lower limbs ● Gait changes ● Muscle weakness ● Impaired coordination ● Paresthesia ● Sensory loss ● Hypoactive or hyperactive DTRs ● Sore tongue ● Positive Babinski's reflex ● Fatigue	Anemia, pernicious

NEUROLOGIC SYSTEM: INTERPRETING YOUR FINDINGS *(continued)*

SIGN/SYMPTOM & FINDINGS	PROBABLE CAUSE

ROMBERG'S SIGN *(continued)*

- Blurred vision
- Light-headedness

● Positive Romberg's sign ● Vertigo ● Nystagmus ● Nausea and vomiting	Vestibular disorders

SEIZURES, GENERALIZED TONIC-CLONIC OR SIMPLE PARTIAL

● Generalized seizures depending on location and type of tumor ● Slowly decreasing LOC ● Morning headache ● Dizziness, confusion ● Focal seizures ● Vision loss ● Motor and sensory disturbances ● Aphasia ● Ataxia	Brain tumor
● Generalized seizures ● Severe frontal headache ● Nausea and vomiting ● Increased blood pressure ● Fever ● Peripheral edema ● Sudden weight gain ● Oliguria ● Irritability ● Hyperactive DTRs	Eclampsia

SEIZURES, GENERALIZED TONIC-CLONIC OR SIMPLE PARTIAL *(continued)*

- Decreased LOC

● Seizures early on ● Fever ● Headache ● Photophobia ● Nuchal rigidity ● Neck pain ● Vomiting ● Aphasia ● Ataxia ● Hemiparesis ● Nystagmus ● Irritability ● Cranial nerve palsies ● Myoclonic jerks	Encephalitis
● Generalized seizures possible immediately after injury with partial seizures occurring months later ● Decreased LOC ● Soft tissue injury to the face, head, or neck ● Clear or bloody drainage from the mouth, nose, or ears ● Battle's sign ● Lack of response to oculocephalic and oculovestibular stimulation ● Possible motor and sensory deficits along with altered respirations	Head trauma

(continued)

NEUROLOGIC SYSTEM: INTERPRETING YOUR FINDINGS (continued)

SIGN/SYMPTOM & FINDINGS	PROBABLE CAUSE	SIGN/SYMPTOM & FINDINGS	PROBABLE CAUSE
SEIZURES, GENERALIZED TONIC-CLONIC OR SIMPLE PARTIAL (continued)		**TREMORS (continued)**	
● Partial and generalized seizures ● Café-au-lait spots ● Multiple skin tumors ● Scoliosis ● Kyphoscoliosis ● Dizziness ● Ataxia ● Monocular blindness ● Nystagmus	Neurofibromatosis	● Slow, rhythmic resting tremor in the form of flexion-extension or abduction-adduction of the fingers or hand or pronation-supination of the hand—characteristic pill-rolling tremor ● Cogwheel rigidity ● Bradykinesia ● Propulsive gait with forward leaning posture ● Monotone voice ● Masklike facies ● Drooling ● Dysphagia ● Dysarthria ● Occasionally, oculogyric crisis	
TREMORS			
● Intention tremor ● Ataxia ● Nystagmus ● Incoordination ● Muscle weakness and atrophy ● Hypoactive or absent DTRs	Cerebellar tumor		
● Tremors beginning in fingers and possibly affecting foot, eyelids, jaw, lips, and tongue	Parkinson's disease	● Mild cases with fever, headache, and body aches accompanied by rash and swollen lymph nodes ● More severe cases with headache, high fever, neck stiffness, stupor, disorientation, coma, tremors, occasional seizures, paralysis	West Nile encephalitis

may be unreliable. Also, recognize that dysarthria or speech apraxia may accompany aphasia, so speak slowly and distinctly, and allow the patient ample time to respond. Assess the patient's pupillary response; eye movements; motor function, especially mouth and tongue movement; swallowing ability; and spontaneous movements and gestures. To best assess motor function, first demonstrate the motions, and then have the patient imitate them.

ANALYSIS

Aphasia reflects damage to one or more of the brain's primary language centers, which are normally located in the left hemisphere. It can be classified as Broca's, Wernicke's, anomic, or global aphasia. Anomic aphasia eventually resolves in more than 50% of patients, but global aphasia is generally irreversible. Some causes include stroke, encephalitis, brain tumor or abscess, and head trauma.

AGE AWARE The term "childhood aphasia" is sometimes mistakenly applied to children who fail to develop normal language skills but who aren't considered mentally retarded or developmentally delayed. Aphasia refers solely to loss of previously developed communication skills. Brain damage associated with aphasia in children usually follows anoxia, the result of near drowning or airway obstruction.

Apraxia

Apraxia is the inability to perform purposeful movements in the absence of significant weakness, sensory loss, poor coordination, or lack of comprehension or motivation. Its onset, severity, and duration vary.

HISTORY

If apraxia is detected, ask about previous neurologic disease. Inquire about previous cerebrovascular disease, atherosclerosis, neoplastic disease, infection, or hepatic disease. Ask the patient if he has recently experienced headaches or dizziness. Then assess the apraxia further to help determine its type.

PHYSICAL ASSESSMENT

If the patient fails to report apraxia, begin a neurologic assessment. First, take the patient's vital signs and assess his LOC. Be alert for evidence of aphasia or dysarthria.

Test the patient's motor function, observing for weakness and tremors. Next, use a small pin or other pointed object to test sensory function. Check DTRs for quality and symmetry. Finally, test the patient for visual field deficits.

RED FLAG Be alert for signs and symptoms of increased ICP, such as headache and vomiting. If present, elevate the head of the bed 30 degrees and monitor the patient closely for altered pupil size and reactivity, bradycardia, widened pulse pressure, and irregular respirations. Be prepared to implement emergency resuscitation measures.

ANALYSIS

Apraxia is a neurologic sign that usually indicates a lesion in the cerebral hemisphere. It's classified as ideational, ideomotor, or kinetic, depending on the stage at which voluntary movement is impaired. It can also be classified by type of motor or skill impairment. For example, facial and gait apraxia involve specific motor groups and are easily perceived. Constructional apraxia refers to the inability to copy simple drawings or patterns. Dressing apraxia refers to the inability to correctly dress oneself. Callosal apraxia refers to normal motor function on one side of the body accompanied by the inability to reproduce movements on the other side.

AGE AWARE In children, detecting apraxia can be difficult. However, any sudden inability to perform a previously accomplished movement warrants prompt neurologic evaluation because brain tumor — the most common cause of apraxia in children — can be treated effectively if detected early. Brain damage in young children may cause developmental apraxia, which interferes with the ability to learn activities that require sequential movement, such as hopping, jumping, hitting or kicking a ball, or dancing.

Babinski's reflex

Babinski's reflex — dorsiflexion of the great toe with extension and fanning of the other toes — is an abnormal reflex elicited by firmly stroking the lateral aspect of the sole with a blunt object.

HISTORY

Obtain a complete health history from the patient. Ask about previous neurologic disease. Inquire about previous cerebrovascular disease, atherosclerosis, neoplastic disease, infection, or hepatic disease. Ask the patient if he has recently experienced changes in mental status or consciousness.

PHYSICAL ASSESSMENT

After eliciting a positive Babinski's reflex, evaluate the patient for other neurologic signs. Evaluate muscle strength in each extremity by having the patient push or pull against your resistance. Passively flex and extend the extremity to assess muscle tone. Intermittent resistance to flexion and extension indicates spasticity, and a lack of resistance indicates flaccidity.

Next, check for evidence of incoordination by asking the patient to perform a repetitive activity. Test DTRs in the patient's elbow, antecubital area, wrist, knee, and ankle by striking the tendon with a reflex hammer. An exaggerated muscle response indicates hyperactive DTRs; little or no muscle response indicates hypoactivity.

Evaluate pain sensation and proprioception in the feet. As you move the patient's toes up and down, ask him to identify the direction in which the toes have been moved without looking at his feet.

ANALYSIS

In some patients, Babinski's reflex can be triggered by noxious stimuli, such as pain, noise, or even bumping the bed. An indicator of corticospinal damage, Babinski's reflex may occur unilaterally or bilaterally. It may also be temporary or permanent. A temporary Babinski's reflex commonly occurs during the postictal phase of a seizure, whereas a permanent Babinski's reflex occurs with corticospinal damage. A positive Babinski's reflex usually occurs with incoordination, weakness, and spasticity, all of which increase the patient's risk of injury.

AGE AWARE Babinski's reflex occurs normally in infants up to age 2, reflecting immaturity of the corticospinal tract. After age

2, Babinski's reflex is pathologic and may result from hydrocephalus or any of the causes more commonly seen in adults.

Brudzinski's sign

A positive Brudzinski's sign — flexion of the hips and knees in response to passive flexion of the neck — signals meningeal irritation. Passive flexion of the neck stretches the nerve roots, causing pain and involuntary flexion of the knees and hips.

HISTORY

If the patient is alert, ask him about headache, neck pain, nausea, and vision disturbances, such as blurred or double vision and photophobia — all indications of increased ICP. Next, observe the patient for signs and symptoms of increased ICP, such as an altered LOC, as evidenced by restlessness, irritability, confusion, lethargy, personality changes, and coma; pupillary changes; bradycardia; widened pulse pressure; irregular respiratory patterns, such as Cheyne-Stokes or Kussmaul's respirations; vomiting; and moderate fever.

Ask the patient or his family, if necessary, about a history of hypertension, spinal arthritis, or recent head trauma. Also ask about dental work and abscessed teeth (a possible cause of meningitis), open-head injury, endocarditis, and I.V. drug abuse. Ask about sudden onset of headaches, which may be associated with subarachnoid hemorrhage.

PHYSICAL ASSESSMENT

Continue the neurologic examination by evaluating the patient's cranial nerve function and noting any motor or sensory deficits. Be sure to look for Kernig's sign as evidenced by resistance to knee extension after flexion of the hip, which is a further indication of meningeal irritation. Also, look for signs of central nervous system (CNS) infection, such as fever and nuchal rigidity.

ANALYSIS

Brudzinski's sign is a common and important early indicator of life-threatening meningitis and subarachnoid hemorrhage. It can be elicited in children as well as adults, although more reliable indicators of meningeal irritation exist for infants. Testing for Brudzinski's sign isn't part of the routine examination, unless meningeal irritation is suspected.

AGE AWARE In infants, Brudzinski's sign may not be a useful indicator of meningeal irritation because more reliable signs — such as bulging fontanels, a weak cry, fretfulness, vomiting, and poor feeding — appear early.

Many patients with a positive Brudzinski's sign are critically ill. They need constant ICP monitoring and frequent neurologic checks, in addition to intensive assessment and monitoring of vital signs, intake and output, and cardiorespiratory status.

Corneal reflex, absent

The corneal reflex is tested bilaterally by drawing a fine-pointed wisp of sterile cotton from a corner of each eye to the cornea. Normally, even though only one eye is tested at a time, the patient blinks bilaterally each time either cornea is touched — this is the corneal reflex. When this reflex is absent, neither eyelid closes when the cornea of one is touched.

HISTORY

Because an absent corneal reflex may signify such progressive neurologic disorders as Guillain-Barré syndrome, ask the patient about associated symptoms — facial pain, dysphagia, and limb weakness. Obtain a thorough health history from the patient or his family members.

PHYSICAL ASSESSMENT

If you can't elicit the corneal reflex, look for other signs of trigeminal nerve dysfunction. To test the three sensory portions of the nerve, touch each side of the patient's face on the

brow, cheek, and jaw with a cotton wisp, and ask him to compare the sensations.

If you suspect facial nerve involvement, note if the upper
face (the brow and eyes) and lower face (the cheek, mouth,
and chin) are weak bilaterally. Lower-motor-neuron facial
weakness affects the face on the same side as the lesion, whereas upper-motor-neuron weakness affects the side opposite the
lesion — predominantly the lower facial muscles.

ANALYSIS

The site of the afferent fibers for this reflex is in the ophthalmic branch of the trigeminal nerve (cranial nerve [CN] V);
the efferent fibers are located in the facial nerve (CN VII). Unilateral or bilateral absence of the corneal reflex may result from
damage to these nerves.

RED FLAG When the corneal reflex is absent, protect the patient's affected eye from injury by lubricating it with artificial
tears to prevent drying.

AGE AWARE In children, brain stem lesions and injuries are
the most common causes of absent corneal reflexes; Guillain-
Barré syndrome and trigeminal neuralgia occur less commonly. Infants, especially those born prematurely, may have an absent corneal
reflex due to anoxic damage to the brain stem.

Deep tendon reflexes, hyperactive

A hyperactive DTR is an abnormally brisk muscle contraction
that occurs in response to a sudden stretch induced by sharply
tapping the muscle's tendon of insertion. This elicited sign may
be graded as brisk or pathologically hyperactive.

HISTORY

After eliciting hyperactive DTRs, take the patient's health history. Ask about spinal cord injury or other trauma and about
prolonged exposure to cold, wind, or water. Find out if the patient could be pregnant. A positive response to any of these
questions requires prompt evaluation to rule out life-threaten-

ing autonomic hyperreflexia, tetanus, preeclampsia, or hypothermia.

Ask about the onset and progression of associated signs and symptoms. Ask about vomiting or altered bladder habits.

PHYSICAL ASSESSMENT

Perform a neurologic examination. Obtain the patient's vital signs. Evaluate his LOC, and test motor and sensory function in the limbs. Ask about paresthesia. Check for ataxia or tremors and for speech and vision deficits. Test for Chvostek's sign, an abnormal spasm of the facial muscles elicited by light taps on the facial nerve in a patient with hypocalcemia. Also check for Trousseau's sign, a carpal spasm induced by inflating a sphygmomanometer cuff on the upper arm to a pressure exceeding systolic blood pressure for 3 minutes in the patient who has hypocalcemia or hypomagnesemia. Finally, check for carpopedal spasm.

ANALYSIS

Hyperactive DTRs are commonly accompanied by clonus. The corticospinal tract and other descending tracts govern the reflex arc — the relay cycle that produces any reflex response. A corticospinal lesion above the level of the reflex arc being tested may result in hyperactive DTRs. Abnormal neuromuscular transmission at the end of the reflex arc may also cause hyperactive DTRs. For example, a deficiency of calcium or magnesium may cause hyperactive DTRs because these electrolytes regulate neuromuscular excitability. Although hyperactive DTRs typically accompany other neurologic findings, they usually lack specific diagnostic value. For example, they're an early, cardinal sign of hypocalcemia.

AGE AWARE In neonates, hyperreflexia may be a normal sign. After age 6, reflex responses are similar to those of adults. When testing DTRs in small children, use distraction techniques to promote reliable results. In children, cerebral palsy commonly causes hyperactive DTRs. Reye's syndrome causes generalized hyperactive

DTRs in stage II; in stage V, DTRs are absent. Adult causes of hyperactive DTRs may also appear in children.

Deep tendon reflexes, hypoactive

A hypoactive DTR is an abnormally diminished muscle contraction that occurs in response to a sudden stretch induced by sharply tapping the muscle's tendon of insertion. It may be graded as minimal (+) or absent (0). Symmetrically reduced (+) reflexes may be normal.

HISTORY

After eliciting hypoactive DTRs, obtain a thorough history from the patient or a family member. Have him describe current signs and symptoms in detail. Ask about nausea, vomiting, constipation, and incontinence. Then take a family and drug history.

PHYSICAL ASSESSMENT

Evaluate the patient's LOC. Test motor function in his limbs, and palpate for muscle atrophy or increased mass. Test sensory function, including pain, touch, temperature, and vibration sense. Ask about paresthesia. To observe gait and coordination, have the patient take several steps.

Check for Romberg's sign by asking him to stand with his feet together and his eyes closed. During conversation, evaluate his speech. Check for signs of vision or hearing loss.

Look for ANS effects by taking the patient's vital signs and monitoring for increased heart rate and blood pressure. Also, inspect the skin for pallor, dryness, flushing, or diaphoresis. Auscultate for hypoactive bowel sounds, and palpate for bladder distention.

ANALYSIS

Normally, a DTR depends on an intact receptor, an intact sensory-motor nerve fiber, an intact neuromuscular-glandular junction, and a functional synapse in the spinal cord. Hypoactive DTRs may result from damage to the reflex arc involving the specific muscle, the peripheral nerve, the nerve roots, or the spinal cord at that level. Hypoactive DTRs are an important sign of many disorders, especially when they appear with other neurologic signs and symptoms.

Abrupt onset of hypoactive DTRs accompanied by muscle weakness may occur with life-threatening Guillain-Barré syndrome, botulism, or spinal cord lesions with spinal shock. Drugs, such as barbiturates, and paralyzing drugs, such as pancuronium, may cause hypoactive reflexes.

AGE AWARE Hypoactive DTRs commonly occur in patients with muscular dystrophy, Friedreich's ataxia, syringomyelia, and spinal cord injury. They also accompany progressive muscular atrophy, which affects preschoolers and adolescents.

Fasciculations

Fasciculations are local muscle contractions representing the spontaneous discharge of a muscle fiber bundle innervated by a single motor nerve filament. These contractions cause visible dimpling or wavelike twitching of the skin, but they aren't strong enough to cause a joint to move. They occur irregularly at frequencies ranging from once every several seconds to two or three times per second; less commonly, myokymia — continuous, rapid fasciculations that cause a rippling effect — may occur. Because fasciculations are brief and painless, they commonly go undetected or are ignored.

HISTORY

Begin taking the history by asking the patient about the nature, onset, and duration of the fasciculations. If the onset was sudden, ask about any precipitating events such as exposure to pesticides.

RED FLAG Pesticide poisoning, although uncommon, is a medical emergency requiring prompt and vigorous intervention.

If the patient isn't in severe distress, find out if he has experienced any sensory changes, such as paresthesia, or difficulty speaking, swallowing, breathing, or controlling bowel or bladder function. Ask him if he's in pain.

Explore the patient's medical history for neurologic disorders, cancer, and recent infections. Also, ask him about his lifestyle, especially stress at home, in his occupation, or at school. Ask the patient about his dietary habits and for a recall of recent food and fluid intake because electrolyte imbalances may also cause muscle twitching.

PHYSICAL ASSESSMENT

Perform a physical examination, looking for fasciculations while the affected muscle is at rest. Observe and test for motor and sensory abnormalities, particularly muscle atrophy and weakness, and decreased DTRs. If these signs and symptoms are noted, suspect motor neuron disease, and perform a comprehensive neurologic examination.

ANALYSIS

Benign, nonpathologic fasciculations are common and normal. They commonly occur in tense, anxious, or overtired people and typically affect the eyelid, thumb, or calf. However, fasciculations may also indicate a severe neurologic disorder, most notably a diffuse motor neuron disorder that causes loss of control over muscle fiber discharge.

 RED FLAG Fasciculations, particularly of the tongue, are an important early sign of Werdnig-Hoffmann disease.

Headache

The most common neurologic symptom, a headache may be localized or generalized, producing mild to severe pain. About 90% of headaches are benign and can be described as vascular, muscle-contraction, or both.

HISTORY

Ask the patient to describe the headache's characteristics and location. Find out how often he gets a headache and how long it typically lasts. Try to identify precipitating factors, such as certain foods and exposure to bright lights. Ask the patient if he's under stress and if he has trouble sleeping. Take a drug history, and ask about head trauma within the past 4 weeks. Find out if the patient has recently experienced nausea, vomiting, photophobia, or vision changes. Ask him if he feels drowsy, confused, or dizzy. Find out if he has recently developed seizures or if he has a history of seizures.

PHYSICAL ASSESSMENT

Begin the physical examination by evaluating the patient's LOC. While checking his vital signs, stay alert for signs of increased ICP — widened pulse pressure, bradycardia, altered respiratory pattern, and increased blood pressure. Check pupil size and response to light, and note any neck stiffness.

AGE AWARE If a child is too young to describe his symptom, suspect a headache if you see him banging or holding his head. In an infant, a shrill cry or bulging fontanels may indicate increased ICP and headache.

ANALYSIS

If not benign, headaches can indicate a severe neurologic disorder associated with intracranial inflammation, increased ICP, or meningeal irritation. They may also result from ocular or sinus disorders and the effects of drugs, tests, and treatments.

Other causes of headache include fever, eyestrain, dehydration, stress, and systemic febrile illnesses. Headaches may occur with certain metabolic disturbances — such as hypoxemia, hypercapnia, hyperglycemia, and hypoglycemia — but they aren't a diagnostic or prominent symptom. Some individuals get headaches after seizures or from coughing, sneezing, heavy lifting, or stooping.

Kernig's sign

A reliable early indicator and tool used to diagnose meningeal irritation, Kernig's sign elicits resistance and hamstring muscle pain when the health care provider attempts to extend the knee while the hip and knee are flexed 90 degrees. However, when the patient's thigh isn't flexed on the abdomen, he can usually completely extend his leg.

HISTORY

If you don't suspect meningeal irritation, ask the patient if he feels back pain that radiates down one or both legs. Find out if he also feels leg numbness, tingling, or weakness. Ask about other signs and symptoms, and find out if he has a history of cancer or back injury.

PHYSICAL ASSESSMENT

Perform a physical examination, concentrating on observing and testing for motor and sensory abnormalities, particularly muscle atrophy and weakness, and decreased DTRs.

ANALYSIS

RED FLAG If a positive Kernig's sign is elicited, suspect life-threatening meningitis or subarachnoid hemorrhage, and immediately prepare for emergency intervention.

With these potentially life-threatening disorders, hamstring muscle resistance results from stretching the blood- or exudate-irritated meninges surrounding spinal nerve roots.

Kernig's sign can also indicate a herniated disk or spinal tumor. With these disorders, sciatic pain results from disk or tumor pressure on spinal nerve roots.

AGE AWARE In children, Kernig's sign is considered ominous because of the greater potential for rapid deterioration.

Level of consciousness, decreased

A decrease in LOC can range from lethargy to stupor to coma. LOC can deteriorate suddenly or gradually and can remain altered temporarily or permanently.

The most sensitive indicator of decreased LOC is a change in the patient's mental status. The Glasgow Coma Scale, which measures ability to respond to verbal, sensory, and motor stimulation, can be used to quickly evaluate a patient's LOC.

HISTORY

Try to obtain health history information from the patient if he's lucid and from his family. Find out if the patient complained of headache, dizziness, nausea, vision or hearing disturbances, weakness, fatigue, or other problems before his LOC decreased. Ask his family if they noticed changes in the patient's behavior, personality, memory, or temperament.

Ask about a history of neurologic disease, cancer, or recent trauma; drug and alcohol use; and the development of other signs and symptoms.

PHYSICAL ASSESSMENT

Because decreased LOC can result from disorders that affect any body system, tailor the remainder of the evaluation according to the patient's associated symptoms. Start by using the Glasgow Coma Scale.

ANALYSIS

Decreased LOC usually results from a neurologic disorder and commonly signals life-threatening complications of hemorrhage, trauma, or cerebral edema. However, this sign can also result from a metabolic, GI, musculoskeletal, urologic, or cardiopulmonary disorder; severe nutritional deficiency; exposure to toxins; or use of certain drugs.

Consciousness is affected by the reticular activating system (RAS), an intricate network of neurons whose axons extend from the brain stem, thalamus, and hypothalamus to the cerebral cortex. A disturbance in any part of this integrated system prevents the intercommunication that makes consciousness possible. Loss of consciousness can result from a bilateral cerebral disturbance, an RAS disturbance, or both. Cerebral dysfunction characteristically produces the least dramatic decrease in a patient's LOC. In contrast, dysfunction of the RAS produces the most dramatic decrease in LOC — coma.

AGE AWARE In children, the primary cause of decreased LOC is head trauma, which commonly results from physical abuse or a motor vehicle accident. Other causes include accidental poisoning, hydrocephalus, and meningitis or brain abscess following an ear or respiratory tract infection.

Muscle flaccidity

Flaccid muscles are profoundly weak and soft, with decreased resistance to movement, increased mobility, and greater than normal range of motion (ROM).

HISTORY

If the patient isn't in distress, ask about the onset and duration of muscle flaccidity and any precipitating factors. Ask about associated symptoms, notably weakness, other muscle changes, and sensory loss or paresthesia.

RED FLAG If the patient has experienced trauma resulting in muscle flaccidity, make sure that his cervical spine has been stabilized and quickly determine his respiratory status. Be prepared to institute emergency measures, as necessary.

PHYSICAL ASSESSMENT

Perform a thorough neurologic examination, focusing on motor and sensory function. Examine the affected muscles for atrophy, which indicates a chronic problem. Test muscle strength and DTRs in all limbs.

AGE AWARE When assessing an infant or a young child, observe the positioning. An infant or a young child with generalized flaccidity may lie in a froglike position, with his hips and knees abducted.

ANALYSIS

The result of disrupted muscle innervation, muscle flaccidity can be localized to a limb or muscle group or generalized over the entire body. Its onset may be acute, as in trauma, or chronic, as in neurologic disease.

AGE AWARE Pediatric causes of muscle flaccidity include myelomeningocele, Lowe's disease, Werdnig-Hoffmann disease, and muscular dystrophy.

Muscle spasticity

Spasticity is a state of excessive muscle tone manifested by increased resistance to stretching and heightened reflexes. It's commonly detected by evaluating a muscle's response to passive movement; a spastic muscle offers more resistance when the passive movement is performed quickly.

HISTORY

When you detect spasticity, ask the patient about its onset, duration, and progression. Find out what, if any, events precipitate the onset. Ask the patient if he has experienced other muscular changes or related symptoms. Find out if his medical history reveals any incidence of trauma or degenerative or vascular disease.

PHYSICAL ASSESSMENT

Take the patient's vital signs, and perform a complete neurologic examination. Test reflexes and evaluate motor and sensory function in all limbs. Evaluate muscles for wasting contractures.

ANALYSIS

Caused by an upper-motor-neuron lesion, spasticity usually occurs in the arm and leg muscles. Long-term spasticity results in muscle fibrosis and contractures.

 RED FLAG Generalized spasticity and trismus in a patient with a recent skin puncture or laceration indicates tetanus.

 AGE AWARE In children, muscle spasticity may be a sign of cerebral palsy.

Paralysis

Paralysis, the total loss of voluntary motor function, results from severe cortical or pyramidal tract damage. Paralysis can be local or widespread, symmetrical or asymmetrical, transient or permanent, and spastic or flaccid. It's usually classified according to location and severity as paraplegia, quadriplegia, or hemiplegia. Incomplete paralysis with profound weakness, or paresis, may precede total paralysis in some patients.

HISTORY

If the patient is in no immediate danger, perform a complete neurologic assessment. Start with the health history, relying on family members for information, if necessary.

Ask about the onset, duration, intensity, and progression of paralysis and about the events leading up to it. Focus medical history questions on the incidence of degenerative neurologic or neuromuscular disease, recent infectious illness, sexually transmitted disease, cancer, or recent injury.

Explore related signs and symptoms, noting fever, headache, vision disturbances, dysphagia, nausea and vomiting, bowel or bladder dysfunction, muscle pain or weakness, and fatigue.

PHYSICAL ASSESSMENT

Perform a complete neurologic examination, testing cranial nerve, motor, and sensory function and DTRs. Assess strength in all major muscle groups, and note any muscle atrophy.

ANALYSIS

Paralysis can occur in patients with a cerebrovascular disorder, degenerative neuromuscular disease, trauma, a tumor, or a CNS infection. Acute paralysis may be an early indicator of a life-threatening disorder such as Guillain-Barré syndrome.

AGE AWARE In children, paralysis may result from trauma, infection, tumors, or a hereditary or congenital disorder such as Tay-Sachs disease, Werdnig-Hoffmann disease, spina bifida, or cerebral palsy.

Pupils, nonreactive or sluggish

Nonreactive, or fixed, pupils fail to constrict in response to light or to dilate when the light is removed. A sluggish pupillary reaction is an abnormally slow pupillary response to light. It can occur in one pupil or both, unlike the normal reaction, which is always bilateral.

HISTORY

If the patient is conscious, obtain a brief health history. Ask him what type of eyedrops he's using, if any, and when they were last instilled. Also ask if he's experiencing pain and, if so, try to determine its location, intensity, and duration.

PHYSICAL ASSESSMENT

Check the patient's visual acuity in both eyes. To evaluate pupillary reaction to light, first test the patient's direct light reflex. Darken the room, and cover one of the patient's eyes while you hold open the opposite eyelid. Using a bright penlight, bring the light toward the patient from the side and shine it directly into his opened eye. If normal, the pupil will promptly constrict. Next, test the consensual light reflex. Hold the patient's eyelids open and shine the light into one eye while watching the pupil of the opposite eye. If normal, both pupils will promptly constrict. Repeat both procedures in the opposite eye.

Also check the pupillary reaction to accommodation. Normally, both pupils constrict equally as the patient shifts his glance from a distant to a near object. Next, hold a penlight at the side of each eye and examine the cornea and iris for any abnormalities. Measure intraocular pressure (IOP) with a manometer, or estimate IOP by placing your second and third fingers over the patient's closed eyelid. If the eyeball feels rock-hard, suspect elevated IOP. Ophthalmoscopic and slit-lamp examinations of the eye will need to be performed.

RED FLAG If the patient has experienced ocular trauma, don't manipulate the affected eye. After the examination, cover the affected eye with a protective metal shield, but don't let the shield rest on the globe.

ANALYSIS

The development of a unilateral or bilateral nonreactive response indicates an important change in the patient's condition and may signal a life-threatening emergency and possibly brain death. A unilateral or bilateral nonreactive response indicates dysfunction of CNs II and III, which mediate the pupillary light reflex. It also occurs with the use of certain drugs. Instillation of a topical mydriatic and a cycloplegic may induce a temporarily nonreactive pupil in the affected eye. Opiates, such as heroin and morphine, cause pinpoint pupils with a minimal light response that can be seen only with a magnifying glass. Atropine poisoning produces widely dilated, nonreactive pupils.

A sluggish reaction accompanies degenerative disease of the CNS and diabetic neuropathy.

AGE AWARE Children have nonreactive or sluggish pupils for the same reasons as adults. The most common cause of nonreactive pupils in children is oculomotor nerve palsy from increased ICP. Sluggish pupils can occur normally in elderly people, whose pupils become smaller and less responsive with age.

Romberg's sign

A positive Romberg's sign refers to a patient's inability to maintain balance when standing erect with his feet together and his eyes closed. Normally, the patient should be able to stand with his feet together and his eyes closed with minimal swaying for about 20 seconds.

HISTORY

Obtain a thorough health history, focusing on areas of problems with coordination and balance. Question the patient about any problems involving dizziness or vertigo and recent ear problems such as infection. Ask the patient if he can sit and stand without support. Note if he uses any assistive devices to maintain his balance or aid in walking.

PHYSICAL ASSESSMENT

After you detect a positive Romberg's sign, perform other neurologic screening tests. A positive Romberg's sign indicates only the presence of a defect; it doesn't pinpoint its cause or location. First, test proprioception. If the patient can't maintain his balance with his eyes open, ask him to hop on one foot and then on the other. Next, ask him to do a knee bend and to walk a straight line, placing heel to toe. Last, ask him to walk a short distance so you can evaluate his gait.

Test the patient's awareness of body part position by changing the position of one of his fingers, or another joint, while his eyes are closed. Ask him to describe the change you've made.

Next, test the patient's direction of movement. Ask him to close his eyes and to touch his nose with the index finger of one hand and then with the other. Ask him to repeat this movement several times, gradually increasing his speed. Then test the accuracy of his movement by having him rapidly touch each finger of one hand to the thumb. Next, test sensation in all dermatomes, using a pin to assess differentiation between sharp and dull. Also test two-point discrimination by touching two pins, one in each hand, to his skin simultaneously. Ask him if he feels one or two pinpricks. Finally, test and characterize the patient's DTRs.

To test the patient's vibratory sense, ask him to close his eyes, and then apply a mildly vibrating tuning fork to a bony prominence such as the medial malleolus. If the patient doesn't feel the stimulus initially, increase the vibration, and then test the knee or hip. This procedure can also be done to test the fingers, the elbow, and the shoulder. Record and compare all test results. Also, ask the patient if he has noticed sensory changes, such as numbness and tingling in his limbs. If so, find out when these changes began.

ANALYSIS

If positive, Romberg's sign indicates a vestibular or proprioceptive disorder or a disorder of the spinal tracts (the posterior columns) that carry proprioceptive information — the perception of one's position in space, of joint movements, and of pressure sensations — to the brain. Insufficient vestibular or proprioceptive information causes an inability to execute precise movements and maintain balance without visual cues. Difficulty performing this maneuver with the eyes open or closed may indicate a cerebellar disorder.

AGE AWARE In children, Romberg's sign can't be tested until they can stand without support and follow commands. However, a positive sign in children commonly results from spinal cord disease.

Seizures, generalized tonic-clonic or simple partial

Like other types of seizures, generalized tonic-clonic seizures are caused by the paroxysmal, uncontrolled discharge of CNS neurons, leading to neurologic dysfunction. Unlike most other types of seizures, however, this cerebral hyperactivity isn't confined to the original focus or to a localized area but extends to the entire brain.

GENERALIZED TONIC-CLONIC SEIZURES

A generalized tonic-clonic seizure may begin with or without an aura. As seizure activity spreads to the subcortical structures, the patient loses consciousness, falls to the ground, and may utter a loud cry that's precipitated by air rushing from the lungs through the vocal cords. His body stiffens in the tonic phase, and then undergoes rapid, synchronous muscle jerking and hyperventilation in the clonic phase. Tongue biting, incontinence, diaphoresis, profuse salivation, and signs of respiratory distress may also occur. The seizure usually stops after 2 to 5 minutes. The patient then regains consciousness but displays confusion. He may complain of headache, fatigue, muscle soreness, and arm and leg weakness.

SIMPLE PARTIAL SEIZURES

Resulting from an irritable focus in the cerebral cortex, simple partial seizures typically last about 30 seconds and don't alter the patient's LOC. The type and pattern reflect the location of the irritable focus.

Simple partial seizures may be classified as motor, including jacksonian seizures and epilepsia partialis continua, or somatosensory, including visual, olfactory, and auditory seizures.

A focal motor seizure is a series of unilateral clonic, or muscle jerking, and tonic, or muscle stiffening, movements of one part of the body. The patient's head and eyes characteristically turn away from the hemispheric focus — usually the frontal lobe near the motor strip. A tonic-clonic contraction of the trunk or extremities may follow.

A jacksonian motor seizure typically begins with a tonic contraction of a finger, the corner of the mouth, or one foot. Clonic movements follow, spreading to other muscles on the same side of the body, moving up the arm or leg, and eventually involving the whole side. Alternatively, clonic movements may spread to the opposite side, becoming generalized and leading to loss of consciousness. In the postictal phase, the patient may experience paralysis (Todd's paralysis) in the affected limbs, usually resolving within 24 hours.

Epilepsia partialis continua causes clonic twitching of one muscle group, usually in the face, arm, or leg. Twitching occurs every few seconds and persists for hours, days, or months without spreading. Spasms usually affect the distal arm and leg muscles more than the proximal ones; in the face, they affect the corner of the mouth, one or both eyelids and, occasionally, the neck or trunk muscles unilaterally.

A focal somatosensory seizure affects a localized body area on one side. Usually, this type of seizure initially causes numbness, tingling, or crawling or "electric" sensations; occasionally, it causes pain or burning sensations in the lips, fingers, or toes. A visual seizure involves sensations of darkness or of stationary or moving lights or spots, usually red at first, then blue, green, and yellow. It can affect both visual fields or the visual field on the side opposite the lesion. The irritable focus is in the occipital lobe. In contrast, the irritable focus in an auditory or olfactory seizure is in the temporal lobe.

HISTORY

If the patient isn't experiencing a generalized seizure at the moment, obtain a description from a witness, if possible. Ask when the seizure started and how long it lasted. Find out if the patient reported any unusual sensations before the seizure began. Ask the witness if the seizure started in one area of the body and spread, or if it affected the entire body right away. Find out if the patient fell on a hard surface and if his eyes or head turned. Find out if he turned blue and lost bladder control. Ask about any other seizures before he recovered.

If the patient may have sustained a head injury, observe him closely for loss of consciousness, unequal or nonreactive pupils, and focal neurologic signs. Ask the patient if he has a headache and muscle soreness. Note if he's increasingly difficult to arouse when you check on him at 20-minute intervals. Examine his arms, legs, and face, including his tongue, for injury, residual paralysis, or limb weakness.

Next, obtain a health history. Find out if the patient has ever had generalized or focal seizures before. If so, find out if they occurred frequently. Ask him if other family members also have them. Find out if the patient is receiving drug therapy and if he's compliant. Also, ask about sleep deprivation and emotional or physical stress at the time the seizure occurred.

For a partial seizure, note whether the patient turns his head and eyes. If so, note to which side he turns them. Observe where movement first starts and if it spreads. Because a partial seizure may become generalized, watch closely for loss of consciousness, bilateral tonicity and clonicity, cyanosis, tongue-biting, and urinary incontinence

Ask the patient to describe exactly what he remembers, if anything, about the seizure and its aftermath. Ask the patient what happened before the seizure. Also ask him if he can describe an aura or if he recognized its onset. If so, find out how, such as if it was by a smell, a vision disturbance, or a sound or visceral phenomenon such as an unusual sensation in his stomach. Ask him how this seizure compares with others he has had. Also, explore fully any history, recent or remote, of head trauma. Check for a history of stroke or recent infection, especially with a fever, headache, or stiff neck.

PHYSICAL ASSESSMENT

Perform a complete neurologic examination, focusing on the patient's mental status and LOC. Also observe for residual deficits, such as weakness in the involved extremity, and sensory disturbances.

ANALYSIS

Generalized tonic-clonic seizures usually occur singly. The patient may be asleep or awake and active. Possible complications include respiratory arrest due to airway obstruction from secretions, status epilepticus (occurring in 5% to 8% of patients), head or spinal injuries and bruises, Todd's paralysis and, rarely, cardiac arrest. Life-threatening status epilepticus is marked by prolonged seizure activity or by rapidly recurring seizures with no intervening periods of recovery. It's most commonly triggered by abrupt discontinuation of anticonvulsant therapy.

Generalized seizures may be caused by a brain tumor, vascular disorder, head trauma, infection, metabolic defect, barbiturates, alcohol withdrawal syndrome, exposure to toxins such as arsenic, or a genetic defect. Contrast agents used in radiologic tests may cause generalized seizures. Toxic blood levels of some drugs, such as theophylline, lidocaine, meperidine, penicillins, and cimetidine, may cause generalized seizures. Phenothiazines, tricyclic antidepressants, amphetamines, isoniazid, and vincristine may cause seizures in patients with preexisting epilepsy. Generalized seizures may also result from a focal seizure. With recurring seizures, or epilepsy, the cause may be unknown.

AGE AWARE In children, generalized seizures are common. In fact, 75% to 90% of patients with epilepsy experience their first seizure before age 20. Many children ages 3 months to 3 years experience generalized seizures associated with fever; some of these children later develop seizures without fever. Generalized seizures may also stem from inborn errors of metabolism, perinatal injury, brain infection, Reye's syndrome, Sturge-Weber syndrome, arteriovenous malformation, lead poisoning, hypoglycemia, and idiopathic causes. The pertussis component of the diphtheria and tetanus toxoids and pertussis vaccine also may cause seizures, although this is rare. Affecting more children than adults, focal seizures are likely to spread and become generalized. They typically cause the eyes, or the head and eyes, to turn to the side; in neonates, they cause mouth twitching, staring, or both. Focal seizures in children can result from hemiplegic cerebral palsy, head trauma, child abuse, arteriovenous malformation, or Sturge-Weber syndrome.

Tremors

The most common type of involuntary muscle movement, tremors are regular, rhythmic oscillations that result from alternating contraction of opposing muscle groups. Tremors can be characterized by their location, amplitude, and frequency.

HISTORY

Begin the patient history by asking him about the tremor's onset, and about its duration, progression, and any aggravating or alleviating factors. Find out if the tremor interferes with the patient's normal activities. Ask him if he has other symptoms. Find out if he has noticed behavioral changes or memory loss — the patient's family or his friends may provide more accurate information about this.

Explore the patient's personal and family medical history for a neurologic (especially seizures), endocrine, or metabolic disorder. Obtain a complete drug history, noting especially the use of phenothiazines or herbal remedies. Also, ask about alcohol use.

PHYSICAL ASSESSMENT

Assess the patient's overall appearance and demeanor, noting mental status. Test ROM and strength in all major muscle groups while observing for chorea, athetosis, dystonia, and other involuntary movements. Check DTRs and, if possible, observe the patient's gait.

ANALYSIS

Tremors are classified as resting, intention, or postural. Resting tremors occur when an extremity is at rest and subside with movement. They include the classic pill-rolling tremor of Parkinson's disease. Conversely, intention tremors occur only with movement and subside with rest. Postural (or action) tremors appear when an extremity (or the trunk) is actively held in a particular posture or position. A common type of postural tremor is called an *essential tremor.*

Tremorlike movements may also be elicited, such as aster-ixis — the characteristic flapping tremor seen in hepatic fail-ure. Stress or emotional upset tends to aggravate a tremor. Al-cohol commonly diminishes postural tremors.

Tremors are typical signs of extrapyramidal or cerebellar disorders and can also result from certain drugs. Phenoth-iazines, particularly piperazine derivatives, such as fluphenazine and other antipsychotics, may cause resting and pill-rolling tremors. Less commonly, metoclopramide and metyrosine may also cause these tremors. Lithium toxicity; sympathomimetics, such as terbutaline and pseudoephedrine; amphetamines; and phenytoin can all cause tremors that dis-appear with dose reduction. Manganese toxicity and mercury poisoning also may cause tremors.

RED FLAG Herbal products, such as ephedra (ma huang), have been known to cause serious adverse reactions, which may include tremors.

AGE AWARE A normal neonate may display coarse tremors with stiffening — an exaggerated hypocalcemic startle reflex — in response to noises and chills. Pediatric-specific causes of pathologic tremors include cerebral palsy, fetal alcohol syndrome, and maternal drug addiction.

3

Diagnostic tests and procedures

Diagnostic tests are performed to detect such brain diseases or disorders as congenital defects and anomalies, perinatal defects, ventricular abnormalities, epilepsies, degenerative diseases, and space-occupying lesions. This last category includes neoplasms, infections, and vascular lesions such as arteriovenous malformations. (See *Neuropsychological testing.*)

Infectious diseases may also be diagnosed, including those caused by bacteria, such as meningitis; viruses, such as encephalitis or polioencephalomyelitis; spirochetes, such as neurosyphilis; parasitic infestations, such as toxoplasmosis (common in patients with acquired immunodeficiency syndromes); and fungal and related infections. Demyelinating diseases, such as multiple sclerosis; cerebrovascular disorders, including stroke, transient ischemic attacks, aneurysms of the blood vessels, and subdural and subarachnoid hemorrhages; and disorders of the skull, vertebral column, and other nonneural tissues may also be diagnosed using the tests presented in this chapter.

These tests may also detect such disorders of the brain stem and cranial nerves as vascular insufficiency due to obstruction to specific regions of the brain stem, cranial nerve syndromes (such as trigeminal neuralgia), headache disorders, and congenital disorders that occur as distortions of normal relationships between the skull and vertebral column or as abnormal formations of the skull base.

NEUROPSYCHOLOGICAL TESTING

Rather than documenting physiologic changes in the nervous system, neuropsychological testing evaluates the effects of neurologic disorders on a patient's ability to function.

Indications

Neuropsychological tests can evaluate cognitive functioning, including general intelligence, attention span, memory, and judgment as well as motor, sensory, and speech ability. Certain tests can assess emotional lability, quality of language production, abstraction, distractibility, persistence, or the ability to sequence learned activities. The neuropsychologist chooses the appropriate test based on the reason for the assessment and the skills being assessed.

Besides determining the type and extent of functional deficits in the patient with a known neurologic illness, neuropsychological tests can diagnose organic brain dysfunction and dementia. They're also used to determine whether an injured patient can return to a previous occupation or should be declared disabled. What's more, these tests can assess the extent of rehabilitation or vocational training required before the patient can fully function again. Neuropsychological tests may be performed before and after a major neurosurgical or radiologic procedure to obtain baseline information for comparison with postprocedural information. A neuropsychologist administers the series of paper-and-pencil tests, possibly in combination with other tests using puzzles, blocks, or word or recall games. The neuropsychologist explains each test to the patient before administration.

Precautions

Because these tests are mentally demanding and lengthy, they may tire the patient. If possible, withdraw medications that affect his ability to concentrate before the test. The patient should be well rested and free from sedatives, if possible, before testing. Any physiologic problem that may interfere with mental function or level of consciousness, such as fever or electrolyte imbalance, should be treated before testing to ensure that results are as accurate as possible.

The spinal cord may be affected by metastasis from non-central nervous system primary tumors that spread to the vertebrae and meninges, producing extradural tumors that distort the spinal cord or interrupt cerebrospinal fluid (CSF) flow in the spinal subarachnoid spaces. This, in turn, causes a block in CSF circulation accompanied by spinal cord dysfunction. In addition to the spinal cord, the brain stem may also be affected by Guillain-Barré syndrome, which is typically a myeloradiculopathy.

Because disorders of the peripheral nervous system are in many cases toxic or metabolic in origin, the tests covered in this chapter are generally not as useful for investigating exposure to toxins or as a systemic metabolic workup. In addition, the diagnosis of peripheral neuropathies commonly depends on nerve biopsy, which allows the identification of specific pathologic change in the nerve fibers. Similarly, when attempting to identify myopathies or muscle disorders, muscle biopsy is commonly the preferred diagnostic tool.

The patient's ability to function with neurologic disorders can be evaluated by other tests.

LABORATORY TESTS
BACTERIAL MENINGITIS ANTIGEN

The bacterial meningitis antigen test can detect specific antigens of *Streptococcus pneumoniae, Neisseria meningitidis, Haemophilus influenzae* type B, or group B streptococci, the principal etiologic agents in meningitis. Although cerebrospinal fluid (CSF) and urine are the preferred sample for analysis, the test may also be performed using samples of serum, pleural fluid, and joint fluid. Positive results identify the specific bacterial antigen: *S. pneumoniae, N. meningitidis, H. influenzae* type B, or group B streptococci.

Nursing considerations
- Explain the purpose of the test to the patient and his family, as appropriate.
- Inform the patient that this test requires a specimen of urine or CSF. Explain who will perform the procedure and when.
- If a CSF specimen is required, describe how it will be obtained by a lumbar puncture procedure.

- Explain to the patient that he may experience discomfort from the needle puncture.
- Advise the patient that headache is the most common complication of lumbar puncture, but that his cooperation during the test minimizes such an effect.
- Verify that the patient or a family member has signed an informed consent form for the lumbar puncture.
- Collect a 10-ml urine specimen or a 1-ml CSF specimen in a sterile container.
- Maintain specimen sterility during collection.
- Wear gloves when obtaining or handling the specimen.
- Make sure the cap is tightly fastened on the specimen container.
- Place the specimen on a refrigerated coolant, and send it to the laboratory immediately.

CEREBROSPINAL FLUID ANALYSIS

Cerebrospinal fluid (CSF), a clear substance that circulates in the subarachnoid space, has many vital functions. It protects the brain and spinal cord from injury and transports products of neurosecretion, cellular biosynthesis, and cellular metabolism through the central nervous system (CNS).

For qualitative analysis, CSF is most commonly obtained by lumbar puncture (usually between the third and fourth lumbar vertebrae) and, rarely, by cisternal or ventricular puncture. A CSF specimen may also be obtained during other neurologic tests, such as myelography or from a ventriculostomy tube. CSF analysis aids the diagnosis of viral or bacterial meningitis, subarachnoid or intracranial hemorrhage, tumors, brain abscesses, neurosyphilis, and chronic CNS infections. (See *Findings in cerebrospinal fluid analysis,* pages 106 and 107.)

Normally, the CSF pressure is recorded and the appearance of the specimen is checked. Three tubes are collected routinely and are sent to the laboratory for protein, sugar, and

(Text continues on page 108.)

FINDINGS IN CEREBROSPINAL FLUID ANALYSIS

TEST	NORMAL	ABNORMALITY
Pressure	50 to 180 mm H_2O	Increase
		Decrease
Appearance	Clear, colorless	Cloudy
		Xanthochromic or bloody
		Brown, orange, or yellow
Protein	15 to 50 mg/dl (SI, 0.15 to 0.5 g/L)	Marked increase
		Marked decrease
Gamma globulin	3% to 12% of total protein	Increase
Glucose	50 to 80 mg/dl (SI, 2.8 to 4.4 mmol/L)	Increase
		Decrease
Cell count	0 to 5 white blood cells	Increase
	No RBCs	RBCs
Venereal Disease Research Laboratories test for syphilis and other serologic tests	Nonreactive	Positive
Chloride	118 to 130 mEq/L (SI, 118 to 130 mmol/L)	Decrease
Gram stain	No organisms	Gram-positive or gram-negative organisms

IMPLICATIONS

Increased intracranial pressure

Spinal subarachnoid obstruction above puncture site

Infection

Subarachnoid, intracerebral, or intraventricular hemorrhage; spinal cord obstruction; traumatic tap (usually noted only in initial specimen)

Elevated protein levels, red blood cell (RBC) breakdown (blood present for at least 3 days)

Tumors, trauma, hemorrhage, diabetes mellitus, polyneuritis, blood in cerebrospinal fluid (CSF)

Rapid CSF production

Demyelinating disease, neurosyphilis, Guillain-Barré syndrome

Systemic hyperglycemia

Systemic hypoglycemia, bacterial or fungal infection, meningitis, mumps, postsubarachnoid hemorrhage

Active disease: meningitis, acute infection, onset of chronic illness, tumor, abscess, infarction, demyelinating disease

Hemorrhage or traumatic lumbar puncture

Neurosyphilis

Infected meninges

Bacterial meningitis

cell analysis as well as for serologic testing, such as the Venereal Disease Research Laboratory test for neurosyphilis. A separate specimen is also sent to the laboratory for culture and sensitivity testing. Electrolyte analysis and Gram stain may be ordered as supplementary tests. CSF electrolyte levels are of
special interest in the patient with abnormal serum electrolyte
levels or CSF infection and in the patient receiving hyperos-
molar agents.

Nursing considerations

- Describe the procedure to the patient and explain that CSF
  analysis analyzes the fluid around the spinal cord.
- Inform the patient that he need not restrict food and fluids.
- Tell the patient who will perform the procedure and where
  and when it will take place.
- Advise the patient that headache is the most common complication of lumbar puncture, but reassure him that his cooperation during the test helps minimize such an effect.
- If the specimen will be obtained by an invasive procedure,
  verify that the patient or a family member has signed an informed consent form for the proceudre. A consent form isn't
  necessary if the specimen is obtained from an existing ventriculostomy.
- If the patient is unusually anxious, assess and report his vital signs.
- If CSF pressure is elevated, assess the patient's neurologic
  status every 15 minutes for 4 hours. If he's stable, assess
  him every hour for 2 hours and then every 4 hours or according to the pretest schedule.

RED FLAG Watch the patient for complications of lumbar
puncture, such as reaction to the anesthetic, meningitis, bleeding into the spinal canal, and cerebellar tonsillar herniation and
medullary compression. Signs of meningitis include fever, neck rigidity, and irritability; signs of herniation include decreased level of consciousness, changes in pupil size and equality, altered vital signs (including widened pulse pressure, decreased pulse rate, and irregular
respirations), and respiratory failure.

- During the procedure, closely observe the patient for adverse reactions, such as elevated pulse rate, pallor, or clammy skin. Report any significant changes immediately.
- Record the collection time on the test request form. Send the form and labeled specimens to the laboratory immediately after collection.

SERUM ANTIDIURETIC HORMONE

Antidiuretic hormone (ADH), also called *vasopressin,* promotes water reabsorption in response to increased osmolality (water deficiency with high concentration of sodium and other solutes). In response to decreased osmolality (water excess), reduced secretion of ADH allows increased excretion of water to maintain fluid balance. Along with aldosterone, ADH helps regulate sodium, potassium, and fluid balance. It also stimulates vascular smooth-muscle contraction, causing an increase in arterial blood pressure.

This relatively rare test may be ordered as part of dehydration or hypertonic saline infusion testing, which determines the body's response to states of hyperosmolality. It may also identify pituitary diabetes insipidus, nephrogenic diabetes insipidus (congenital or familial), and syndrome of inappropriate antidiuretic hormone (SIADH).

ADH values range from 1 to 5 pg/ml (SI, 1 to 5 mg/L). For example, if serum osmolality is less than 285 mOsm/kg, ADH is normally less than 2 pg/ml (SI, < 2 mg/L); if it's greater than 290 mOsm/kg, ADH may range from 2 to 12 pg/ml (SI, 2 to 12 mg/L). Absent or below-normal ADH levels indicate pituitary diabetes insipidus, resulting from a neurohypophyseal or hypothalamic tumor, viral infection, metastatic disease, sarcoidosis, tuberculosis, Hand-Schüller-Christian disease, syphilis, neurosurgical procedures, or head trauma.

Normal ADH levels in the presence of signs of diabetes insipidus (such as polydipsia, polyuria, and hypotonic urine) may indicate the nephrogenic form of the disease, marked by renal tubular resistance to ADH; however, levels may rise if the pituitary gland tries to compensate.

Elevated ADH levels may also indicate SIADH, possibly as a result of bronchogenic carcinoma, acute porphyria, hypothyroidism, Addison's disease, cirrhosis of the liver, infectious hepatitis, severe hemorrhage, or circulatory shock.

Nursing considerations

- Explain to the patient that the test is going to measure his hormonal secretion levels and may aid in pinpointing the cause of his symptoms.
- Instruct the patient to fast and limit physical activity for 10 to 12 hours before the test.
- Tell the patient that the test requires a blood sample. Explain who will perform the venipuncture and when.
- Explain to the patient that he may experience slight discomfort from the tourniquet and the needle puncture.
- Withhold medications that may cause SIADH before the test, as ordered. If they must be continued, note this on the laboratory request.
- Make sure the patient is relaxed and recumbent for 30 minutes before the test.
- Perform a venipuncture and collect the sample in a plastic collection tube (without additives) or a chilled EDTA tube. Make sure you use a syringe and collection tube made of plastic because the fragile ADH degrades on contact with glass.
- Immediately send the sample to the laboratory, where serum must be separated from the clot within 10 minutes.
- Perform a serum osmolality test at the same time to help interpret the results.
- Apply direct pressure to the venipuncture site until bleeding stops.
- If a hematoma develops at the venipuncture site, apply warm soaks.

- Instruct the patient that he may resume his usual diet, activities, and medications discontinued before the test, as ordered.

COMPUTED TOMOGRAPHY SCAN, INTRACRANIAL

An intracranial computed tomography (CT) scan records a series of tomograms, which are translated by a computer and displayed on a monitor, representing cross-sectional images of various layers of the brain. This technique can reconstruct cross-sectional, horizontal, sagittal, and coronal plane images. Hundreds of thousands of readings of radiation levels absorbed by brain tissues may be combined to depict anatomic slices of varying thickness. Specificity and accuracy are enhanced by the degree of resolution, which depends on the number of radiation density calculations made by the computer, and through the use of contrast medium. Although magnetic resonance imaging (MRI) has surpassed CT scanning in diagnosing neurologic anatomy and pathology, the CT scan is more widely available and cost-effective and can be performed more easily in acute situations.

In addition to accurately diagnosing intracranial lesions and bleeding, CT scans may also be used to monitor the effects of surgery, radiation therapy, chemotherapy on intracranial tumors, or to serve as a guide for cranial surgery.

The tissue density (water content) depends on the amount of radiation that has passed through it. For example, normal tissue densities appear as white, black, or shades of gray on the computed image. Bone, the densest tissue, appears white; ventricular and subarachnoid cerebrospinal fluid, the least dense, appears black. Brain matter appears in shades of gray.

In addition to examining density, structures are also evaluated according to their size, shape, and position. Areas of altered density (may appear lighter or darker) or displaced vasculature or other structures may indicate an intracranial tumor, a hematoma, cerebral atrophy, an infarction, edema, or congenital anomalies such as hydrocephalus.

Intracranial tumors vary significantly in appearance and characteristics. Metastatic tumors generally cause extensive edema in early stages and can usually be defined by contrast enhancement. Primary tumors vary in density and in their capacity to cause edema, displace ventricles, and absorb the contrast medium in contrast enhancement. Astrocytomas, for example, usually have low densities; meningiomas have higher densities and can generally be defined with contrast enhancement; glioblastomas, usually ill defined, are also enhanced after injection of a contrast medium.

Because the high density of blood contrasts markedly with low-density brain tissue, it's normally easy to detect subdural and epidural hematomas and other acute hemorrhages with contrast enhancement.

Cerebral atrophy customarily appears as enlarged ventricles with large sulci. Cerebral infarction may appear as low-density areas at the obstruction site or may not be apparent, especially within the first 24 hours or if the infarction is small or doesn't cause edema. With contrast enhancement, the infarcted area may not show in the acute phase, but will show clearly after resolution of the lesion. Cerebral edema usually appears as an area of marked generalized decreased density. In children, enlargement of the fourth ventricle generally indicates hydrocephalus.

Normally, the cerebral vessels don't appear on CT images. However, in the patient with arteriovenous malformation, cerebral vessels may appear with slightly increased density. Contrast enhancement allows a better view of the abnormal area, but MRI is now the preferred procedure for imaging cerebral vessels. Another technology for obtaining brain images is positron emission tomography. (See *Understanding PET and SPECT*.)

UNDERSTANDING PET AND SPECT

Like computed tomography (CT) scanning and magnetic resonance imaging, positron emission tomography (PET) and single-photon emission computed tomography (SPECT) provide brain images through sophisticated computer reconstruction algorithms. However, PET and SPECT images detail brain function as well as structure and thus differ significantly from the images provided by these other advanced techniques. PET and SPECT combine elements of CT scanning and conventional radionuclide imaging. For example, they measure the emissions of injected radioisotopes and convert them to a tomographic image of the brain. PET scanning uses radioisotopes of biologically important elements—oxygen, nitrogen, carbon, and fluorine—that emit particles called positrons; whereas SPECT scanning uses gamma radiation with radionuclides within the brain.

How it works

During PET and SPECT, pairs of gamma rays are emitted; the scanner detects them and relays the information to a computer for reconstruction as an image. PET scanners omit positrons that can be chemically "tagged" to biologically active molecules, such as carbon monoxide, neurotransmitters, hormones, and metabolites (especially glucose), enabling study of their up

take and distribution in brain tissue. For example, blood tagged with 11C-carbon monoxide allows study of hemodynamic patterns in brain tissue; tagged neurotransmitters, hormones, and drugs allow mapping of receptor distribution. SPECT scanners use radionucleotides labeled with iodine or hexamethylpropylene amine oxime to detect blood flow.

Isotope-tagged glucose (which penetrates the blood-brain barrier rapidly) allows dynamic study of brain function because PET scans can pinpoint the sites of glucose metabolism in the brain under various conditions. Researchers expect PET and SPECT scanning to prove useful in the diagnosis of psychiatric disorders, transient ischemic attacks, amyotrophic lateral sclerosis, Parkinson's disease, Wilson's disease, multiple sclerosis, seizure disorders, cerebrovascular disease, and Alzheimer's disease. The rationale behind this theory is that all of these disorders may alter the location and patterns of cerebral glucose metabolism.

Cost factors

PET scanning is a costly test because the radioisotopes used have very short half-lives and must be produced at an on-site cyclotron and attached quickly to the desired tracer molecules.

Nursing considerations

■ Tell the patient that a series of images will be taken of his brain. Describe who will perform the test and where it will take place. Explain that the test will cause minimal discomfort.

■ Explain to the patient that intracranial CT permits assessment of the brain.

■ Make sure that any paperwork required by the facility concerning CT scans is complete.

■ Unless contrast enhancement is scheduled, inform the patient that there are no food or fluid restrictions. If contrast enhancement is scheduled, instruct him to fast for 4 hours before the test.

■ Tell the patient that he'll be positioned on a moving CT bed with his head immobilized and his face uncovered. The head of the table will then be moved into the scanner, which rotates around his head and makes a swirling sound.

■ If a contrast medium is used, tell the patient that he may feel flushed and warm and may experience a transient headache, a salty or metallic taste, or nausea and vomiting after the contrast medium is injected. Reassure him that these reactions are normal.

■ Instruct the patient to wear a gown (outpatients may wear comfortable clothing) and to remove all metal objects from the CT scan field.

■ If the patient is restless or apprehensive, a sedative may be prescribed.

■ If a contrast medium will be used, check the patient's history for hypersensitivity to shellfish, iodine, or contrast media, and mark your findings in his chart. Inform the physician of any sensitivities because he may order prophylactic medications or may choose not to use contrast enhancement.

■ After administration of a contrast medium, watch the patient for residual adverse reactions (headache, nausea, and vomiting) and inform him that he may resume his usual diet.

COMPUTED TOMOGRAPHY SCAN, SPINAL

Much more versatile than conventional radiography, a spinal computed tomography (CT) scan records detailed high-resolution images in the cross-sectional, longitudinal, sagittal, and lateral planes. Multiple X-ray beams from a computerized body scanner are directed at the spine from different angles; these pass through the body and strike radiation detectors, producing electrical impulses. A computer then converts these impulses into digital information, which is displayed as a three-dimensional image on a monitor. Storage of the digital information allows electronic recreation and manipulation of the image, creating a permanent record of the images to enable reexamination without repeating the procedure.

CT scans are helpful in defining the lesions causing spinal cord compression. Metastatic disease and discogenic disease with osteophyte formation and calcification are examples of pathologic processes diagnosed by CT scans. Since the advent of magnetic resonance imaging, CT scans are used less frequently to diagnose infection, abscesses, hematomas, and some disk herniations. However, they continue to be useful in monitoring the effects of spinal surgery or therapy.

In the spinal CT image, normal tissue appears white, black, or gray, depending on its density. Vertebrae, the densest tissues, are white; cerebrospinal fluid is black; and soft tissues appear in shades of gray.

By highlighting areas of altered density and depicting structural malformation, CT scanning can reveal all types of spinal lesions and abnormalities. It's particularly useful in detecting and localizing tumors, which appear as masses varying in density. Measuring this density and noting the configuration and location relative to the spinal cord can usually identify the type of tumor. For example, a neurinoma (schwannoma) appears as a spherical mass dorsal to the cord. A darker, wider mass lying more laterally or ventrally to the cord may be a meningioma.

CT scans also reveal degenerative processes and structural changes in detail. Herniated nucleus pulposus shows as an obvious herniation of disk material with unilateral or bilateral nerve root compression; if the herniation is midline, spinal cord compression is evident. Cervical spondylosis shows as cervical cord compression due to bony hypertrophy of the cervical spine; lumbar stenosis, as hypertrophy of the lumbar vertebrae, causing cord compression by decreasing space within the spinal column. Facet disorders show as soft-tissue changes, bony overgrowth, and spurring of the vertebrae, which result in nerve root compression. Fluid-filled arachnoidal and other paraspinal cysts show as dark masses displacing the spinal cord. Vascular malformations, evident after contrast enhancement, show as masses or clusters, usually on the dorsal aspect of the spinal cord.

Congenital spinal malformations, such as meningocele, myelocele, and spina bifida, show as abnormally large, dark gaps between the white vertebrae.

Nursing considerations

- Tell the patient that a series of scans will be taken of his spine. Explain who will perform the procedure and where it will take place.
- Explain that spinal CT allows visualization of his spine.
- Make sure that any paperwork required by the facility concerning CT scans is complete.
- If contrast medium isn't ordered, tell the patient that he need not restrict food and fluids. If contrast medium is ordered, instruct him to fast for 4 hours before the test.
- Reassure the patient that the procedure is painless, but that he may find having to remain still for a prolonged period uncomfortable.
- For the patient with significant back pain, administer prescribed analgesics before the scan.

- Explain to the patient that he'll be positioned on an X-ray table inside a CT body scanning unit and he'll be told to lie still because movement during the procedure may cause distorted images. The computer-controlled scanner will revolve around him, taking multiple scans.
- If a contrast medium is used, tell the patient that he may feel flushed and warm and may experience a transient headache, a salty or metallic taste, and nausea or vomiting after injection of the contrast medium. Reassure him that these reactions are normal.
- Instruct the patient to wear a radiologic examining gown and to remove all metal objects and jewelry.
- Check the patient's history for hypersensitivity reactions to iodine, shellfish, or contrast media. If such reactions have occurred, note them in the patient's chart and notify the physician, who may order prophylactic medications or choose not to use contrast enhancement.
- If the patient appears restless or apprehensive about the procedure, a mild sedative may be prescribed.

RED FLAG Observe the patient for signs and symptoms of a hypersensitivity reaction, including pruritus, rash, and respiratory difficulty, for 30 minutes after the contrast medium has been injected.

- If a contrast medium was used, watch the patient for residual adverse reactions (headache, nausea, and vomiting) and inform him that he may resume his usual diet.

ELECTROENCEPHALOGRAM

An EEG records the brain's electrical activity through electrodes attached to the patient's scalp. This information is then transmitted to an electroencephalograph, which records the resulting brain waves on recording paper. The procedure may be performed in a special laboratory or by a portable unit at the bedside. Ambulatory recording EEGs are available for the patient to wear at home or at the workplace to record the patient as he performs his normal daily activities. Continuous-video EEG recording is available on an inpatient basis for identifying epileptic discharges during clinical events or for localization of a seizure focus during surgical evaluation of epilepsy. An EEG can help determine the presence and type of seizure disorder; aid in the diagnosis of intracranial lesions, such as abscesses and tumors; evaluate the brain's electrical activity in metabolic disease, cerebral ischemia, head injury, meningitis, encephalitis, mental retardation, psychological disorders, and effects of certain drugs; and evaluate altered states of consciousness or brain death

EEG records a portion of the brain's electrical activity as waves; some are irregular, whereas others demonstrate frequent patterns. Among the basic waveforms are the alpha, beta, theta, and delta rhythms.

Alpha waves occur at a frequency of 8 to 11 cycles/second in a regular rhythm. They're present only in the waking state when the patient's eyes are closed; usually, they disappear with visual activity or mental concentration. *Beta waves* occur at a frequency of 13 to 30 cycles/second. They're generally associated with anxiety, depression, and use of sedatives and are seen most readily in the frontal and central regions of the brain. *Theta waves* occur at a frequency of 4 to 7 cycles/second. They're most common in children and young adults and appear in the frontal and temporal regions. *Delta waves* occur at a frequency of 0.5 to 3.5 cycles/second. They normally occur only in young children and during sleep. (See *Comparing EEG tracings*.)

In the patient with epilepsy, EEG patterns may identify the specific disorder. In *absence seizures,* the EEG shows spikes and waves at a frequency of 3 cycles/second. In *generalized tonic-clonic seizures,* it generally shows multiple, high-voltage, spiked waves in both hemispheres. In *temporal lobe epilepsy,* the EEG usually shows spiked waves in the affected temporal region. In the patient with *focal seizures,* it usually shows localized, spiked discharges.

COMPARING EEG TRACINGS

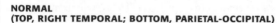

The following tracings are examples of regular and irregular brain electrical activity as recorded by an EEG.

NORMAL
(TOP, RIGHT TEMPORAL; BOTTOM, PARIETAL-OCCIPITAL)

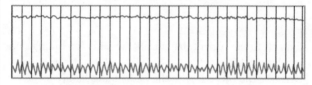

ABSENCE SEIZURES (SPIKES AND WAVES, 3 PER SECOND)

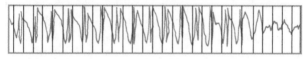

GENERALIZED TONIC-CLONIC SEIZURES
(MULTIPLE HIGH-VOLTAGE SPIKED WAVES)

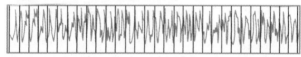

RIGHT TEMPORAL LOBE EPILEPSY (FOCAL SPIKED WAVES)

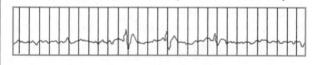

In the patient with an intracranial lesion, such as a tumor or abscess, the EEG may show slow waves (usually delta waves but possibly unilateral beta waves). Vascular lesions, such as cerebral infarcts and intracranial hemorrhages, generally produce focal abnormalities in the injured area.

Generally, any condition that causes a diminishing level of consciousness alters the EEG pattern in proportion to the degree of consciousness lost. For example, in a patient with a metabolic disorder, an inflammatory process (such as meningitis or encephalitis), or increased intracranial pressure, the EEG shows generalized, diffuse, and slow brain waves.

The most pathologic finding of all is an absent EEG pattern — a "flat" tracing (except for artifacts), which may indicate brain death.

Nursing considerations

- Explain to the patient that an EEG records the brain's electrical activity.
- Describe the procedure to the patient and family members and answer all questions.
- Explain that he must withhold caffeine before the test; other than this, there are no food or fluid restrictions. However, tell him that skipping the meal before the test can cause relative hypoglycemia and alter the brain wave pattern.
- Inform the patient that smoking is prohibited for at least 8 hours before the test.
- Thoroughly wash and dry the patient's hair to remove hair sprays, creams, and oils.
- Explain to the patient that during the test, he'll relax in a reclining chair or lie on a bed and that electrodes will be attached to his scalp with a special paste. Assure him that the electrodes won't shock him.
- If needle electrodes are used, explain to the patient that he'll feel a pricking sensation as they're inserted; however, flat electrodes are more commonly used.
- Do your best to allay the patient's fears because nervousness can affect brain wave patterns.
- Check the patient's medication history for drugs that may interfere with test results. Anticonvulsants, tranquilizers, barbiturates, and other sedatives should be withheld for 24 to 48 hours before the test, as ordered by the physician. Infants and very young children occasionally require sedation

to prevent crying and restlessness during the test, but sedation itself may alter test results.

■ A patient with a seizure disorder may require a "sleep EEG." In this case, keep the patient awake the night before the test and administer a sedative (such as chloral hydrate) to help him sleep during the test.

■ After the procedure, reinstate anticonvulsant medication or other drugs withheld before the test.

■ Carefully observe the patient for seizure activity and provide a safe environment.

■ Help the patient remove electrode paste from his hair.

■ If the patient received a sedative before the test, take safety precautions such as raising the bed's side rails.

■ If brain death is confirmed, provide the patient's family members with emotional support.

■ If clinical events are found to be nonepileptic, a psychological evaluation may be needed.

EVOKED POTENTIAL STUDIES

Evoked potential studies measure the brain's electrical response to stimulation of the sensory organs or peripheral nerves. Evoked potentials are recorded as electronic impulses by surface electrodes attached to the scalp and skin over various peripheral sensory nerves. A computer extracts these low-amplitude impulses from background brain wave activity and averages the signals from repeated stimuli. (See *Visual and somatosensory evoked potentials*, pages 122 and 123.)

Three types of responses are measured:

■ *Visual evoked potentials*, produced by exposing the eye to a rapidly reversing checkerboard pattern, help evaluate demyelinating diseases, traumatic injury, and puzzling visual complaints.

■ *Somatosensory evoked potentials*, produced by electrically stimulating a peripheral sensory nerve, help diagnose pe-

(Text continues on page 124.)

VISUAL AND SOMATOSENSORY EVOKED POTENTIALS

Visual (patternshift) evoked potentials

In the visual (pattern-shift) evoked potentials test, visual neural impulses are recorded as they travel along the pathway from the eye to the occipital cortex. Wave P100 is the most significant component of the resultant waveform. Normal P100 latency is about 100 msec after the application of a visual stimulus, as shown in the top diagram. Increased P100 latency, shown in the bottom diagram, is an abnormal finding, indicating a lesion along the visual pathway.

NORMAL TRACING

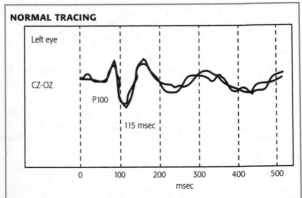

TRACING IN MULTIPLE SCLEROSIS

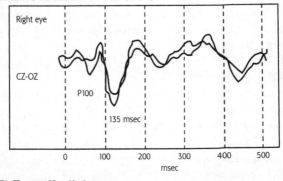

KEY: CZ = vertex; OZ = midocciput

VISUAL AND SOMATOSENSORY EVOKED POTENTIALS *(continued)*

Somatosensory evoked potentials

The somatosensory evoked potentials test measures the conduction time of an electrical impulse traveling along a somatosensory pathway to the cortex. Inter-wave latency is the most significant component of the resultant waveform. On the set of upper- and lower-limb tracings shown below, the top tracings represent normal interwave latencies; the bottom tracings, typical abnormal latencies found in a patient with multiple sclerosis. Because of the close correlation between waveforms and the anatomy of somatosensory pathways, such tracings allow precise location of lesions that produce conduction defects.

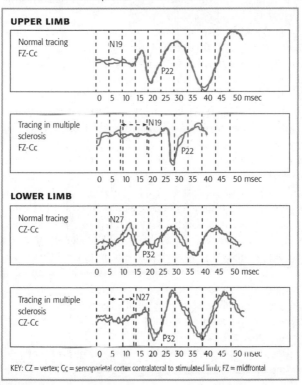

UPPER LIMB

Normal tracing
FZ-Cc
N19
P22
0 5 10 15 20 25 30 35 40 45 50 msec

Tracing in multiple sclerosis
FZ-Cc
N19
P22
0 5 10 15 20 25 30 35 40 45 50 msec

LOWER LIMB

Normal tracing
CZ-Cc
N27
P32
0 5 10 15 20 25 30 35 40 45 50 msec

Tracing in multiple sclerosis
CZ-Cc
N27
P32
0 5 10 15 20 25 30 35 40 45 50 msec

KEY: CZ = vertex; Cc = sensoparietal cortex contralateral to stimulated limb; FZ = midfrontal ripheral nerve disease and locate brain and spinal cord lesions.

- *Auditory brain stem evoked potentials,* produced by delivering clicks to the ear, help locate auditory lesions and evaluate brain stem integrity.

Evoked potential studies help diagnose nervous system lesions and abnormalities and assess the patient's neurologic function. They are also useful for monitoring comatose or anesthetized patients, monitoring spinal cord function during spinal cord surgery, and evaluating neurologic function in an infant whose sensory system normally can't be adequately assessed. However, information from evoked potential studies is insufficient to confirm a specific diagnosis. Test data must be interpreted in light of clinical information.

On the waveform of *visual evoked potentials,* the most significant wave is P100, a positive wave appearing about 100 msec after the pattern-shift stimulus is applied. The most clinically significant measurements are absolute P100 latency (the time between stimulus application and peaking of the P100 wave) and the difference between the P100 latencies of each eye. Because many physical and technical factors affect P100 latency, normal results vary greatly among laboratories and patients. Generally, abnormal (extended) P100 latencies confined to one eye indicate a visual pathway lesion anterior to the optic chiasm. A lesion posterior to the optic chiasm usually doesn't produce abnormal P100 latencies. Because each eye projects to both occipital lobes, the unaffected pathway transmits sufficient impulses to produce a normal latency response. Bilateral abnormal P100 latencies have been found in patients with multiple sclerosis, optic neuritis, retinopathies, amblyopia (although abnormal latencies don't correlate well with impaired visual acuity), spinocerebellar degeneration, adrenoleukodystrophy, sarcoidosis, Parkinson's disease, and Huntington's disease.

With *somatosensory evoked potentials,* waveforms vary, depending on locations of the stimulating and recording electrodes. The positive and negative peaks are labeled in sequence, based on normal time of appearance. For example, N19 is a negative peak normally recorded 19 msec after application of the stimulus. Each wave peak arises from a discrete location: N19 is generated mainly from the thalamus, P22 from the parietal sensory cortex, and so forth. Interwave latencies (time between waves), rather than absolute latencies, are used as a basis for clinical interpretation. Latency differences between sides are significant. Because somatosensory evoked potential components are assumed to be linked in series, an abnormal interwave latency indicates a conduction defect between the generators of the two peaks involved. This commonly identifies a precise location of a neurologic lesion. Abnormal upper-limb interwave latencies may indicate cervical spondylosis, intracerebral lesions, or sensorimotor neuropathies. Abnormalities in the lower limb demonstrate peripheral nerve and root lesions, such as those in Guillain-Barré syndrome, compressive myelopathies, multiple sclerosis, transverse myelitis, and traumatic spinal cord injury.

With *auditory evoked potentials,* normal hearing can detect frequencies between 20 Hz and 20 KHz. These results can vary with age, occupational hearing damage, and gender. Abnormal findings may indicate such conditions as multiple sclerosis and stroke.

Nursing considerations

- Tell the patient that evoked potential studies measure the electrical activity of his nervous system. Explain who will perform the test and where it will take place.
- Tell the patient that he'll sit in a reclining chair or lie on a bed. If visual evoked potentials will be measured, electrodes will be attached to his scalp; if somatosensory evoked potentials will be measured, electrodes will be placed on his scalp, neck, lower back, wrist, knee, and ankle. For auditory evoked potentials, electrodes will be attached to his scalp and earlobes.

- Assure the patient that the electrodes won't hurt him. Encourage him to relax; tension can affect neurologic function and interfere with test results.
- Have the patient remove all jewelry and other metal objects.

MAGNETIC RESONANCE IMAGING, INTRACRANIAL

An intracranial magnetic resonance imaging (MRI) records highly detailed, cross-sectional images of the brain and spine in multiple planes. The primary advantage of MRI is its ability to "see through" bone and to delineate fluid-filled soft tissue. It has proved useful in the diagnosis of cerebral infarction, tumors, abscesses, edema, hemorrhage, nerve fiber demyelination (as in multiple sclerosis), and other disorders that increase the fluid content of affected tissues. It can also show irregularities of the spinal cord with a resolution and detail previously unobtainable. It can also produce images of organs and vessels in motion.

Exposed to an external magnetic field, positively charged atomic nuclei and their negatively charged electrons align uniformly in the field. Radiofrequency energy is then directed at the atoms, knocking them out of this magnetic alignment and causing them to precess, or spin. When the radiofrequency pulse is discontinued, the atoms realign themselves with the magnetic field, emitting radiofrequency energy as a tissue-specific signal based on the relative density of nuclei and the realignment time. These signals are monitored by the MRI computer, which processes them and displays the information on a video monitor as a high-resolution image.

No harmful effects have been documented through the use of MRI. However, research continues on determining the optimal magnetic fields and radiofrequency waves for each type of tissue. (See *New methods of monitoring cerebral function*. Also see *MRI techniques,* page 128.)

NEW METHODS OF MONITORING CEREBRAL FUNCTION

Optical imaging

Optical imaging uses fiber-optic light and a camera to produce visual images of the brain as it responds to stimulation. This technique produces higher-resolution pictures of the brain than magnetic resonance imaging (MRI) or positron emission tomography scans. Researchers believe it may be valuable during neurosurgery to minimize damage to crucial areas of the brain that control speech, movement, and other activities. Because the procedure scans only the brain's surface, it's meant to be used in combination with other diagnostic techniques.

Fast MRI

Fast MRI produces pictures less than a second apart. These images display blood flow through the brain and the changes that occur in blood flow when the patient performs different tasks. Neuroscientists believe that active areas of the brain must consume more oxygen and that areas of the brain that are currently working become laden with oxygen. Fast MRI can distinguish between oxygen-laden and oxygen-depleted blood. Thus, this test may be used to help identify which areas of the normal brain are involved in certain activities and emotions. Possible applications for fast MRI include guiding neurosurgeons during surgery and helping researchers better understand epilepsy, brain tumors, and even psychiatric illnesses.

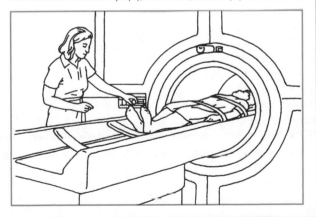

MRI TECHNIQUES

Magnetic resonance imaging (MRI) is used to provide clear images of parts of the brain, such as the brain stem and cerebellum, which are difficult to image by other methods. Four MRI techniques are available to examine other aspects of the brain.

Magnetic resonance angiography

Magnetic resonance angiography allows the visualization of blood flowing through the cerebral vessels. Although images of blood vessels done with magnetic resonance angiography aren't as clear as those obtained by angiography, this technique is less invasive.

Magnetic resonance spectroscopy

Magnetic resonance spectroscopy creates images over time that show the metabolism of certain chemical markers in a specific area of the brain. Some researchers have dubbed this test a "metabolic biopsy" because it reveals pathologic neurochemistry over time.

Diffusion-perfusion imaging

Diffusion-perfusion imaging uses a stronger-than-normal magnetic gradient to reveal areas of focal cerebral ischemia within minutes. Currently used in stroke research, this MRI technique may be used to distinguish permanent from reversible ischemia.

Neurography

Neurograms provide a three-dimensional image of nerves and may be used to find the exact location of nerves that are damaged, crimped, or in disarray.

An MRI can show normal anatomic details of the central nervous system in any plane, without bone interference. Brain and spinal cord structures should appear distinct and sharply defined. Tissue color and shading will vary, depending on the radiofrequency energy, magnetic strength, and degree of computer enhancement.

Because an MRI depicts the density of tissue, it clearly shows structural changes resulting from disorders that increase tissue water content, such as cerebral edema, demyelinating disease, and pontine and cerebellar tumors. Edematous fluid, for example, generally appears cloudy or gray, whereas blood generally appears dark. Lesions of multiple sclerosis appear as areas of demyelination (curdlike, gray or gray-white areas) around the edges of ventricles. Tumors appear as changes in normal anatomy, which computer enhancement may further delineate.

Nursing considerations

- Explain to the patient that an intracranial MRI assesses bone and soft tissue. Tell him who will perform the test and where it will take place.
- Verify that the patient or a responsible family member has signed an informed consent form and any other paperwork required by the facility.
- Explain to the patient that MRI is painless and involves no exposure to radiation from the scanner. A radioactive contrast dye may be used, depending on the type of tissue being studied. This dye may cause a temporary flushing sensation when injected.
- Advise the patient that he'll have to remain still for the entire procedure.
- Inform the patient that the opening for the head and body is quite small and deep. Tell him that he'll hear the scanner clicking, whirring, and thumping as it moves inside its housing.
- Explain to the patient that sedation may be administered if he suffers from claustrophobia or if extensive time is required for scanning.
- Reassure the patient that he'll be able to communicate with the technician at all times.
- Instruct the patient to remove all metallic objects and jewelry.
- Tell the patient that he may resume his usual activity after the test.
- If the patient was sedated, ensure that he remains safe after the procedure.

- If the test took a long time and the patient was lying flat for an extended period, observe him for orthostatic hypotension.

RED FLAG Because MRI works through a powerful magnetic field, it can't be performed on the patient with surgically implanted joints, pins, valves, pumps, pacemaker, an intracranial aneurysm clip, or other ferrous metal implants or on a patient with gunshot wounds to the head. Metallic or computer-based equipment (for example, ventilators and I.V. pumps) can't enter the MRI area.

OCULOPLETHYSMOGRAPHY

An important cerebrovascular test, oculoplethysmography (OPG) indirectly measures blood flow in the ophthalmic artery. Because the ophthalmic artery is the first major branch of the internal carotid artery, its blood flow accurately reflects carotid blood flow and ultimately that of cerebral circulation. Two techniques are used for this test. In OPG, pulse arrival times in the eyes and ears are measured and compared to detect carotid occlusive disease. In ocular pneumoplethysmography (OPG-Gee), ophthalmic artery pressures are measured indirectly and compared with the higher brachial pressure and with each other.

Indications for both of these tests include symptoms of transient ischemic attacks, asymptomatic carotid bruits, and nonhemispheric neurologic symptoms, such as dizziness, ataxia, or syncope. This test aids in the detection and evaluation of carotid occlusive disease and may also be performed as a follow-up procedure after carotid endarterectomy or with transcranial Doppler studies or carotid imaging. If indicated, it may be followed by cerebral angiography. Carotid phonoangiography is also a valuable complement to OPG. (See *Carotid phonoangiography*.)

With normal OPG results, all pulses should occur simultaneously. Carotid occlusive disease reduces the rate of blood flow during systole and delays the arrival of a pulse in the ipsi-

CAROTID PHONOANGIOGRAPHY

Carotid phonoangiography graphically records the intensity of carotid bruits during systolic and diastolic phases, thus helping to identify the presence, site, and severity of carotid artery occlusive disease.

For this test, the patient assumes a supine position and holds his breath while a transducer is placed at several sites along the carotid artery. Soundings are made directly over the clavicle (common carotid artery), midway up the neck (carotid bifurcation), and directly below the mandible (internal carotid artery). Oscillographic recordings are obtained and stored on Polaroid film and magnetic tape for later study.

Absence of bruits generally indicates an absence of significant carotid artery disease. However, bruits may also be absent when stenosis nears total occlusion. Bruits heard at all three sites, but loudest over the clavicle, usually originate in the aortic arch or in the heart. Blood flow in the carotid artery itself is unobstructed. Bruits heard over the carotid bifurcation and internal carotid sites, but louder over the latter, indicate turbulent blood flow in the internal carotid artery and the probability of more than 40% occlusion.

Carotid phonoangiography is a quick test and relatively simple to perform, but it's less sensitive and less specific than other noninvasive techniques such as carotid imaging with Doppler ultrasound. Nevertheless, this test is approximately 85% accurate in detecting carotid artery stenosis of more than 40%.

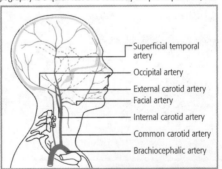

- Superficial temporal artery
- Occipital artery
- External carotid artery
- Facial artery
- Internal carotid artery
- Common carotid artery
- Brachiocephalic artery

In this phonoangiogram of a patient with an internal carotid artery bruit, the bruit is loudest directly below the mandible (A), present midway up the neck (B), and absent directly over the clavicle (C).

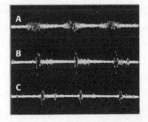

UNDERSTANDING CAROTID IMAGING

Carotid imaging is a diagnostic test that assesses the carotid arteries for occlusive disease. In this test, a pulsed Doppler ultrasonic flow transducer or a real-time imager produces images of the carotid artery and records them.

Real-time imaging (photo below) uses the echo technique to visualize the carotid artery. In this technique, a Doppler signal can be directed to specific points along the vessel. The audio signal is then evaluated.

Pulsed Doppler technique (photos at right) uses a transducer with a range-gating system that allows alternate transmission and reception of ultrasonic signals. The sound reflected from moving red blood cells within the lumen is then collected and stored in a computer for subsequent image reconstruction.

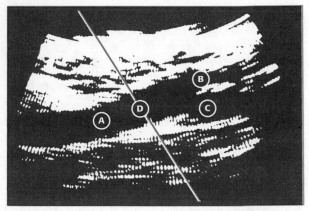

This normal real-time image shows the common carotid artery (A), external carotid artery (B), internal carotid artery (C), and Doppler beam (D).

lateral eye or ear. When all pulses are compared, any delay can be measured and the degree of carotid artery stenosis is estimated as mild, moderate, or severe. This test only estimates the extent of stenosis; it can't provide an exact percentage. (See *Understanding carotid imaging.*)

For normal OPG-Gee results, the difference between ophthalmic artery pressures should be less than 5 mm Hg. Oph-

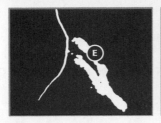
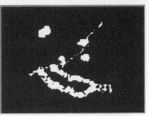

The abnormal pulsed Doppler image above left shows total occlusion (E) of the internal carotid artery. Compare this to the normal pulsed Doppler image above right.

Procedure

The patient is placed in the supine position, and the probe is placed on his neck and moved slowly from the vicinity of the common carotid artery to that of the bifurcation and then to the site of the internal and external carotid arteries.

Advantages and disadvantages

Carotid imaging detects ulcerating plaques that can't be detected by other methods; it can also differentiate between total and near-total arterial occlusion.

However, intramural calcification prevents sound penetration and may lead to false-positive results.

thalmic artery pressure divided by the higher brachial systolic pressure should be greater than 0.67. A difference between ophthalmic artery pressures of more than 5 mm Hg suggests the presence of carotid occlusive disease on the side with the lower pressure. A ratio between the ophthalmic artery pressure and the higher brachial systolic pressure of less than 0.67 reinforces this finding. In other words, the ratio is related to the

OPG EXAMINATION AND TRACINGS

The patient shown here is undergoing oculoplethysmography (OPG). The eyecups on the patient's corneas detect ocular pulsations, which are compared with each other and with the blood flow in the ear. Blood flow in the ear is detected by a small photo-electric cell (not shown).

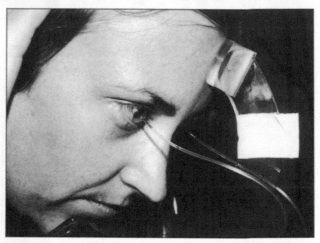

degree of stenosis: The lower the ratio, the more severe the stenosis. As with OPG, OPG-Gee only estimates the degree of stenosis present; angiography may be necessary to provide a precise evaluation. (See *OPG examination and tracings.*)

Nursing considerations

- Explain to the patient that this test evaluates carotid artery function.
- Inform the patient that he need not restrict food and fluids.
- Tell the patient who will perform the test, where it will take place, and that the procedure takes only a few minutes.

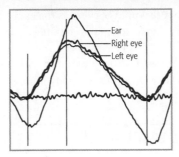

The OPG tracing at left is normal, showing simultaneous pulsations in the right and left eyes and in the right ear. The differential waveform of ocular pulses (horizontal waveform), which amplifies pulse differences, and the vertical lines drawn on valleys and peaks of pulses to indicate pulse delays confirm simultaneous pulsation.

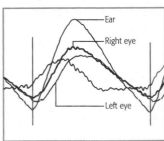

The OPG tracing at left is abnormal; the left-eye pulsation (vertical lines) arrives later than the other two pulsations, indicating left internal carotid artery stenosis. Note the elevation of the differential waveform.

- Inform the patient that anesthetic eyedrops are instilled to minimize patient discomfort during the test but that his eyes may burn slightly after the eyedrops are instilled.
- If OPG-Gee is scheduled, warn the patient that he may experience transient loss of vision when suction is applied to the eyes.
- Instruct the patient not to blink or move during the procedure.
- If the patient wears contact lenses, tell him to remove them before the test.
- The patient with glaucoma may take his usual medications and eyedrops.

- To prevent corneal abrasion, instruct the patient not to rub his eyes for 2 hours after the test. Observe for symptoms of corneal abrasion, such as pain or photophobia, and report them to the physician.
- Advise the patient that he may feel mild burning as the eye-drops wear off and that this normal. Tell him to report severe burning, however.
- If the patient wears contact lenses, instruct him not to reinsert them for about 2 hours after OPG; this will allow the effect of the anesthetic drops to wear off.

SKULL RADIOGRAPHY

Skull radiography evaluates the three groups of bones that comprise the skull: the calvaria (vault), the mandible (jawbone), and the facial bones. The calvaria and the facial bones are closely connected by immovable joints with irregular serrated edges called sutures. The skull bones form an anatomic structure so complex that a complete skull examination requires several radiologic views of each area. (See *Positioning the skull for radiography*.)

Although skull radiography is of limited value in assessing patients with head injuries, they're extremely valuable for studying abnormalities or fractures of the skull base and cranial vault (although basilar fractures may not show on the film if the bone is dense), congenital and perinatal anomalies, and systemic diseases that produce bone defects of the skull. For more accurate assessment of head injuries as well as of skull and head abnormalities, nonenhanced computed tomography studies of the head may be performed.

A radiologist interprets the X-rays, evaluating the size, shape, thickness, and position of the cranial bones as well as the vascular markings, sinuses, and sutures.

This test may show erosion, enlargement, or decalcification of the sella turcica that result from increased intracranial pressure (ICP). A marked rise in ICP may cause the brain to

POSITIONING THE SKULL FOR RADIOGRAPHY

Right lateral and left lateral

The sagittal plane is parallel to the tabletop and the film. A support, such as a folded towel or the patient's clenched fist, is placed under the chin. (Adequate film shows both halves of the mandible directly superimposed.)

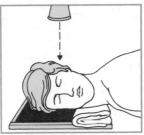

Anteroposterior Towne's

The patient lies in a supine position with his chin flexed toward the neck; the canthomeatal line is perpendicular to the tabletop and the film. The X-ray beam is angled 30 degrees toward the feet.

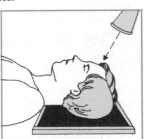

Posteroanterior Caldwell

The patient lies in a prone position; his chin may be supported by a folded towel or his fist. The sagittal plane and the canthomeatal line are perpendicular to the tabletop and the film. The X-ray beam is angled 15 degrees toward the feet.

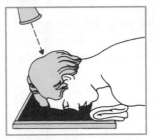

Axial (base)

The patient lies in a prone position with his chin fully extended; his head rests in such a way that the line of the face is perpendicular and the canthomeatal line is parallel to the tabletop and the film.

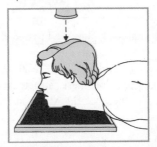

expand and press against the inner bony table of the skull, yielding visible marks or impressions.

In conditions such as osteomyelitis (with possible skull calcification) and chronic subdural hematomas, skull radiography may show abnormal areas of calcification. The test can detect neoplasms within brain substances that contain calcium (such as oligodendrogliomas or meningiomas) or the midline shifting of a calcified pineal gland caused by a space-occupying lesion.

Skull radiography may also detect other changes in bone structure — for example, those that arise from metabolic disorders, such as acromegaly or Paget's disease.

Nursing considerations

- Tell the patient that skull radiography helps to determine the presence of anomalies and helps establish a diagnosis.
- Explain to the patient that his head will be immobilized and that several X-rays of his skull will be taken from various angles.
- Tell the patient who will perform the test and when and where it will take place.
- Explain to the patient that he need not restrict food and fluids and that the test will cause no discomfort.
- Tell the patient to remove glasses, dentures, jewelry, or any metallic objects that would be in the X-ray field.

SPINAL RADIOGRAPHY

Spinal X-rays are used to detect spinal fracture; displacement and subluxation due to partial dislocation; destructive lesions, such as primary and metastatic bone tumors; arthritic changes or spondylolisthesis; structural abnormalities, such as kyphosis, scoliosis, and lordosis; and congenital abnormalities.

Nursing considerations

- Explain to the patient that a spinal X-ray provides a picture of the spine. Tell him who will perform the test and where it will take place.
- Reassure the patient that X-rays are painless.
- As ordered, administer an analgesic before the procedure if the patient has existing pain.
- Remove the patient's cervical collar if cervical X-rays reveal no fracture and the physician permits it.

TRANSCRANIAL DOPPLER STUDIES

Transcranial Doppler studies provide information about the presence, quality, and changing nature of circulation to an area of the brain by measuring the velocity of blood flow through cerebral arteries. Narrowed blood vessels produce high velocities, indicating possible stenosis or vasospasm. High velocities may also indicate an arteriovenous malformation. Transcranial Doppler studies also help determine whether collateral blood flow exists before surgical ligation or radiologic occlusion of diseased vessels.

The type of waveforms and velocities obtained indicate whether pathology exists, possible warranting further testing. (See *Comparing velocity waveforms,* page 140.)

After the transcranial Doppler study and before surgery, the patient may undergo cerebral angiography to further define cerebral blood flow patterns and locate the exact vascular abnormality.

Nursing considerations

- Explain the purpose of the transcranial Doppler study to the patient (or to his family).
- Tell the patient who will perform the test and when and where it will take place.
- Tell the patient that he need not restrict food and fluids.

COMPARING VELOCITY WAVEFORMS

A normal transcranial Doppler signal is usually characterized by mean velocities that fall within the normal reported values. Additional information can be gathered by evaluating the shape of the velocity waveform.

Effect of significant proximal vessel obstruction

A delayed systolic upstroke can be seen in a waveform when significant proximal vessel obstruction is present.

NORMAL

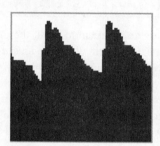

PROXIMAL VESSEL OBSTRUCTION

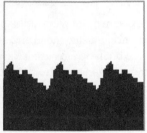

Effect of increased cerebrovascular resistance

Changes in cerebrovascular resistance, as occur with increased intracranial pressure, cause a decrease in diastolic flow.

NORMAL

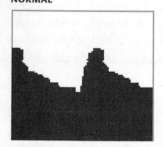

INCREASED RESISTANCE

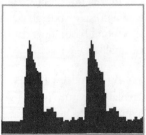

- Tell the patient that the test will be done while he lies on a bed or stretcher or sits in a reclining chair (or it can be performed at the bedside if he's too ill to be moved to the laboratory).
- Explain that a small amount of gel will be applied to his skin and that a probe will be used to transmit a signal to the artery being studied. Tell the patient that it usually takes less than 1 hour, depending on the number of vessels to be examined and any interfering factors.

INVASIVE TESTS AND PROCEDURES
CEREBRAL ANGIOGRAPHY

Cerebral angiography involves injecting a contrast medium to allow radiographic examination of the cerebral vasculature. Possible injection sites include the femoral, carotid, and brachial arteries. Because it allows visualization of four vessels (the carotid and the vertebral arteries), the femoral artery is used most commonly.

This test is usually performed on patients with a suspected abnormality of the cerebral vasculature, such as with an aneurysm or arteriovenous malformation (AVM), thrombosis, narrowing, or occlusion. These abnormalities may be suggested by intracranial computed tomography, lumbar puncture, magnetic resonance imaging, or magnetic resonance angiography findings, thus warranting this test. It may also be used to study vascular displacement caused by tumor, hematoma, edema, herniation, vasospasm, increased intracranial pressure (ICP), or hydrocephalus, or to locate clips applied to blood vessels during surgery and to evaluate the postoperative status of affected vessels.

During the arterial phase of perfusion, contrast medium fills and opacifies in the superficial and deep arteries and arterioles; during the venous phase, it opacifies superficial and deep veins. The finding of apparently normal (symmetrical) cerebral vasculature must be correlated with the patient's history and clinical status.

Changes in the caliber of vessel lumina suggest vascular disease, possibly due to spasms, plaques, fistulas, AVM, or arteriosclerosis. Diminished blood flow to vessels may be related to increased ICP.

Vessel displacement may reflect the presence and size of a tumor, areas of edema, or obstruction of the cerebrospinal fluid pathway. Cerebral angiography may also show circulation within a tumor, usually giving precise information on its position and nature. Meningeal blood supply originating in the external carotid artery may indicate an extracerebral tumor, but usually designates a meningioma. Such a tumor may arise outside the brain substance, but it may still be within the cerebral hemisphere.

Nursing considerations

- Explain to the patient that cerebral angiography shows blood circulation in the brain.
- Describe the test, including who will administer it and where and when it will take place.
- Verify that the patient has signed an informed consent form.
- Tell the patient to fast for 8 to 10 hours before the test.
- Make sure that any pretest blood work results are on the chart to determine bleeding tendency or kidney function.
- Explain to the patient that he'll wear a gown and that he must remove all jewelry, dentures, hairpins, and other metallic objects in the radiographic field.
- If ordered, administer a sedative and an anticholinergic drug 30 to 45 minutes before the test.
- Make sure the patient voids before leaving his room.
- Tell the patient that he'll be positioned on an X-ray table with his head immobilized and that he should remain still.
- Explain that a local anesthetic will be administered (some patients, especially children, receive a general anesthetic).

- Explain to the patient that he'll feel a transient burning sensation as the medium is injected; a warm, flushed feeling; a transient headache; a salty or metallic taste; or nausea and vomiting after the dye is injected. Reassure him that these are normal reactions.

RED FLAG Check the patient's history for hypersensitivity to iodine, iodine-containing substances (such as shellfish), or other contrast media. Note any hypersensitivities on his chart and report them, as appropriate.

- After the test, observe the patient for bleeding and frequently check distal pulses.
- Have the patient maintain bed rest for 6 to 8 hours. Administer prescribed pain medications and monitor his vital signs and neurologic status for 6 hours.
- Observe the puncture site for signs of extravasation (redness, swelling) and apply an ice bag to ease the patient's discomfort and minimize swelling. If bleeding occurs, apply firm pressure to the puncture site and inform the physician.

RED FLAG If the femoral approach was used, keep the patient's affected leg straight for 6 hours or longer and routinely check pulses distal to the site (dorsalis pedis, popliteal). Monitor the leg for temperature, color, and sensation. Thrombosis or hematoma can occlude blood flow; extravasation can also impede blood flow by exerting pressure on the artery.

- Monitor the patient for disorientation and weakness or numbness in the extremities (signs of thrombosis or hematoma) and for arterial spasms, which may produce symptoms of transient ischemic attacks.
- If the brachial approach was used, immobilize the affected arm for 6 hours or longer and routinely check the radial pulse.
- Place a sign near the patient's bed warning personnel not to take blood pressure readings from the affected arm.
- Observe the patient's arm and hand for changes in color, temperature, or sensation. If they become pale, cool, or numb, report these changes immediately.

- After the test, tell the patient he may resume his usual diet. Encourage him to drink fluids to help him pass the contrast medium.

RED FLAG Monitor the catheter puncture site frequently and closely for hemorrhage or hematoma formation. If either occurs, notify the physician immediately.

DIGITAL SUBTRACTION ANGIOGRAPHY

Digital subtraction angiography (DSA) is a sophisticated radiographic technique that uses video equipment and computer-assisted image enhancement to examine the vascular systems. As in conventional angiography, X-ray images are obtained after injecting a contrast medium. However, unlike conventional angiography, in which images of bone and soft tissue commonly obscure vascular detail, DSA provides a high-contrast view of blood vessels without interfering images or shadows.

Fluoroscopic images are taken before and after injection of a contrast medium. A computer converts these images into digital information and then "subtracts" the first image from the second, eliminating most information (mainly bone and soft tissue) common to both images. The result is a better image of the contrast-enhanced vasculature.

In addition to superior image quality, DSA has other advantages over conventional angiography. Indeed, DSA allows I.V., rather than intra-arterial, injection of the contrast medium; avoids the risk of stroke associated with conventional angiography; and reduces the pain and discomfort associated with arterial catheterization.

Although DSA has been used to study peripheral and renal vascular disease, it's probably most useful in diagnosing cerebrovascular disorders, such as carotid stenosis and occlusion, arteriovenous malformation, aneurysms, and vascular tumors. It's also useful in visualizing displacement of vasculature by other intracranial abnormalities or traumatic injuries and in detecting lesions typically missed by CT scans, such as thrombosis of the superior sagittal sinus. It may also be used to aid postoperative evaluation of cerebrovascular surgery, such as with arterial grafts and endarterectomies.

The contrast medium should fill and opacify all superficial and deep arteries, arterioles, and veins, allowing visualization of normal cerebral vasculature. Vascular filling defects, seen as areas of increased vascular opacity, may indicate arteriovenous occlusion or stenosis, possibly due to vasospasm, vascular malformation or angiomas, arteriosclerosis, or cerebral embolism or thrombosis. Outpouchings in vessel lumina may reflect cerebral aneurysms that frequently rupture, causing subarachnoid hemorrhage. Vessel displacement or vascular masses may indicate an intracranial tumor. DSA can clearly depict the vascular supply of some tumors, reflecting the tumor's position, size, and nature.

Nursing considerations

- Explain to the patient that DSA visualizes cerebral blood vessels.
- Tell the patient who will perform the procedure and where and when it will take place.
- Tell the patient that he'll need to fast for 4 hours before the test, but he need not restrict fluids.
- Explain to the patient that he'll receive an injection of a contrast medium, either by needle or through a venous catheter inserted in his arm, and that a series of X-rays will be taken of his head. Tell him who will perform the test, where it will take place, and that it takes 30 to 90 minutes.
- Inform the patient that he'll be positioned on an X-ray table with his head immobilized and will be asked to lie still. (Some patients, especially children, may be given a sedative to prevent movement during the procedure.)
- Instruct the patient to remove all jewelry, dentures, and other radiopaque objects from the X-ray field.

- Tell the patient that he'll probably feel some transient pain from insertion of the needle or catheter and that he may experience a feeling of warmth, a headache, a metallic or salty taste, and nausea or vomiting after the contrast medium is injected. Reassure him that these reactions are normal.
- Verify that the patient or a responsible family member has signed an informed consent form.
- Check the patient's history for hypersensitivity to iodine; iodine-containing substances, such as shellfish; and contrast media. If he's had such reactions, note them on the chart and inform the physician, who may order prophylactic medications or choose not to perform the test.
- Because the contrast medium acts as a diuretic, encourage the patient to increase his fluid intake for 24 hours after this test. Advise him that extra fluid intake will also speed excretion of the contrast medium. Monitor his intake and output, as ordered.
- Check the venipuncture site for signs of extravasation, such as redness or swelling. If bleeding occurs, apply firm pressure to the puncture site. If a hematoma develops, elevate the arm and apply warm soaks.
- Observe the patient for a delayed hypersensitivity reaction to the contrast medium, which can occur up to 18 hours after the procedure.
- Tell the patient that he may resume his usual diet.

ELECTROMYOGRAPHY

Electromyography (EMG) records the electrical activity of selected skeletal muscle groups at rest and during voluntary contraction. An EMG is performed to aid in differentiating between primary muscle disorders, such as the muscular dystrophies, and secondary disorders. It may also help assess diseases characterized by central neuronal degeneration such as amyotrophic lateral sclerosis (ALS); aid in the diagnosis of

NERVE CONDUCTION STUDIES

Nerve conduction studies help diagnose peripheral nerve injuries and diseases affecting the peripheral nervous system, such as peripheral neuropathies. To measure nerve conduction time, a nerve is stimulated electrically through the skin and underlying tissues. The patient experiences a mild electric shock with each stimulation. At a known distance from the point of stimulation, a recording electrode detects the response from the stimulated nerve.

The time between stimulation of the nerve and the detected response is measured on an oscilloscope. The speed of conduction along the nerve is then calculated by dividing the distance between the point of stimulation and the recording electrode by the time between stimulus and response. In peripheral nerve injuries and diseases, nerve conduction time is abnormal.

neuromuscular disorders, such as myasthenia gravis; and aid in the diagnosis of radiculopathies.

EMG involves percutaneous insertion of a needle electrode into a muscle. The electrical discharge of the muscle is then measured by an oscilloscope. Nerve conduction time is often measured simultaneously. (See *Nerve conduction studies*.)

At rest, a normal muscle exhibits minimal electrical activity. During voluntary contraction, electrical activity increases markedly. A sustained contraction or one of increasing strength causes a rapid "train" of motor unit potentials that can be heard as a crescendo of sounds over the audio amplifier.

At the same time, the monitor displays a sequence of waveforms that vary in amplitude (height) and frequency. Waveforms that are close together indicate a high frequency, whereas waveforms that are far apart signify a low frequency.

In primary muscle diseases, such as muscular dystrophy, motor unit potentials are short (low amplitude), with frequent, irregular discharges. In such disorders as ALS and those involving the peripheral nerve, motor unit potentials are isolated and irregular, but show increased amplitude and duration. In myasthenia gravis, motor unit potentials initially may be normal, but progressively diminish in amplitude with continuing contractions.

The interpreter distinguishes between waveforms that indicate a muscle disorder and those that indicate denervation. Findings must be correlated with the patient's history, clinical features, and the results of other neurodiagnostic tests.

Nursing considerations

- Explain to the patient that EMG measures the electrical activity of his muscles.
- Describe the test, including who will perform it and where and when it will take place.
- Tell the patient that there are usually no restrictions on food and fluids; however, in some cases, cigarettes, coffee, tea, and cola may be restricted for 2 to 3 hours before the test.
- Tell the patient that he may wear a hospital gown or comfortable clothing that permits access to the muscles to be tested.
- Advise the patient that a needle will be inserted into selected muscles and that he may experience discomfort. Reassure him that adverse effects and complications are rare.
- Verify that the patient or a responsible family member has signed an informed consent form.
- Check the patient's history for medications that may interfere with the results of the test — for example, cholinergics, anticholinergics, and skeletal muscle relaxants. If the patient is receiving such medications, note this on the chart and withhold medications, as ordered.
- If the patient experiences residual pain, apply warm compresses and administer prescribed analgesics.
- Tell the patient that he may resume his usual medications, as ordered.

INTRACRANIAL PRESSURE MONITORING

Intracranial pressure (ICP) monitoring measures pressure exerted by the brain, blood, and cerebrospinal fluid (CSF) against the inside of the skull. ICP monitoring enables prompt intervention, which can avert damage caused by cerebral hypoxia and shifts of brain mass.

Indications for ICP monitoring include head trauma with bleeding or edema, overproduction or insufficient absorption of CSF, cerebral hemorrhage, and space-occupying lesions.

There are four basic types of ICP monitoring systems. (See *Monitoring ICP,* pages 150 and 151.) Regardless of which system is used, the insertion procedure is always performed by a neurosurgeon in the operating room, emergency department, or critical care unit. Insertion of an ICP monitoring device requires sterile technique to reduce the risk of central nervous system infection.

The neurosurgeon inserts a ventricular catheter or subarachnoid screw through a twist-drill hole created in the skull. Both devices have built-in transducers that convert ICP to electrical impulses that allow constant monitoring. The ventricular catheter may also be used to drain CSF fluid if needed.

Nursing considerations

- Tell the patient and family that a catheter will be inserted into the skull and attached to the monitor in order to assess cerebral perfusion and fluid status.
- Tell him who will perform the procedure, when it will occur, and where it will take place.
- Verify that the patient or a responsible family member has signed an informed consent form.
- Explain that the information obtained from the monitor readings is monitored by the intensive care nurses and reported to the neurologist or neurosurgeon.

(Text continues on page 153.)

MONITORING ICP

Intracranial pressure (ICP) can be monitored using one of four systems.

Intraventricular catheter monitoring

Intraventricular catheter monitoring, which is used to monitor ICP directly, involves insertion of a small polyethylene or silicone rubber catheter into the lateral ventricles through a burr hole.

Although this method is most accurate for measuring ICP, it carries the greatest risk of infection. This is the only type of ICP monitoring that allows evaluation of brain compliance and significant drainage of cerebrospinal fluid (CSF).

Contraindications usually include stenotic cerebral ventricles, cerebral aneurysms in the path of catheter placement, and suspected vascular lesions.

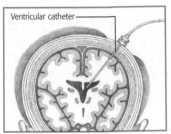

Ventricular catheter

Subarachnoid bolt monitoring

Subarachnoid bolt monitoring involves insertion of a special bolt into the subarachnoid space through a twist-drill burr hole in the front of the skull, behind the hairline.

Placing the bolt is easier than placing an intraventricular catheter, especially if a computed tomography scan reveals that the cerebrum has shifted or the ventricles have collapsed. This type of ICP monitoring also carries less risk of infection and parenchymal damage because the bolt doesn't penetrate the cerebrum.

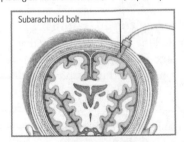

Subarachnoid bolt

Epidural or subdural sensor monitoring

ICP can also be monitored from the epidural or subdural space. For epidural monitoring, a fiber-optic sensor is inserted into the epidural space through a burr hole. However, this system's main drawback is its questionable accuracy because ICP isn't being measured directly from a CSF-filled space.

For subdural monitoring, a fiber-optic transducer-tipped catheter is tunneled through a burr hole and is placed on brain tissue under the dura mater. The main drawback to this method is its inability to drain CSF.

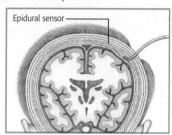

Epidural sensor

Intraparenchymal monitoring

With intraparenchymal monitoring, a catheter is inserted through a small sub-arachnoid bolt and, after punctuating the dura, advanced a few centimeters into the brain's white matter. There's no need to balance or calibrate the equipment after insertion.

This method doesn't provide direct access to CSF, but measurements are accurate because brain tissue pressure correlates well with ventricular pressures. Intraparenchymal monitoring may be used to obtain ICP measurements in patients with compressed or dislocated ventricles.

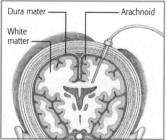

Dura mater   Arachnoid
White matter

INTERPRETING ICP WAVEFORMS

Three waveforms—A, B, and C—are used to monitor intracranial pressure (ICP). A waves are an ominous sign of intracranial decompensation and poor compliance, B waves correlate with changes in respiration, and C waves correlate with changes in arterial pressure.

Normal waveform

A normal ICP waveform typically shows a steep upward systolic slope followed by a downward diastolic slope with a dicrotic notch. In most cases, this waveform is continuous and indicates an ICP between 0 and 15 mm Hg (normal pressure).

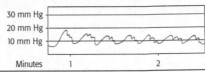

A waves

The most clinically significant ICP waveforms are A waves, which may reach elevations of 50 to 100 mm Hg, persist for 5 to 20 minutes, then drop sharply, signaling exhaustion of the brain's compliance mechanisms.

A waves may come and go, spiking from temporary increases in thoracic pressure or from any condition that increases ICP beyond the brain's ability to comply. Activities, such as sustained coughing or straining during defecation, can cause temporary elevations in thoracic pressure.

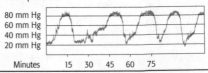

B waves

B waves, which appear sharp and rhythmic with a sawtooth pattern, occur every 1½ to 2 minutes and may reach an elevation of 50 mm Hg. The clinical significance of B waves isn't clear; however, the waves correlate with respiratory changes and may occur more frequently with decreasing compensation. Because B waves sometimes precede A waves, notify the physician if B waves occur frequently.

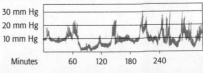

INTERPRETING ICP WAVEFORMS *(continued)*

C waves
Like B waves, C waves are rapid and rhythmic, but they aren't as sharp. They're clinically insignificant and may fluctuate with respirations or systemic blood pressure changes.

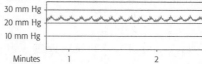

Waveform showing equipment problem
A waveform like the one shown at right signals a problem with the transducer or monitor. Check for line obstruction, and determine whether the transducer needs rebalancing.

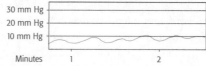

- After the catheter is inserted, observe and document digital ICP readings and waveforms. (See *Interpreting ICP waveforms.*)
- Assess the patient's clinical status and monitor routine and neurologic vital signs every hour, or as ordered.
- Calculate cerebral perfusion pressure (CPP) hourly. To calculate CPP, subtract ICP from mean arterial pressure.
- Inspect the insertion site at least every 24 hours for redness, swelling, and drainage.

LUMBAR PUNCTURE

A lumbar puncture, also known as a *spinal tap,* obtains cerebral spinal fluid (CSF) for qualitative analysis. It also measures CSF pressure and may be useful in detecting an obstruction of CSF circulation. A lumbar puncture also aids in the diagnoses of viral or bacterial meningitis; subarachnoid or intracranial hemorrhage; tumors and brain abscesses; and neurosyphilis and chronic central nervous system infections.

Normal results of CSF analysis include:

- pressure is 50 to 180 mm H_2O
- appearance is clear and colorless
- protein is 15 to 45 mg/dl
- gamma globulin is 3% to 12% of total protein
- glucose is 50 to 80 mg/dl
- cell count, 0 to 5 white blood cells with no red blood cells (RBCs)
- Venereal Disease Research Laboratories test nonreactive
- chloride is 118 to 130 mEq/L
- Gram stain showing no organisms.

   Increased intracranial pressure (ICP) indicates tumor, hemorrhage, or edema caused by trauma; decreased ICP, spinal subarachnoid obstruction. Cloudy CSF suggests infection; yellow or bloody appearance, intracranial hemorrhage or spinal cord obstruction; brown or orange appearance, increased protein levels or RBC breakdown. If CSF analysis reveals increased protein, it suggests tumor, trauma, diabetes mellitus, or blood in CSF; decreased protein, rapid CSF production. The presence of gram-positive or gram-negative organisms indicates bacterial meningitis.

Nursing considerations

- Explain the procedure to the patient. Tell him who will perform the test and where and when it will take place.
- Verify that the patient has signed an informed consent form.
- Note and report all allergies.
- Inform the patient that he need not restrict food and fluids.
- Explain that the test takes at least 15 minutes and that he will need to lie on his side with his knees drawn up to his chest.
- Explain that headache is the most common adverse effect.
- Tell the patient that he will need to lie flat for 4 to 6 hours, but that he can turn from side to side.

- Encourage the patient to drink fluids and assist him, as needed.
- Assess pain level, and give analgesics, as prescribed. Evaluate effect of treatment.
- Monitor the patient's vital signs, neurologic status, and intake and output.
- Monitor the puncture site for redness, swelling, and drainage.

MUSCLE BIOPSY

A muscle biopsy is a procedure in which a piece of muscle tissue is extracted from somewhere on the body for analysis. It's helpful in distinguishing between nerve and muscle disorders and diagnosing metabolic muscle defects and connective tissue diseases. It may also be used to identify diseases of the blood vessels and infections that affect the muscles.

Nursing considerations

- Explain to the patient that a muscle biopsy can help detect abnormalities with the muscle or nerves.
- Describe the test, including who will perform it and where and when it will take place.
- Tell the patient that his food and fluid intake need not be restricted.
- Verify that the patient or a responsible family member has signed an informed consent form.
- Explain to the patient that a local anesthetic will be injected before the sample is obtained. Tell them that this may cause a transient burning sensation.
- Explain that the procedure is not painful, but that they may feel a pulling sensation as the sample is obtained.
- After the procedure, observe the biopsy site for bleeding.
- Tell the patient that the area tested may feel sore for about 1 week.

MYELOGRAPHY

Myelography uses fluoroscopy and radiography to evaluate the spinal subarachnoid space after injection of a contrast medium. Because the contrast medium is heavier than cerebrospinal fluid (CSF), it flows through the subarachnoid space to the dependent area when the patient, lying prone on a fluoroscopic table, is tilted up or down. The fluoroscope allows the physician to see the flow of the contrast medium and the outline of the subarachnoid space. X-rays are taken to provide a permanent record.

Myelography can help evaluate and determine the cause of neurologic symptoms, such as numbness, pain, or weakness; identify lesions, such as tumors and herniated intervertebral disks that partially or totally block the flow of CSF in the subarachnoid space; and help detect arachnoiditis, spinal nerve root injury, or tumors in the posterior fossa of the skull. Sometimes it's performed to confirm the need for surgery; in such cases, a neurosurgeon may stand by. If this test confirms a spinal tumor, the patient may be taken directly to the operating room. Immediate surgery may also be necessary when the contrast medium causes a total block of the subarachnoid space.

Test results must be correlated with the patient's history and clinical status.

Nursing considerations

- Explain to the patient that myelography reveals obstructions in the spinal cord.
- Tell the patient that his food and fluid intake will be restricted for 8 hours before the test. If the test is scheduled for the afternoon and facility policy permits, the patient may have clear liquids before the test.
- Describe the test, including who will administer it and where and when and when it will take place.

- Explain to the patient that he may feel a transient burning sensation as the contrast medium is injected; a warm, flushed feeling; transient headache; a metallic or salty taste; or nausea and vomiting. Reassure him that these reactions are normal. Also explain that he may feel some pain caused by his positioning, needle insertion and, in some cases, removal of the contrast medium.
- Verify that the patient or a responsible family member has signed an informed consent form.

RED FLAG Check the patient's history for hypersensitivity to iodine and iodine-containing substances (for example, shellfish), radiographic contrast media, and associated medications. Notify the radiologist if the patient has a history of epilepsy or phenothiazine use. If metrizamide is to be used as a contrast medium, discontinue phenothiazine 48 hours before the test.

- Tell the patient to remove all jewelry and other metallic objects in the X-ray field.
- If metrizamide was used, tell the patient that the head of his bed must be elevated for 6 to 8 hours after the test and that that he'll remain on bed rest for an additional 6 to 8 hours. If an oil-based contrast agent is used, inform the patient that it will be manually removed after the test and that he'll need to remain flat in bed for 6 to 24 hours.
- Perform pretest procedures and administer prescribed medications. If the puncture is to be performed in the lumbar region, an enema may be prescribed. A sedative and anticholinergic (such as atropine sulfate) may be prescribed to reduce swallowing during the procedure. Make sure that pretest laboratory work (may include coagulation and kidney function studies) is in the chart.
- After the procedure, monitor the patient's vital signs and neurologic status at least every 15 minutes for the first hour, every 30 minutes for the next 2 hours, and then every 4 hours for 24 hours.
- Encourage the patient to drink extra fluids. He should void within 8 hours after the procedure.

- If there are no complications or adverse reactions, tell the patient that he may resume his usual diet and activities the day after the test.
- Monitor the patient for radicular pain, fever, back pain, or signs of meningeal irritation, such as headache, irritability, or stiff neck. If these signs or symptoms occur, keep the room quiet and dark and administer an analgesic or antipyretic, as needed.

TENSILON TEST

The Tensilon test involves careful observation of the patient after I.V. administration of Tensilon (edrophonium chloride), a rapid, shortacting anticholinesterase that improves muscle strength by increasing muscle response to nerve impulses.

It's especially useful in diagnosing myasthenia gravis, an abnormality of the myoneural junction in which nerve impulses fail to induce normal muscular responses. Patients with myasthenia gravis experience extreme fatigue at the end of the day and after repetitive activity or stress. This test may also aid in differentiating between myasthenic and cholinergic crises and be used to monitor oral anticholinesterase therapy.

Someone who doesn't have myasthenia gravis usually develops fasciculation in response to Tensilon. If the patient has myasthenia gravis, muscle strength should improve promptly after administration of Tensilon; if the patient responds only slightly, the test may need to be repeated to confirm the diagnosis. The degree of improvement depends on the muscle group being tested; improvement is usually obvious within 30 seconds. Although the maximum benefit lasts only several minutes, lingering effects may persist — for example, up to 2 hours in a patient receiving prednisone. The test may yield inconsistent results if myasthenia gravis affects only the ocular muscles, as in mild or early forms of the disorder. It may produce a positive response in motor neuron disease and in some neuropathies and myopathies. The response is usually less dramatic and less consistent than in myasthenia gravis.

Unlike the patient in myasthenic crisis showing brief improvement in muscle strength after Tensilon administration, the patient in cholinergic crisis (anticholinesterase overdose) may experience exaggerated muscle weakness. If Tensilon increases the patient's muscle strength without increasing adverse effects, oral anticholinesterase therapy can be increased. If Tensilon decreases muscle strength in a person with severe adverse reactions, therapy should be reduced. If the test shows no change in muscle strength and only mild adverse effects occur, therapy should remain the same.

Nursing considerations

- Explain to the patient that the Tensilon test helps determine the cause of muscle weakness.
- Describe the test, including who will perform it and where and when it will take place.
- Don't describe the exact response that will be evaluated; foreknowledge can affect the test's objectivity.
- Explain to the patient that a small tube will be inserted into a vein in his arm and that a drug will be administered periodically. He'll be asked to make repetitive muscle movements and his reactions will be observed. To ensure accuracy, the test may be repeated several times.
- Advise the patient that Tensilon may produce some adverse effects, but reassure him that someone will be with him at all times and that any reactions will quickly disappear.
- Check the patient's history for medications that affect muscle function, anticholinesterase therapy, drug hypersensitivities, and respiratory disease. Withhold medications, as ordered. If the patient is receiving anticholinesterase therapy, note this on the requisition request; include the time of the most recent dose.
- Verify that the patient or a responsible family member has signed an informed consent form.

■ When the test is complete, discontinue the I.V. and check the patient's vital signs.
■ Check the puncture site for hematoma, excessive bleeding, and swelling.
■ Tell the patient that he may resume his usual medications, as ordered.

4

Treatments

Treatments for patients with neurologic disorders may include medication therapy, surgery, and other forms of treatment.

MEDICATION THERAPY

For many of your patients with neurologic disorders, medication or drug therapy is essential. For example:
- thrombolytics are used to treat patients with acute ischemic stroke
- anticonvulsants are used to control seizures
- corticosteroids are used to reduce inflammation.

Other types of drugs commonly used to treat patients with neurologic disorders include:
- analgesics
- anticoagulants and antiplatelets
- barbiturates
- benzodiazepines
- calcium-channel blockers
- corticosteroids
- diuretics. When caring for a patient receiving medication therapy, be alert for severe adverse reactions and interactions with other drugs. Some drugs such as barbiturates also carry a high risk of toxicity. (See *Common neurologic drugs*, pages 162 to 167.)

(Text continues on page 166.)

COMMON NEUROLOGIC DRUGS

Use this table to find out about common neurologic drugs, their indications and adverse effects, and related monitoring measures.

DRUG	INDICATIONS	ADVERSE EFFECTS
ANALGESICS, NONOPIOID		
Acetaminophen	● Mild pain, headache	● Severe liver damage, neutropenia, thrombocytopenia
ANALGESICS, OPIOID		
Codeine	● Mild to moderate pain	● Respiratory depression, bradycardia, sedation, constipation
Morphine	● Severe pain	● Respiratory depression, apnea, bradycardia, seizures, sedation
ANTICONVULSANTS		
Carbamazepine	● Generalized tonic-clonic seizures, complex partial seizures, mixed seizures	● Heart failure, worsening of seizure, atrioventricular block, hepatitis, thrombocytopenia, Stevens-Johnson syndrome
Fosphenytoin	● Status epilepticus, seizures during neurosurgery	● Increased ICP, cerebral edema, somnolence, bradycardia, QT prolongation, heart block
Phenytoin	● Generalized tonic-clonic seizures, status epilepticus, nonepileptic seizures after head trauma	● Agranulocytosis, thrombocytopenia, toxic hepatitis, slurred speech, Stevens-Johnson syndrome
Primidone	● Generalized tonic-clonic seizures, focal seizures, and complex partial seizures	● Thrombocytopenia, drowsiness, ataxia
Valproic acid, valproate	● Complex partial seizures, simple and complex absence seizures	● Thrombocytopenia, pancreatitis, toxic hepatitis, sedation, ataxia

PRACTICE POINTERS

● Monitor total daily intake of acetaminophen because of risk of liver toxicity. Use with caution in elderly patients and those with liver disease.

● Monitor for respiratory depression. Use with caution in elderly patients and those with head injury, seizures, or increased ICP.

● Monitor for respiratory depression. Use with caution in elderly patients and those with head injury, seizures, or increased ICP. Contraindicated in patients with acute bronchial asthma.

● Use cautiously in patients with mixed seizure disorders because it can increase the risk of seizure. Use cautiously in patients with hepatic dysfunction. Obtain baseline liver function studies, complete blood count, and blood urea nitrogen level. Monitor blood levels of the drug; therapeutic level is 4 to 12 mcg/ml.

● Stop drug with acute hepatotoxicity. May cause hyperglycemia; monitor blood glucose in diabetic patients. Fosphenytoin should be prescribed and dispensed in PE units. Monitor for cardiac arrhythmias and QT prolongation.

● Abrupt withdrawal can trigger status epilepticus. Contraindicated in patients with heart block. Use cautiously in patients with hepatic disease and myocardial insufficiency. Monitor blood levels of the drug; therapeutic range is 10 to 20 mcg/ml. If rash appears, stop the drug.

● Abrupt withdrawal can cause status epilepticus. Reduce dosage in elderly patients.

● Obtain baseline liver function tests. Avoid use in patients at high risk for hepatotoxicity. Abrupt withdrawal may worsen seizures. Monitor blood levels of the drug; therapeutic range is 50 to 100 mcg/ml.

(continued)

COMMON NEUROLOGIC DRUGS *(continued)*

DRUG	INDICATIONS	ADVERSE EFFECTS
ANTICOAGULANTS Heparin	• Embolism prophylaxis after cerebral thrombosis in evolving stroke	• Hemorrhage, thrombocytopenia
ANTIPLATELETS Aspirin	• Transient ischemic attacks, thromboembolic disorders	• GI bleeding, acute renal insufficiency, thrombocytopenia, liver dysfunction
Sulfinpyrazone	• Thrombotic stroke prophylaxis	• Blood dyscrasia, thrombocytopenia, bronchoconstriction
Ticlopidine	• Thrombotic stroke prophylaxis	• Thrombocytopenia, agranulocytosis
BARBITURATES Phenobarbital	• All types of seizures except absence seizures and febrile seizures in children; also used for status epilepticus, sedation, and drug withdrawal	• Respiratory depression, apnea, bradycardia, angioedema, Stevens-Johnson syndrome
BENZODIAZEPINES Clonazepam	• Absence and atypical seizures, generalized tonic-clonic seizures, status epilepticus, panic disorders	• Respiratory depression, thrombocytopenia, leukopenia, drowsiness, ataxia
Diazepam	• Status epilepticus, anxiety, acute alcohol withdrawal, muscle spasm	• Respiratory depression, bradycardia, cardiovascular collapse, drowsiness, acute withdrawal syndrome
Lorazepam	• Status epilepticus, anxiety, agitation	• Drowsiness, acute withdrawal syndrome

PRACTICE POINTERS

● Monitor for bleeding. Obtain baseline prothrombin time/International Normalized Ratio (PT/INR), and partial thromboplastin time (PTT). Monitor PTT at regular intervals. Protamine sulfate reverses the effects of heparin.

● Monitor for bleeding. Avoid use in patients with active peptic ulcer and GI inflammation.

● Monitor for bleeding. Avoid use in patients with active peptic ulcer and GI inflammation.

● Monitor for bleeding. Avoid use in patients with hepatic impairment and peptic ulcer disease.

● Monitor for respiratory depression and bradycardia. Keep resuscitation equipment on hand when administering I.V. dose; monitor respirations.

● Abrupt withdrawal may precipitate status epilepticus. Elderly patients are at a greater risk for central nervous system (CNS) depression and may require a lower dose.

● Monitor for respiratory depression and cardiac arrhythmia. Don't stop suddenly; can cause acute withdrawal in physically dependent persons.

● Don't stop abruptly; can cause withdrawal. Monitor for CNS depressant effects in elderly patients.

(continued)

COMMON NEUROLOGIC DRUGS (continued)

DRUG	INDICATIONS	ADVERSE EFFECTS
CALCIUM CHANNEL BLOCKERS		
Nimodipine	● Neurologic deficits caused by cerebral vasospasm after congenital aneurysm rupture	● Decreased blood pressure, tachycardia, edema
CORTICOSTEROIDS		
Dexamethasone, methylprednisolone	● Cerebral edema, severe inflammation	● Heart failure, cardiac arrhythmias, edema, circulatory collapse, thromboembolism, pancreatitis, peptic ulceration
DIURETICS		
Furosemide (loop)	● Edema, hypertension	● Renal failure, thrombocytopenia, agranulocytosis, volume depletion, dehydration
Mannitol (osmotic)	● Cerebral edema, increased intracranial pressure (ICP)	● Heart failure, seizures, fluid and electrolyte imbalance
THROMBOLYTICS		
Alteplase (recombinant tissue plasminogen activator)	● Acute ischemic stroke	● Cerebral hemorrhage, spontaneous bleeding, allergic reaction
Streptokinase	● Acute ischemic stroke	● Cerebral hemorrhage, spontaneous bleeding, allergic reaction

Successful therapy hinges on strict adherence to the medication schedule. Compliance is especially critical for drugs that require steady blood levels for therapeutic effectiveness such as anticonvulsants.

PRACTICE POINTERS

● Use cautiously in hepatic failure. Monitor for hypotension and tachycardia.

● Use cautiously in patients with recent myocardial infarction, hypertension, renal disease, and GI ulcer. Monitor blood pressure and blood glucose levels.

● Monitor blood pressure, pulse, and intake and output. Monitor serum electrolyte levels, especially potassium levels. Monitor for cardiac arrhythmias.

● Contraindicated in severe pulmonary congestion and heart failure. Monitor blood pressure, heart rate, and intake and output. Monitor serum electrolyte levels. Use with caution in patients with renal dysfunction.

● Contraindicated in patients with intracranial or subarachnoid hemorrhage. The patient must meet criteria for thrombolytic therapy before initiation of therapy. Monitor baseline laboratory values: hemoglobin level, hematocrit, PTT, PT/INR. Monitor vital signs. Monitor for signs of bleeding. Monitor puncture sites for bleeding.

● Contraindicated in patients with intracranial or subarachnoid hemorrhage. The patient must meet criteria for thrombolytic therapy before initiation of therapy. Monitor baseline laboratory values: hemoglobin level, hematocrit, PTT, PT/INR. Monitor vital signs. Monitor for signs of bleeding. Monitor puncture sites for bleeding.

ANTIBIOTICS

Antibiotics may be ordered as prophylaxis to neurosurgical treatments or to treat existing infection, as with a brain or spinal abscess or meningitis. The type of antibiotic ordered is based on patient allergies and type of infection. The patient should be monitored for response to treatment and adverse effects.

Patient preparation

- Explain what type of antibiotic is being administered and why. Be sure to ask the patient or family about allergies before administering the first dose.

Monitoring and aftercare

- Monitor the patient for signs of allergic response. Other adverse signs to watch for include nausea and vomiting, diarrhea, and continued signs of infection.

BARBITURATE COMA

The neurologist may order barbiturate coma when conventional treatments, such as fluid restriction, diuretic or corticosteroid therapy, or ventricular shunting, don't control sustained or acute episodes of increased intracranial pressure (ICP).

During barbiturate coma, the patient receives high I.V. doses of a short-acting barbiturate (such as pentobarbital) to produce a comatose state. The drug reduces the patient's metabolic rate and cerebral blood flow.

The goal of barbiturate coma is to relieve increased ICP and protect cerebral tissue by increasing cerebral perfusion pressures. It's used for patients with:

- acute ICP elevation, over 40 mm Hg
- persistent ICP elevation, over 20 mm Hg
- rapidly deteriorating neurologic status that's unresponsive to other treatments.

If barbiturate coma doesn't reduce ICP, the patient's prognosis for recovery is poor.

Patient (and family) preparation

■ Focus your attention on the patient's family. The patient's condition and apprehension about the treatment is likely to frighten them. Provide clear explanations of the procedure and its effects, and encourage them to ask questions. Convey a sense of optimism but provide no guarantees as to the treatment's success.

■ Prepare the family for expected changes in the patient during therapy, such as decreased respirations, hypotension, and loss of muscle tone and reflexes.

Monitoring and aftercare

■ Closely monitor the patient's ICP, electrocardiogram, and vital signs. Notify the neurologist of increased ICP, arrhythmias, or hypotension.

■ Check serum barbiturate levels frequently, as ordered.

■ Because the patient is in a drug-induced coma, provide skin care to prevent pressure ulcers.

CHEMOTHERAPY

Chemotherapy may be used in conjunction with surgery and radiation therapy to treat brain tumors. The purpose of chemotherapy is to kill cancer cells left behind after surgery and to prevent cancer cells from dividing. Many different chemotherapeutic agents are available and treatment is tailored specifically for the individual based on the type of cancer being treated.

Patient preparation

■ Explain to the patient the type of chemotherapy that he'll receive. Answer all questions regarding amount of time it will take to infuse the drug and the expected adverse effects.

■ Reassure the patient that he'll be monitored closely during the infusion. Tell the patient that he'll be given medication to decrease the adverse effect of nausea.

Monitoring and aftercare

- After the chemotherapeutic treatment, monitor the patient for adverse effects. Teach the patient signs and symptoms to watch for and report after discharge, such as infection, bleeding, constipation, skin rash, decreased urine output, and nausea and vomiting.
- Tell the patient when the next chemotherapy session is scheduled.

NEUROMUSCULAR BLOCKADE

Neuromuscular blockade (NMB) may be necessary when intracranial pressure (ICP) can't be controlled through other measures. It may also be necessary to increase cerebral perfusion pressures in the patient with acute respiratory failure whose oxygenation is not improving secondary to inverted inspiratory-expiratory ratio.

Patient preparation

- Explain to the patient and family the reason for NMB and how it works. Answer any questions and provide emotional support.
- Explain that the patient's respirations will be controlled by a ventilator while receiving NMB. Reassure them that the patient will be continually monitored.
- Tell the patient and family that sedation will be administered continually while the NMB is being administered. Reassure them that analgesia will also be administered, if indicated.

Monitoring and aftercare

- NMB dosage should be titrated to administer the lowest dose possible to achieve desired effects. A peripheral nerve stimulator should be utilized to elicit a "train of four" response to guide dosage. (See *Using a peripheral nerve stimulator*.)

USING A PERIPHERAL NERVE STIMULATOR

A nerve stimulator is a device utilized to evaluate nerve response to neuromuscular (NMB) blockade administration.

How the nerve stimulator works

The nerve stimulator has a positive and negative electrode. The negative electrode should be placed as close to a nerve as possible, commonly the ulnar nerve at the wrist. The positive electrode can be placed anywhere along the nerve on the forearm. The nerve stimulator supplies a decreasing current that causes muscle contraction (usually the thumb).

"Train of four"

The train of four (TOF) is four stimuli or "twitches" sent to the electrodes at 0.5-second intervals. These twitches cause muscle response and are assessed to evaluate the amount of blockade that's needed to suppress muscle contraction. When only one or two twitches are evident (usually the thumb), the NMB is at an adequate dosage. If no twitches occur, the NMB dosage should be decreased until one or two twitches occur with stimulation. Each TOF should be documented as to how many twitches occurred (such as TOF 2/4).

■ NMB should be stopped every shift to assess neurologic status.

SURGERY

Neurologic disorders may call for surgery, which may be classified nonemergent, as with some brain tumors; and emergent, as with cerebral hemorrhage.

You may be responsible for the patient's care before and after surgery. Here are some general preoperative and postoperative guidelines:

■ The prospect of surgery usually causes fear and anxiety, so give ongoing emotional support to the patient and his family. Make sure that you're ready to answer all of their questions.

- Postoperative care may include teaching about diverse topics, such as ventricular shunt care and tips about cosmetic care after craniotomy. Be ready to give thorough patient and family teaching.

CEREBRAL ANEURYSM REPAIR

Surgical intervention is the only sure way to prevent rupture or rebleeding of a cerebral aneurysm.

With cerebral aneurysm repair, a craniotomy is performed to expose the aneurysm. Depending on the shape and location of the aneurysm, the surgeon then uses one of several corrective techniques, such as:

- clamping the affected artery
- wrapping the aneurysm wall with a biologic or synthetic material
- clipping the aneurysm.

An alternative to open aneurysm repair is called inventional neuroradiology. It's less invasive and requires less recovery time. (See *Interventional neuroradiology*.)

Patient preparation

- Explain the procedure. Encourage the patient and his family members to ask questions about the procedure. Provide clear, honest answers to reduce their confusion and anxiety and to enhance effective coping.
- Tell the patient and his family members that monitoring is done in the critical care unit before and after surgery. Explain that several I.V. lines, endotracheal intubation, and mechanical ventilation and intracranial pressure (ICP) monitoring may be needed.

Monitoring and aftercare

- Monitor the incision site for signs of infection or drainage.
- Monitor the patient's neurologic status and vital signs, and report acute changes immediately. Watch for signs of in-

INTERVENTIONAL NEURORADIOLOGY

Interventional neuroradiology, also known as *endovascular radiology,* utilizes fluoroscopic angiography to place small coils (Guglielmi detachable coils) within the neck of the aneurysm. Up to thirty coils may be used to block circulation to the aneurysm; the aneurysm is then obliterated through electrothrombosis.

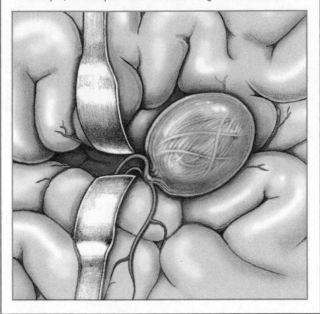

creased ICP, such as pupil changes, weakness in extremities, headache, a change in level of consciousness, and elevated ICP readings.
- Assess the patient's pain level, and provide analgesics, as indicated.
- Provide emotional support to the patient and his family members. Answer all questions regarding recovery, remaining treatment, and neurologic deficits (if any).

CRANIECTOMY

A craniectomy is a surgical procedure that removes part of the skull. It's performed to remove bone fragments from a skull fracture or for decompression of the brain and is usually performed after a traumatic head injury.

Patient preparation

- Encourage the patient and his family members to ask questions about the procedure. Provide clear, honest answers to reduce their confusion and anxiety and to enhance effective coping.
- Explain that the patient's head will be shaved before surgery.
- Tell the patient and his family that monitoring is done in the critical care unit before and after surgery. Explain that several I.V. lines, endotracheal intubation, and mechanical ventilation and intracranial pressure (ICP) monitoring may be needed.
- Discuss the recovery period so the patient and his family understand what to expect. Explain that he'll awaken with a dressing on his head to protect the incision and may have a surgical drain.
- Tell him to expect a headache and facial swelling for 2 to 3 days after surgery, and reassure him that he'll receive pain medication.

Monitoring and aftercare

- Monitor the patient's neurologic status and vital signs, and report any acute change immediately. Watch for signs of increased ICP, such as pupil changes, weakness in extremities, headache, and change in level of consciousness.
- Monitor ICP readings and report increased ICP measurements not responsive to treatment. Note cerebral perfusion pressures.
- Monitor the incision site for signs of infection, bleeding, or drainage.

- Assess the patient's pain level, and provide analgesics, as indicated. Evaluate effect of medication.
- Provide emotional support to the patient and his family members. Answer all questions regarding recovery, remaining treatment, and neurologic deficits (if any).

CRANIOTOMY

A craniotomy is a surgical procedure to open the skull and expose the brain. This procedure allows for various treatments, such as ventricular shunting, excision of a tumor or abscess, hematoma aspiration, and aneurysm clipping. After the procedure, the opening is closed with a bone flap.

The degree of risk depends on your patient's condition and the complexity of the surgery.

Possible complications include:

- infection
- hemorrhage
- respiratory compromise
- increased intracranial pressure (ICP).

Patient preparation

- Encourage the patient and his family to ask questions about the procedure. Provide clear, honest answers to reduce confusion and anxiety and to enhance effective coping.
- Explain that the patient's head will be shaved before surgery.
- Tell the patient and his family that monitoring is done in the critical care unit before and after surgery. Explain that several I.V. lines, endotracheal intubation, and mechanical ventilation and ICP monitoring may be needed.
- Discuss the recovery period so the patient understands what to expect. Explain that he'll awaken with a dressing on his head to protect the incision and may have a surgical drain.
- Tell him to expect a headache and facial swelling for 2 to 3 days after surgery, and reassure him that he'll receive pain medication.

Monitoring and aftercare

- Monitor the patient's neurologic status and vital signs, and report any acute change immediately. Watch for signs of increased ICP, such as pupil changes, weakness in extremities, headache, and change in level of consciousness.
- Monitor ICP readings and report increased ICP measurements not responsive to treatment. Note cerebral perfusion pressures.
- Drain cerebrospinal fluid through a ventriculostomy, as ordered.
- Monitor the incision site for signs of infection, bleeding, or drainage.
- Assess the patient's pain level, and provide analgesics, as indicated. Evaluate the effect of the medication.
- Provide emotional support to the patient and his family members. Answer all questions regarding recovery, remaining treatment, and neurologic deficits (if any).

DEEP BRAIN STIMULATION

Deep brain stimulation (DBS) is a procedure where a neurotransmitter is inserted to deliver electrical stimulation to a targeted area to help control disabling neurological symptoms, such as essential tremors. It's also used to treat Parkinson's disease in the patient whose symptoms are not adequately controlled by medication. The DBS system is made up of an electrode, an extension, and a neurotransmitter. The electrode is implanted into the targeted area of the brain through a small hole. The extension is threaded under the skin of the neck and shoulder and connected to the neurotransmitter, which is implanted under the collarbone.

Patient preparation

- Explain the procedure and why it's necessary. Reinforce any information provided by the neurosurgeon. Encourage the patient and his family to ask questions about the procedure and recovery. Provide clear, honest answers to reduce their confusion and anxiety and to enhance effective coping.

■ Tell the patient and his family that monitoring is done in the critical care unit after surgery to ensure proper functioning of the DBS system.

Monitoring and aftercare

■ Monitor the incision site for signs of infection, bleeding, or drainage.

■ Monitor the patient's neurologic status and vital signs, and report acute changes immediately.

■ Assess movement of the extremities. Compare to baseline assessments to evaluate improvement and function of the DBS system. The DBS system programming can be adjusted without the need for further surgery.

■ Give emotional support to the patient and his family members, as needed. Teach them the signs and symptoms of DBS system malfunction to report.

SPINAL SURGERY

Surgery on the spine is performed when a herniated disk causes sensory loss, paresis, loss of sphincter control, compression of the spinal cord, severe, unrelenting pain, or sciatica that interferes with lifestyle. Spinal surgery may also be performed when there's evidence of spinal cord compression, penetrating wound or bone fragment in the spinal canal, or compound fracture of the vertebrae.

Typical procedures include:

■ posterior, anterior, or lateral laminectomy

■ diskectomy

■ hemilaminectomy

■ spinal fusion

■ foraminotomy.

Patient preparation

- Explain the procedure and why it's necessary. Reinforce any information provided by the neurosurgeon. Encourage the patient and his family to ask questions about the procedure and recovery. Provide clear, honest answers to reduce their confusion and anxiety and to enhance effective coping.
- Tell the patient that after the surgery, his vital signs will be monitored closely and that he will also be monitored closely for neurological function and pain. Reassure the patient that pain medication will be given, as needed.

Monitoring and aftercare

- Monitor the incision site for signs of infection or drainage.
- Monitor the patient's neurologic status and vital signs, and report acute changes immediately.
- The patient's activity level will be based on the type and location of surgery. If the patient is required to wear a cervical collar, teach the patient how to remove it and reapply it correctly, and how long he will need to wear it.
- Give emotional support to the patient and his family members, as needed.

VENTRICULAR SHUNT

A ventricular shunt is a tube that's inserted into one of the ventricles of the brain in order to drain cerebrospinal fluid (CSF) to reduce or prevent increased intracranial pressure (ICP) and is also used to treat hydrocephalus. The shunt system is composed of a catheter, a reservoir, a one-way valve, and a terminal catheter. The catheter is inserted into the ventricle, with the reservoir resting on the mastoid bone. The reservoir obtains CSF samples and performs "pumping" of the shunt, which flushes the catheter of exudates that could cause obstruction. The one-way valve prevents CSF reflux and is set to open and drain CSF when the ICP reaches a level determined by the neurologist. The terminal catheter drains the CSF into the subarachnoid space, abdomen, or vena cava.

Patient preparation

- Explain the procedure and why it's necessary. Reinforce any information provided by the neurosurgeon. Encourage the patient and his family to ask questions about the procedure and recovery. Provide clear, honest answers to reduce their confusion and anxiety and to enhance effective coping.
- Tell the patient and his family that monitoring is done in the critical care unit after surgery to ensure proper functioning of the shunt.

Monitoring and aftercare

- Monitor the incision site for signs of infection, bleeding, or drainage. CSF may be tested to ensure that there's no infection present.
- Monitor the patient's neurologic status and vital signs, and report acute changes immediately. Watch for signs of increased ICP, such as pupil changes, weakness in extremities, headache, and a change in level of consciousness. ICP pressure may be checked to ensure that the shunt is functioning properly.
- Give emotional support to the patient and his family members to help them cope with caring for a ventricular shunt. Teach the family how to "pump" the shunt and the signs and symptoms of increased ICP to report.

OTHER TREATMENTS

PLASMAPHERESIS

Plasmapheresis is the process of plasma exchange, in which blood from the patient flows into a cell separator, which separates plasma from formed elements. The plasma is then filtered to remove toxins and disease mediators, such as immune complexes and autoantibodies, from the patient's blood.

The cellular components are then transfused back into the patient using fresh frozen plasma or albumin (in place of the plasma removed).

Plasmapheresis benefits patients with neurologic disorders such as Guillain-Barré syndrome and, especially, myasthenia gravis. In myasthenia gravis, plasmapheresis is used to remove circulating antiacetylcholine receptor antibodies.

Plasmapheresis is used most commonly for patients with long-standing neuromuscular disease, but it may also be used to treat patients with acute exacerbations. Some acutely ill patients require treatment up to four times per week; others about once every 2 weeks. When it's successful, treatment may relieve symptoms for months, but results vary.

Patient preparation

- Discuss the treatment and its purpose with the patient and his family.
- Explain that the procedure can take up to 5 hours. During that time, blood samples are taken frequently to monitor calcium and potassium levels. Blood pressure and heart rate are checked regularly. Tell the patient to report any paresthesia (numbness, burning, tingling, prickling, or increased sensitivity) during treatment.

Monitoring and aftercare

- If possible, give the patient prescribed medications after treatment because they're removed from the blood during treatment.
- Monitor the patient's vital signs according to facility policy.
- Check puncture sites for signs of bleeding or extravasation.

STEREOTACTIC RADIOSURGERY

Stereotactic radiosurgery is a noninvasive procedure that uses radiation to treat brain tumors and other brain abnormalities. It may also treat leftover tumor tissue, following surgery. Three-dimensional computer software is used to plan specific targeting of the radiation beams. There are three types of stereotactic radiotherapy: gamma knife, linear accelerator, and particle beam (proton) or cyclotron. (See *Types of stereotactic radiosurgery*.)

TYPES OF STEREOTACTIC RADIOSURGERY

There are three forms of sterotactic radiosurgery. They differ in the type of instrument used and the source of radiation.

Gamma knife surgery

Gamma knife surgery is used to treat brain tumors of 3.5 cm or less and arteri-ovenous malformations and other brain dysfunctions, such as trigeminal neuralgia and seizures. Gamma knife surgery uses 201 beams of highly focused gamma radiation that targets the lesion, leaving surrounding tissue unharmed. One dose causes the lesion to slowly reduce in size and eventually dissolve.

Linear accelerator

Linear accelerator (LINAC) machines deliver high-energy photons or electrons in curving paths around the patient's head. This type of radiation is effective on large tumors and can be used for fractionation of treatment. LINAC machines are also used for Intensity-Modulated Radiation Therapy (IMRT). IMRT is an advanced type of high-precision radiotherapy that conforms to the shape of the target and utilizes higher radiation doses.

Proton beam radiosurgery

Proton beam radiosurgery uses the quantum wave properties of protons (through use of a cyclotron) to significantly reduce the amount of radiation to tissue surrounding the target. It can be used for unusually shaped tumors, skull base tumors, and vascular malformations of the brain.

This treatment may involve a single session (completed in 1 day); or, may involve fractionated sessions (treatments completed over weeks or months), which is called stereotactic radiotherapy.

Because this surgery is noninvasive, risks and complications are decreased. It's a viable treatment option in cases where invasive surgery isn't recommended due to the patient's age or his condition.

Patient preparation

- Explain the procedure and why it's necessary. Reinforce any information provided by the radiologist and neurosurgeon. Encourage the patient and his family to ask questions about the procedure. Provide clear, honest answers to reduce their confusion and anxiety and to enhance effective coping.
- Explain to the patient that his head will be held in place by a large frame so that the preestablished targeting of the lesion is accurately reached by the radiation beams. The head frame will be removed after the procedure is complete.
- Tell the patient that the session can take several minutes to a few hours, depending on the dose required and the shape of the target.

Monitoring and aftercare

- This procedure is typically done on an outpatient basis or only requires an overnight stay. Monitor vital signs and neurologic status after the procedure. Report any abnormalities.
- Tell the patient that he can return to preprocedure activities, but that he may feel fatigued.
- Explain to the patient that he may have hair loss in the area of radiation and that the scalp may become reddened.

VENTRICULOSTOMY

A ventriculostomy is the placement of a catheter into the lateral ventricle through a burr hole in the patient's skull in order to monitor intracranial pressure (ICP) and drain cerebrospinal fluid (CSF), if needed. (See *CSF closed drainage system,* page 184.) The goal of CSF drainage is to reduce ICP to the desired level and keep it at that level. It may be inserted after brain surgery, with head injury, hydrocephalus, cerebral aneurysms, or arteriovenous malformations.

Patient preparation

- Explain the procedure and why it's necessary. Reinforce any information provided by the neurosurgeon. Encourage the patient and his family members to ask questions about the procedure. Provide clear, honest answers to reduce their confusion and anxiety and to enhance effective coping.
- Tell the patient and his family members that monitoring is done in the critical care unit to ensure proper functioning of the catheter and to monitor ICP closely.

Monitoring and aftercare

- Drain CSF, as ordered, by putting on gloves and turning the main stopcock on to drainage and allowing the CSF to collect in the drip chamber.
- To stop drainage, turn off the stopcock to drainage. Record the time and the amount of collected CSF.
- Check the patient's dressing frequently for drainage.
- Check the tubing for patency by observing the CSF draining into the drip chamber.
- Observe the CSF for color, clarity, amount, blood, and sediment.
- Maintain the patient on bed rest with the head of the bed at 30 to 45 degrees to prevent increased ICP.

CSF CLOSED DRAINAGE SYSTEM

During treatment for traumatic injury or other conditions that cause increased intracranial pressure, the goal of cerebrospinal fluid drainage is to control the increased pressure. Here's one common procedure.

Ventricular drain

For a ventricular drain, the physician makes a burr hole in the patient's skull and inserts the catheter into the ventricle. The distal end of the catheter is connected to a closed drainage system.

CLOSED DRAINAGE SYSTEM

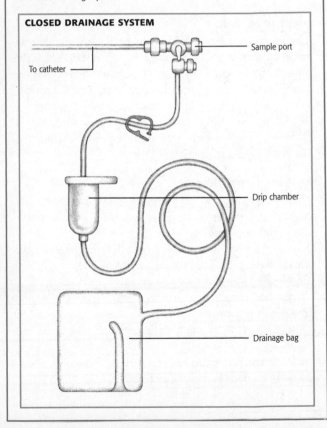

- Sample port
- To catheter
- Drip chamber
- Drainage bag

■ Observe for complications, such as excessive CSF drainage, characterized by headache, tachycardia, diaphoresis, and nausea. Overly rapid accumulation of drainage is a neuro-surgical emergency. Cessation of drainage may indicate clot formation. Monitor for signs and symptoms of infection.

Congenital disorders

Neurologic disorders present at birth can stem from a variety of maternal or fetal causes. For example, arteriovenous malformations result from abnormalities of the blood vessels in the brain. Some, such as cerebral palsy, result from prenatal, perinatal, or postnatal central nervous system damage. Others, such as hydrocephalus, result from cerebrospinal fluid dysfunction. Embryonic neural tube defects during the first trimester of pregnancy can lead to spinal cord malformations.

ARTERIOVENOUS MALFORMATION

Cerebral arteriovenous malformation (AVM) is a congenital disorder of the blood vessels consisting of an abnormal connection between the arteries and the veins in the brain and occur in approximately 3 out of 10,000 people. Although some AVMs may occur as a result of penetrating injuries, such as trauma, most are present at birth. Although subsequent symptoms may occur at any time, they typically occur between ages 10 and 20, with two-thirds of cases occurring before age 40. Evidence suggests that AVMs run in families, equally affecting males and females.

Pathophysiology

An AVM is a tangled mass of thin-walled, dilated blood vessels between arteries and veins that aren't connected by capillaries and primarily occurs in the posterior portion of the cerebral hemispheres. Brain tissue perfusion is inadequate due to abnormal channels between the arterial and venous systems that allow mixing of oxygenated and unoxygenated blood, resulting in increased venous pressure, which causes engorgement and dilation of the venous structures. AVMs range in size from a few millimeters to large malformations that extend from the cerebral cortex to the ventricles. In fact, if the AVM is large enough, the shunting can deprive the surrounding tissue of adequate blood flow, resulting in cardiac decompensation— where the heart can't pump enough blood to compensate for bleeding in the brain (typical in infants and small children). Thin-walled vessels may ooze small amounts of blood—they may even rupture—causing hemorrhage into the brain or subarachnoid space.

Complications

- Development of cerebral aneurysm and subsequent rupture
- Hemorrhage (intracerebral, subarachnoid, or subdural, depending on the location of the AVM)
- Hydrocephalus

Assessment findings

In more than 50% of patients with AVM, hemorrhage (from rupture) from the malformation is the first symptom.

Symptoms that occur before an AVM rupture are related to slower bleeding from the abnormal vessels and may include:

- chronic mild headache, a sudden and severe headache, or a localized or general headache
- seizure
- vision disturbances
- muscle weakness or inability to move a limb or a side of the body
- lack of sensation in part of the body, or abnormal sensations, such as ringing and numbness
- mental status change (sleepy, stuporous, lethargic, confused, disoriented, or irritable)

- stiff neck
- impaired speech or sense of smell
- fainting, dizziness, and decreased level of consciousness
- facial paralysis, eyelid drooping, and tinnitus.

Diagnostic test results
- Magnetic resonance imaging identifies irregular or globoid masses; however, hemorrhage may obscure findings.
- Cerebral arteriogram confirms the presence of AVMs and evaluates blood flow.
- Doppler ultrasonography reveals abnormal, turbulent blood flow.
- Computed tomography scan identifies intracerebral hemorrhage and large AVMs.

Treatment
General support measures include aneurysm precautions to prevent possible rupture, which involves placing the patient on bed rest or limiting activity and maintaining a quiet atmosphere. Analgesics may be given for headache, and sedatives may be given to help calm the patient. Stool softeners may be given to prevent straining at defecation, which increases intracranial pressure. Anticonvulsants, such as phenytoin, may also be administered to prevent seizures.

A bleeding AVM is a medical emergency and requires immediate hospitalization. The goal of treatment is to prevent further complications by limiting bleeding, controlling seizures and, if possible, removing the AVM. Surgical techniques may include block dissection, laser, or ligation to repair the communicating channels and remove the feeding vessels. Surgery is dependent upon the accessibility and size of the lesion and the patient's status.

Open brain surgery, embolization, and stereotactic radiosurgery may also be used separately or in any combination. Open brain surgery involves the actual removal of the malformation through an opening made in the skull. This type of

TEACHING THE PATIENT WITH AN AVM

Before discharge, teach the patient and his family:
- about arteriovenous malformation (AVM) and its implications
- about prescribed medication administration, dosage, possible adverse effects, and when to notify the physician
- postoperative care of any incision
- activity recommendations
- signs and symptoms of complications, such as shunt infection or intracranial bleeding (sudden severe headache, vision changes, decreased movement in extremities, and change in level of consciousness)
- the importance of follow-up care
- the benefits of utilizing available community resources or support groups, especially if neurologic deficits have occurred.

surgery carries a higher risk because the surgery itself may cause the AVM to bleed uncontrollably.

If surgery isn't possible—due to the size or location of the lesion—embolization or stereotactic radiosurgery may be performed to close the communicating channels and feeder vessels, thereby reducing blood flow to the AVM. Embolization involves injecting a gluelike substance into the abnormal vessels to stop aberrant blood flow into the AVM. Stereotactic radiosurgery is particularly useful for small, deep lesions, which are typically difficult to remove by surgery.

Nursing interventions
- Monitor vital signs and titrate medications to control hypertension.
- Monitor neurologic status.
- Monitor for seizure activity and institute seizure precautions.
- Maintain a quiet atmosphere and provide relaxation techniques.

- Provide appropriate education to the parents (and patient if appropriate) before discharge. (See *Teaching the patient with an AVM,* page 189.)

CEREBRAL PALSY

Cerebral palsy (CP)—the most common crippling disease in children—includes several neuromuscular disorders resulting from prenatal, perinatal, or postnatal central nervous system damage. The three major types of CP include spastic, affecting approximately 70% of children; athetoid, affecting approximately 20%; and ataxic, affecting approximately 10%. Some types may occur in mixed forms. Motor impairment may be minimal (sometimes apparent only during physical activities such as running) or severely disabling. Associated defects, such as seizures, speech disorders, and mental retardation, are common.

Prenatal causes include Rh factor or ABO blood type incompatibility, maternal infection (especially rubella in the first trimester), maternal diabetes, irradiation, anoxia, toxemia, malnutrition, abnormal placental attachment, and isoimmunization.

Perinatal causes include trauma during delivery, depressed maternal vital signs from general or spinal anesthesia, asphyxia from the cord wrapping around the neck, prematurity, prolonged or unusually rapid labor, and multiple births (infants born last in a multiple birth have an especially high rate of CP).

Postnatal causes include infections, such as meningitis and encephalitis, head trauma, poisoning, and any condition that results in cerebral thrombus or embolus. (See *Causes of cerebral palsy.*)

Pathophysiology

In the early stages of brain development, a lesion or abnormality causes structural and functional defects that, in turn, cause

CAUSES OF CEREBRAL PALSY

Conditions that result in cerebral anoxia, hemorrhage, or other damage may cause cerebral palsy (CP).

● *Prenatal conditions that may increase risk of CP:* maternal infection (especially rubella), maternal drug ingestion, radiation, anoxia, toxemia, maternal diabetes, abnormal placental attachment, malnutrition, and isoimmunization.

● *Perinatal and birth difficulties that may increase the risk of CP:* forceps delivery, breech presentation, placenta previa, abruptio placentae, metabolic or electrolyte disturbances, abnormal maternal vital signs from general or spinal anesthetic, prolapsed cord with delay in delivery of head, premature birth, prolonged or unusually rapid labor, and multiple birth (especially infants born last in a multiple birth).

● *Infection or trauma during infancy that may increase the risk of CP:* poisoning, severe kernicterus resulting from erythroblastosis fetalis, brain infection, head trauma, prolonged anoxia, brain tumor, cerebral circulatory anomalies causing blood vessel rupture, and systemic disease resulting in cerebral thrombosis or embolus.

impaired motor function and cognition. Even though defects are present at birth, signs and symptoms may not be apparent until months later, when the axons have become myelinated and the basal ganglia are mature.

Complications
- Contracture
- Skin breakdown and ulcer formation
- Muscle atrophy
- Malnutrition
- Seizure disorders (in about 25% of patients)
- Speech, vision, and hearing problems
- Language and perceptual deficits
- Mental retardation (in up to 40% of patients)
- Dental problems
- Aspiration pneumonia

Assessment findings

Shortly after birth, the infant with CP may exhibit some typical signs and symptoms, including:

- excessive lethargy or irritability
- high-pitched cry
- poor head control
- weak sucking reflex
- smaller than normal head circumference
- abnormal postures
- abnormal reflexes
- abnormal muscle tone. (See *Assessing signs of cerebral palsy.*)

   Findings for spastic CP include:
- underdevelopment of affected limbs
- characteristic scissors gait
- hyperactive deep tendon reflexes and increased stretch reflexes
- rapid alternating muscle contraction and relaxation
- muscle weakness
- muscle contraction in response to manipulation with a tendency toward contractures.

   Findings for athetoid CP include:
- involuntary movements, such as grimacing, wormlike writhing, dystonia, and sharp jerks that impair voluntary movement
- involuntary facial movements (affects speech).

   Findings for ataxic CP include:
- lack of leg movement during infancy
- wide gait
- disturbed balance
- incoordination (especially of the arms)
- hypoactive reflexes
- nystagmus
- muscle weakness and tremors
- lack of sudden or fine movements.

ASSESSING SIGNS OF CEREBRAL PALSY

Each type of cerebral palsy (CP) is manifested by specific findings. This chart highlights the major signs and symptoms associated with each type of CP. The manifestations reflect impaired upper motor neuron function and disruption of the normal stretch reflex.

TYPE OF CP	SIGNS AND SYMPTOMS
Spastic CP (due to impairment of the pyramidal tract [most common type])	<ul><li>Hyperactive deep tendon reflexes</li><li>Increased stretch reflexes</li><li>Rapid alternating muscle contraction and relaxation</li><li>Muscle weakness</li><li>Underdevelopment of affected limbs</li><li>Muscle contraction in response to manipulation</li><li>Tendency toward contractures</li><li>Typical walking on toes with a scissors gait, crossing one foot in front of the other</li></ul>
Athetoid CP (due to impairment of the extrapyramidal tract)	<ul><li>Involuntary movements usually affecting arms more severely than legs, including: –grimacing –wormlike writhing –dystonia sharp jerks</li><li>Difficulty with speech due to involuntary facial movements</li><li>Increasing severity of movements during stress; decreased with relaxation and disappearing entirely during sleep</li></ul>
Ataxic CP (due to impairment of the extrapyramidal tract)	<ul><li>Disturbed balance</li><li>Incoordination (especially of arms)</li><li>Hypoactive reflexes</li><li>Nystagmus</li><li>Muscle weakness</li><li>Tremor</li><li>Lack of leg movement during infancy</li><li>Wide gait as child begins to walk</li><li>Sudden or fine movements impossible (due to ataxia)</li></ul>
Mixed CP	<ul><li>Spasticity and athetoid movements</li><li>Ataxic and athetoid movements (resulting in severe impairment)</li></ul>

Findings for children who have mixed forms of CP may include:

- retarded growth and development
- difficulty chewing and swallowing.

Diagnostic test results

- Cranial ultrasound identifies structural abnormalities, hemorrhage and hypoxic-ischemic injury.
- Computed tomography scan and magnetic resonance imaging may show congenital malformations, hemorrhage, and periventricular leukomalacia.
- EEG may identify the source of seizure activity.

Treatment

Although CP can't be cured, proper treatment can help affected children reach their full potential within the limits set by the disorder. Such treatment requires a comprehensive and cooperative effort involving physicians, nurses, teachers, psychologists, the child's family, and occupational, physical, and speech therapists. Children with milder forms of CP may attend regular school; severely afflicted children may need special education classes.

Treatment usually includes:

- braces or splints and special appliances, such as adapted eating utensils and a low toilet seat with arms to help children perform activities independently
- an artificial urinary sphincter for the incontinent child who can use hand controls
- range-of-motion (ROM) exercises to minimize contractures
- phenytoin, phenobarbital, or another anticonvulsant to control seizures
- muscle relaxants, antispasmotics, or neurosurgery to decrease spasticity
- orthopedic surgery to correct contractures (common treatment for spastic CP) (Children with spastic CP are especial-

ly prone to developing equinus deformity because the heel cord shortens.)
■ Achilles tendon lengthening to improve foot function
■ muscle transfer procedures to improve function of the wrist or other joints.

Nursing interventions
■ Provide care in an unhurried manner to avoid increasing muscle spasticity.
■ Encourage the child to ask for things he wants and listen patiently. Speak slowly and distinctly.
■ Encourage family participation in providing care as much as possible. This improves the child's self-esteem and body image and also helps his family continue the care plan at home.
■ Provide an adequate diet to meet the child's high energy needs. During meals, maintain a quiet atmosphere with as few distractions as possible. The child may need special utensils and a chair with a solid footrest. Stroking the throat may aid swallowing.
■ Perform frequent mouth care.
■ Move the child carefully after surgery to reduce muscle spasms that may increase postoperative pain. Give analgesics, as ordered, and monitor for response.
■ Gently rotate a spastic limb inward toward the spasticity and then rotate it outward. Repeating this motion helps relax the spastic extremity. Pressure on the tendons located in the joint socket while rotating increases relaxation. Open a spastic hand by gently grasping the lateral aspects and moving inward and outward.
■ Assist with brace application, as needed.
■ Inspect the skin for areas of pallor or redness that indicate prolonged pressure. Provide meticulous skin care.
■ Administer prescribed medications.
■ Perform passive ROM and assist with active ROM exercises, as ordered. As appropriate, teach parents how to perform

DISCHARGE TEACHING

TEACHING THE PATIENT WITH CEREBRAL PALSY

Before discharge, teach the patient and his family:
- about the disorder and its implications
- treatment options, such as surgery and therapy
- about prescribed medication administration, dosage, possible adverse effects, and when to notify the physician
- the importance of good nutrition and what types of food may be best for the child to handle and swallow
- range-of-motion exercises to improve the child's muscle tonicity and control spasms
- types of therapy that would be beneficial, such as physical therapy, speech therapy, and occupational therapy
- signs and symptoms of complications
- methods to promote the child's independence
- the importance of follow-up care
- the benefits of utilizing available community support groups such as the local chapter of the United Cerebral Palsy Association.

prescribed exercises to maintain muscle tone and joint function.
- Provide emotional support to child and family.
- Provide appropriate education to the parents before the child's discharge. (See *Teaching the patient with cerebral palsy*.)

HYDROCEPHALUS

Hydrocephalus is an excessive accumulation of cerebrospinal fluid (CSF) in the ventricular spaces of the brain. It's most common in neonates but can also occur in adults as a result of injury or disease. In infants, hydrocephalus enlarges the head; in both infants and adults, resulting compression can damage brain tissue. With early detection and surgical intervention, the prognosis improves but remains guarded.

Pathophysiology

Hydrocephalus results from an obstruction in CSF flow (non-communicating hydrocephalus) or from faulty absorption of CSF (communicating hydrocephalus). (See *Normal circulation of CSF,* page 198.)

In noncommunicating hydrocephalus, the obstruction occurs most frequently between the third and fourth ventricles and at the aqueduct of Sylvius. It can also occur at the outlets of the fourth ventricle (foramina of Luschka and Magendie) or, rarely, at the foramen of Monro. This obstruction may result from faulty fetal development (myelomeningocele, congenital arachnoid cysts), infection (syphilis, granulomatous diseases, meningitis), tumor, cerebral aneurysm, or a blood clot.

In communicating hydrocephalus, faulty reabsorption of CSF may result from surgery to repair a myelomeningocele, adhesions between meninges at the base of the brain, or meningeal hemorrhage.

Complications

- Mental retardation
- Impaired motor function
- Vision loss
- Death (as a result of increased intracranial pressure [ICP] in people of all ages or as a result of infection and malnutrition in infants)

Assessment findings

In the infant, findings include:
- an enlarged head that's clearly disproportionate to the infant's growth
- bulging fontanels
- distended scalp veins
- thin, fragile, and shiny scalp skin
- underdeveloped neck muscles (see *Signs of hydrocephalus,* page 199)
- irritability

NORMAL CIRCULATION OF CSF

Cerebrospinal fluid (CSF) is produced from blood in a capillary network (choroid plexus) in the brain's lateral ventricles. From the lateral ventricles, CSF flows through the interventricular foramen (foramen of Monro) to the third ventricle. From there, it flows through the aqueduct of Sylvius to the fourth ventricle and through the foramina of Luschka and Magendie to the cisterna of the subarachnoid space.

The fluid then passes under the base of the brain, upward over the brain's upper surfaces, and down around the spinal cord. Eventually, CSF reaches the arachnoid villi, where it's reabsorbed into venous blood at the venous sinuses.

Normally, the amount of fluid produced (about 500 ml/day) equals the amount absorbed. The average amount circulated at one time is 150 to 175 ml.

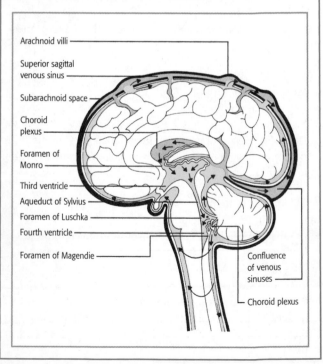

SIGNS OF HYDROCEPHALUS

In infants, characteristic signs of hydrocephalus include marked enlargement of the head; distended scalp veins; thin, shiny, and fragile-looking scalp skin; and weak muscles that can't support the head.

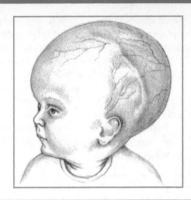

- anorexia with episodes of projectile vomiting
- high-pitched, shrill cry
- depression of the roof of the eye orbit, displacement of the eyes downward, and prominent sclera (sunset sign)
- abnormal muscle tone of the legs.

In adults and older children with a fused cranium, findings include:

- signs of increased ICP (nausea and vomiting that may be projectile)
- diplopia
- restlessness
- decreased level of consciousness (LOC)
- ataxia
- impaired intellect
- incontinence.

Diagnostic test results

- Skull X-rays show thinning of the skull with separation of sutures and widening of the fontanels in infants.

ARNOLD-CHIARI SYNDROME

Arnold-Chiari syndrome frequently accompanies hydrocephalus, especially when a myelomeningocele is also present. In this condition, an elongation or tonguelike downward projection of the cerebellum and medulla extends through the foramen magnum into the cervical portion of the spinal canal, impairing cerebrospinal fluid drainage from the fourth ventricle.

In addition to signs and symptoms of hydrocephalus, infants with Arnold-Chiari syndrome have nuchal rigidity, noisy respirations, irritability, vomiting, weak sucking reflex, and a preference for hyperextension of the neck.

Treatment requires surgery to insert a shunt like that used in hydrocephalus. Surgical decompression of the cerebellar tonsils at the foramen magnum is also sometimes indicated.

■ Angiography, computed tomography scan, and magnetic resonance imaging differentiate between hydrocephalus and intracranial lesions and may also reveal Arnold-Chiari syndrome, which occurs with hydrocephalus. (See *Arnold-Chiari syndrome*.)

Treatment

Surgery is the only treatment for hydrocephalus and is performed either to remove an obstruction to CSF flow or to divert CSF flow; such surgery involves insertion of a ventriculoperitoneal shunt, which drains excess CSF fluid from the brain's lateral ventricle into the peritoneal cavity.

If a concurrent abdominal problem exists, the physician may use a ventriculoatrial shunt, which drains fluid from the brain's lateral ventricle into the right atrium of the heart, where the fluid makes its way into the venous circulation. Endoscopic third ventriculostomy involves creating a passage between the third ventricle and the basal cisterns. This procedure is used for noncommunicating hydrocephalus in patients older than age 2 years.

Nursing interventions

- Check fontanels for tension or fullness, and measure and record head circumference. Mark the forehead so future measurements are consistent.
- Elevate the head of the bed or crib to 30 degrees to help decrease ICP.
- Administer oxygen, as ordered. Have suction equipment at the bedside, and suction as necessary.
- Provide emotional support, and encourage the patient (if appropriate) and his family to express their concerns.
- Encourage maternal-infant bonding when possible. When caring for the infant yourself, hold him on your lap for feeding, stroke and cuddle him, and speak soothingly.

BEFORE SHUNT SURGERY

- Provide small, frequent feedings, if necessary, to ensure adequate nutrition. To help lessen vomiting, decrease movement during and immediately after meals.
- Feed the infant slowly. To lessen strain from the weight of the infant's head on your arm while holding him during feeding, place his head, neck, and shoulders on a pillow. After feedings, place the infant on his side and reposition every 2 hours, or prop him up in an infant seat to prevent aspiration.
- Monitor the infant closely for signs of neurologic complications, such as change in LOC, vomiting, seizure activity, irregular respirations, and bradycardia. Notify the physician immediately if these changes occur.
- Check the infant's growth and development periodically.

AFTER SHUNT SURGERY

- Position the infant on the side opposite the operative site with his head level with his body, unless the physician's orders specify otherwise.
- Monitor intake and output, temperature, pulse rate, blood pressure, and LOC.

DISCHARGE TEACHING

TEACHING THE PATIENT WITH HYDROCEPHALUS

Before discharge, teach the patient and his family:
- about the disorder and its implications
- about prescribed medication administration, dosage, possible adverse effects, and when to notify the physician
- proper postoperative care of the incision
- activity recommendations
- proper shunt care
- signs and symptoms of complications, such as shunt malfunction, infection, and paralytic ileus
- the importance of follow-up care and the need for shunt revision in children to accommodate growth
- the benefits of utilizing available support groups such as the National Hydrocephalus Foundation.

- Assess fontanels for fullness daily. Note any vomiting, which may be an early sign of increased ICP and shunt malfunction.
- Assess for signs of infection, such as fever, stiff neck, irritability, or tense fontanels, which may signal meningitis. Also, watch for redness, swelling, and other signs of local infection over the shunt tract. Check dressing often for drainage. Use strict sterile technique when changing dressing.

RED FLAG Be alert for other postoperative complications, including shunt failure, adhesions, paralytic ileus, migration, peritonitis, and intestinal perforation (with peritoneal shunt).

- Provide appropriate education to the patient (if appropriate) and his family before discharge. (See *Teaching the patient with hydrocephalus*.)

NEURAL TUBE DEFECTS

Neural tube defects are caused by defective embryonic neural tube closure during the first trimester of pregnancy, which may result in the meninges and brain protruding through the skull without proper fusion. (See *Understanding anencephaly and encephalocele*.) These defects usually occur in the lumbosacral area, but they're occasionally found in the sacral, thoracic, and cervical areas. Although the exact cause of neural tube defects isn't known, viruses, radiation, and other environmental factors may be responsible. Additionally, they sometimes occur in offspring of females who have previously had children with similar defects; therefore, the genetic link is a possible factor.

UNDERSTANDING ANENCEPHALY AND ENCEPHALOCELE

Anencephaly occurs when the head (or cephalic) end of the neural tube fails to close during fetal development, resulting in an underdeveloped brain and incomplete skull. Neonates with anencephaly are either stillborn or don't survive more than a few hours after birth.

An encephalocele is a congenital saclike protrusion of the meninges and brain through a defective opening in the skull. It's usually found in the occipital area, but it may occur in the parietal, nasopharyngeal, or frontal area.

Clinical effects

Various clinical effects of encephalocele depend on the defect's location and the degree of tissue involvement. Visual defects may occur because optic tracks are stretched or absent. Often, paralysis and hydrocephalus accompany encephalocele.

Treatment

Surgery is performed during infancy to place protruding tissues back in the skull, excise the sac, and correct associated craniofacial abnormalities.

Always handle an infant with encephalocele carefully and avoid pressure on the sac. Both before and after surgery, watch for signs of increased intracranial pressure (bulging fontanels). As the child grows older, teach his parents to watch for developmental deficiencies that may signal mental retardation.

Research indicates that insufficient folic acid intake in the mother's diet is also a major risk factor.

Spina bifida occulta is an incomplete closure of one or more vertebrae without protrusion of the spinal cord or meninges. It's the least severe neural tube defect. In more severe forms of spina bifida, such as spina bifida cystica, incomplete closure of one or more vertebrae causes protrusion of the spinal contents in an external sac or a cystic lesion.

Spina bifida cystica is classified as myelomeningocele (meningomyelocele) or meningocele. With myelomeningocele, the external sac contains meninges, cerebrospinal fluid (CSF), and a portion of the spinal cord or nerve roots distal to the conus medullaris. When the spinal nerve roots end at the sac, motor and sensory functions below the sac are terminated. With meningocele (less severe form), the sac contains only meninges and CSF. Neurologic symptoms may not occur with meningocele. (See *Types of neural tube defects*.)

Spina bifida and anencephaly are the two most common forms of neural tube defects. The prognosis varies with the degree of accompanying neurologic defect. It's worse in patients with large open lesions, neurogenic bladders (which predispose to infection and renal failure), or total paralysis of the legs. Because such features are usually absent in spina bifida occulta and meningocele, the prognosis is much better for these patients and many of them can lead normal lives.

Pathophysiology

Normally, about 20 days after conception, the embryo develops a neural groove in the dorsal ectoderm. This groove rapidly deepens as the two edges fuse to form the neural tube. By day 23, this tube is completely closed except for an opening at each end. Theoretically, if the posterior portion of the neural tube fails to close by the fourth week of gestation, or if it closes and then splits open from a cause such as an abnormal increase in CSF later in the first trimester, a neural tube defect results.

TYPES OF NEURAL TUBE DEFECTS

The three major types of neural tube defects are illustrated here. Spina bifida occulta is characterized by a depression or raised area and a tuft of hair over the defect. With myelomeningocele, an external sac contains meninges, cerebrospinal fluid (CSF), and a portion of the spinal cord or nerve roots. With meningocele, an external sac contains only meninges and CSF.

SPINA BIFIDA OCCULTA

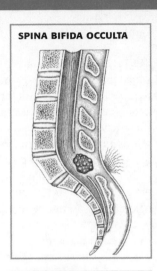

MYELOMENINGOCELE

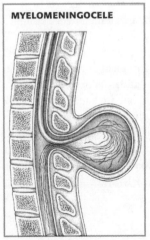

MENINGOCELE

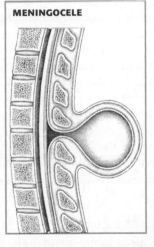

Complications
- Infection
- Paralysis
- Hydrocephalus
- Death

Assessment findings

Maternal history may reveal environmental factors that could have placed the infant at risk for development of neural tube defects. (See *Folic acid supplement recommendations*.)

Inspection of the neonate with spina bifida occulta typically reveals a depression or dimple; a tuft of hair; soft, fatty deposits; port wine nevi; or a combination of these abnormalities over the spinal defect. Palpation may reveal a depression or raised area along the spine over the defect. In many cases, neurologic status is normal because spina bifida occulta doesn't always cause neurologic dysfunction.

In spina bifida cystica, inspection reveals a saclike protrusion over the spinal cord. Transillumination of the protruding sac can sometimes distinguish between meningocele (light typically crosses through the sac) and myelomeningocele (light doesn't cross the sac). Depending on the defect's location, effects of myelomeningocele may include permanent neurologic dysfunction. Neurologic examination may reveal flaccid or spastic paralysis and bowel and bladder incontinence.

Other assessment findings are often related to associated disorders. These findings may include trophic skin disturbances (ulcerations, cyanosis), clubfoot, knee contractures, hydrocephalus (in about 90% of patients) and, possibly, mental retardation, Arnold-Chiari syndrome (in which part of the brain protrudes into the spinal canal), and curvature of the spine.

Diagnostic test results

- Alpha-fetoprotein (AFP) screening indicates the presence of neural tube defects.

FOLIC ACID SUPPLEMENT RECOMMENDATIONS

Folic acid supplementation before and during pregnancy has been found to reduce the risk of neural tube defects by 50% to 70%. The following recommendations for folic acid supplement dosages have been endorsed by the Centers for
Disease Control and Prevention, the U.S. Public Health Service, the March of
Dimes Birth Defects Foundation, and the Spina Bifida Association of America,
among other groups.

All females of childbearing age
All females who are capable of becoming pregnant should:
- consume 0.4 mg of folic acid per day to reduce the risk of having a child with
a neural tube defect such as spina bifida
- continue to consume 0.4 mg of folic acid per day during pregnancy until the
health care provider prescribes other prenatal vitamins.

Females at high risk
Females who have a neural tube defect themselves as well as those who have
previously given birth to an infant with a neural tube defect should:
- receive genetic counseling before their next pregnancy
- consume 0.4 mg of folic acid per day
- when actively trying to become pregnant (at least 2 months before conception), increase the dosage of folic acid to 4 mg per day (by taking a separate folic
acid supplement, not by increasing their intake of multivitamins)
- continue to take 4 mg of folic acid per day during the first 3 months of pregnancy.

- Amniocentesis may reveal the presence of AFP in the amni-
otic fluid.
- Ultrasound may detect open neural tube defects or ventral
wall defects.
- Skull X-rays and computed tomography scan can identify
the defects and detect associated hydrocephalus.

Treatment
Care of the infant with a severe spinal defect requires a team
approach, including the neurosurgeon, orthopedist, urologist,

pediatrician, nurse, social worker, occupational and physical therapists, and family members. Specific measures depend on the severity of the neurologic deficit.

Spina bifida occulta requires little or no treatment. If indicated, surgery is performed soon after birth to release the tethered spinal cord and prevent further neurologic deterioration.

Initial treatment for spina bifida cystica includes surgical closure of the defect as soon as possible after birth, possibly within 48 hours. If the protruding sac is large, plastic surgery is required for skin grafting over the lesion. Usually, a shunt is necessary to relieve associated hydrocephalus. If hydrocephalus isn't apparent at the time of the initial surgery, the child must be frequently reassessed for its occurrence because hydrocephalus occurs in about 90% of children with myelomeningocele.

After surgery, supportive measures are required to promote independence and prevent further complications. Because surgery doesn't actually reverse the neurologic deficit, orthopedic, rehabilitation, and urologic consultations can help determine the extent of the infant's rehabilitation needs, which may be necessary throughout the child's life. They may include:

■ waist supports, leg braces, walkers, crutches, and other orthopedic appliances
■ diet and bowel training to manage fecal incontinence
■ neurogenic bladder management to reduce urinary stasis, possibly intermittent catheterization, and antispasmodics, such as bethanechol or propantheline.

Fetal surgery, typically performed at 24 to 30 weeks' gestation, may be used to correct myelomeningocele in utero; however, premature birth is a major risk factor of this procedure. Although initial research indicates that fetal surgery is beneficial in reducing the incidences of associated hydrocephalus and hind brain herniation, the procedure is still considered experimental and is performed in only a few health care facilities in the United States.

Nursing interventions

- Provide emotional and psychological support. Help parents work through their feelings of fear, guilt, anger, and helplessness.

BEFORE SURGERY

- Clean the defect gently with sterile normal saline solution or other solutions, as ordered. Inspect the defect often for signs of infection and keep it covered with sterile dressings moistened with sterile normal saline solution. Don't use ointments on the defect because they may cause skin maceration.
- Administer prophylactic antibiotics, as ordered.
- Provide skin care. Keep the skin clean and apply lotion to knees, elbows, chin, and other pressure areas.
- Position the infant on his abdomen with the head of the bed slightly elevated to prevent contamination of the sac with urine or stool. If necessary, use pediatric fecal-incontinence bags to protect skin integrity.
- Observe the infant for signs of meningitis, including irritability, fever, feeding intolerance, and seizures. Notify the neurosurgeon if any of these signs occur.
- Provide adequate time for parent-infant bonding.
- Measure head circumference daily and watch for signs of hydrocephalus and meningeal irritation, such as fever and nuchal rigidity. Be sure to mark the place where you measure the infant's head so that consistent readings are obtained.
- Perform passive range-of-motion exercises. Place a pad between the infant's knees or position bags and ankle rolls to abduct the hips while lying in the crib.
- Monitor intake and output. Watch for signs of decreased skin turgor, dryness, or other signs of dehydration.
- Provide meticulous perineal care to prevent infection.
- Provide nutritional feedings and monitor for appropriate weight gain.

TEACHING PARENTS ABOUT NEURAL TUBE DEFECTS

Before discharge, teach the parents:
- about the specific type of defect and its implications
- about treatment options
- about prescribed medications administration, dosage, possible adverse effects, and when to notify the physician
- the importance of a high-fiber diet and increased fluid intake to help prevent urinary tract infections (UTIs) and constipation
- range-of-motion exercises to improve muscle strength
- types of therapy that would be beneficial such as physical therapy
- signs and symptoms of complications, such as hydrocephalus, pressure ulcers, and UTI
- how to help maintain adequate bladder function through use of Credé's maneuver, intermittent catheterization and, if necessary, conduit hygiene
- how to help prevent constipation and bowel obstruction through increased fluid intake, a high-fiber diet, exercise, and use of a stool softener, as ordered (Encourage parents to begin a bowel-training program with the child by age 3.)
- how to recognize developmental delays early (a possible result of hydrocephalus) and to provide stimulation and activities that promote mental development
- the importance of follow-up care
- the significance of genetic counseling and amniocentesis in future pregnancies
- the benefits of utilizing available community support groups such as the local chapter of the Spina Bifida Association of America.

AFTER SURGERY

- Monitor the infant's vital signs often. Watch for signs of shock (decreased blood pressure, tachycardia, lethargy), infection (malaise, elevated temperature, alteration in feeding pattern), and increased intracranial pressure (ICP [projectile vomiting]). Frequently assess the infant's fontanels. Remember that before age 2 months, infants don't show typical signs of increased ICP because suture lines aren't fully closed. In infants, the most telling sign is bulging fontanels.
- Use sterile technique when caring for the wound. Change the dressing regularly, as ordered, or whenever it becomes

soiled with urine or stool. Report any signs of drainage, wound rupture, and infection.

■ Place the infant in a prone position during the first 48 hours after surgery, if a muscle flap has been used to close the defect site.

■ Keep the infant warm in an Isolette. Don't use a diaper.

■ Monitor for signs of hydrocephalus. Measure the infant's head circumference daily and monitor fontanel size and sutures.

■ Observe for fever and neurologic changes. Observe the shunt site for redness or swelling, if a shunt is in place to decrease hydrocephalus.

■ Provide appropriate education to the parents before the infant's discharge. (See *Teaching parents about neural tube defects*.)

Neuromuscular and paroxysmal disorders

Neuromuscular disorders target the nerves, ultimately weakening the muscle. (See *Motor neuron disease*.) Amyotrophic lateral sclerosis, muscular dystrophy, and myasthenia gravis are examples of neuromuscular disorders. Paroxysmal disorders are characterized by an involuntary episodic increase in symptoms that affect the neurologic system and include epilepsy and headache.

NEUROMUSCULAR DISORDERS

AMYOTROPHIC LATERAL SCLEROSIS

Amyotrophic lateral sclerosis (ALS), also known as *Lou Gehrig disease,* is the most common motor neuron disease of muscular atrophy. ALS is a chronic, progressive, and debilitating disease that's invariably fatal and is characterized by progressive degeneration of the anterior horn cells of the spinal cord and cranial nerves and of the motor nuclei in the cerebral cortex and corticospinal tracts.

The exact cause of ALS is unknown; however, about 10% of patients with ALS inherit the disease as an autosomal dominant trait. ALS may also be caused by a virus that creates metabolic disturbances in motor neurons or by immune complexes such as those formed in autoimmune disorders.

MOTOR NEURON DISEASE

In its final stages, motor neuron disease affects both upper and lower motor neuron cells. However, the site of initial cell damage varies according to the specific disease:

- *progressive bulbar palsy:* degeneration of upper motor neurons in the medulla oblongata
- *progressive muscular atrophy:* degeneration of lower motor neurons in the spinal cord
- *amyotrophic lateral sclerosis:* degeneration of upper motor neurons in the medulla oblongata and lower motor neurons in the spinal cord.

Precipitating factors that can cause acute deterioration include severe stress, such as myocardial infarction, traumatic injury, viral infections, and physical exhaustion.

ALS is about three times more common in males than in females and generally affects people ages 40 to 70. Although some patients may live as long as 10 to 15 years, most die within 3 years of diagnosis. Death usually results from such complications as aspiration pneumonia or respiratory failure.

Pathophysiology

ALS progressively destroys the upper and lower motoneurons. However, because it doesn't affect cranial nerves III, IV, and VI, some facial movements such as blinking persist. Intellectual and sensory functions aren't affected.

Some believe that glutamate—the primary excitatory neurotransmitter of the CNS—accumulates to toxic levels at the synapses. In turn, affected motor units are no longer innervated, and progressive degeneration of axons cause loss of myelin. Some nearby motor neurons may sprout axons in an attempt to maintain function, but ultimately, nonfunctional scar tissue replaces normal neuronal tissue.

Complications

- Pneumonia
- Respiratory failure
- Aspiration
- Complications of physical immobility

Assessment findings

Signs and symptoms of ALS depend on the location of the affected motor neurons and the severity of the disease and may include:

- progressive weakness in muscles of the arms, legs, and trunk
- muscle atrophy
- muscle fasciculations (most obvious in the feet and hands)
- difficulty talking, chewing, swallowing and, ultimately, breathing.

Diagnostic test results

Although no diagnostic tests are specific to this disease, the following tests may aid in its diagnosis:

- Electromyography may show abnormalities of electrical activity of involved muscles; however, nerve conduction studies are usually normal.
- Muscle biopsy may disclose atrophic fibers interspersed among normal fibers. Cerebrospinal fluid analysis reveals increased protein content in one-third of patients.
- Computed tomography scan and EEG may help rule out other disorders, including multiple sclerosis, spinal cord neoplasms, syringomyelias, myasthenia gravis, and progressive muscular dystrophy.

Treatment

Because ALS has no cure, treatment focuses on controlling symptoms and providing emotional, psychological, and physical support. Riluzole is a neuroprotective agent that may improve the patient's quality of life and length of survival but doesn't reverse or stop the disease progression. Baclofen or diazepam may be used to control spasticity that interferes with activities of daily living (ADLs). Trihexyphenidyl or amitriptyline may be used for impaired ability to swallow saliva. Gastrostomy may be needed early to prevent choking; referral to an otolaryngologist is advised. Physical therapy, rehabilitation, and use of appliances or orthopedic intervention may be required to maximize function. Devices to assist in breathing at night or mechanical ventilation may also be required.

Nursing interventions

- Provide emotional and psychological support to the patient and his family.
- Assist the patient with active and passive range-of-motion exercises.
- Assist with ADLs and meals.
- Establish a regular bowel and bladder elimination routine.
- Provide good skin care and assess skin integrity every 2 to 4 hours, as appropriate.
- Reposition the patient every 2 hours as the patient's mobility decreases.
- Provide an alternate means of communication if the patient develops difficulty talking.
- Administer prescribed medications, as necessary, to relieve the patient's symptoms.
- Encourage deep-breathing and coughing exercises and use of incentive spirometry every hour while the patient is awake. Perform chest physiotherapy and suctioning every 2 to 4 hours, as appropriate.
- Provide soft, semisolid foods and position the patient upright during meals. Administer tube feedings, as ordered, if the patient can no longer swallow adequately.

MODIFYING THE HOME FOR A PATIENT WITH ALS

To help your patient with amyotrophic lateral sclerosis (ALS) live safely at home:
● explain basic safety precautions, such as keeping stairs and pathways free from clutter; using nonskid mats in the bathroom and in place of loose throw rugs; keeping stairs well lit; installing handrails in stairwells and the shower, tub, and toilet areas; and removing electrical and telephone cords from traffic areas.
● discuss the need for rearranging the furniture, and obtaining such equipment as a hospital bed, a commode, or oxygen equipment.
● recommend devices to ease the patient's and caregiver's work, such as extra pillows or a wedge pillow to help the patient sit up, a draw sheet to help him move up in bed, a lap tray for eating, or a bell for calling the caregiver.
● help the patent adjust to changes in the environment. Encourage independence.
● advise the patient to keep a suction machine handy to reduce the fear of choking due to secretion accumulation and dysphagia. Teach him self-suction.

DISCHARGE TEACHING

TEACHING THE PATIENT WITH ALS

Before discharge, teach the patient and his family:
● about amyotrophic lateral sclerosis (ALS) and its implications
● treatment options, such as physical therapy and ventilation support
● about prescribed medication administration, dosage, possible adverse effects, and when to notify the physician
● the importance of good nutrition and what types of food may be best for the patient to handle and swallow
● range-of-motion exercises to improve muscle tonicity and strength
● about the types of therapy that would be beneficial, such as physical therapy, speech therapy, and occupational therapy
● signs and symptoms of complications
● methods to promote the patient's independence and modify the home environment
● the importance of follow-up care
● the benefit of utilizing available community support groups such as the local chapter of the ALS Association.

- Discuss end-of-life issues, as appropriate.
- Discuss the home environment and provide recommendations for adjustments. (See *Modifying the home for a patient with ALS.*)
- Provide appropriate education to the patient and his family before discharge. (See *Teaching the patient with ALS.*)

MUSCULAR DYSTROPHY

Muscular dystrophy is a group of congenital neuromuscular disorders characterized by progressive symmetrical wasting of skeletal muscles without neural or sensory defects. Paradoxically, these wasted muscles tend to enlarge because of connective tissue and fat deposits, giving an erroneous impression of muscle strength. The main types of muscular dystrophy are Duchenne's (DMD) (pseudohypertrophic), Becker's (BMD) (benign pseudohypertrophic), Landouzy-Dejerine (facioscapulohumeral), and Erb's (limb-girdle) dystrophy.

The prognosis varies. DMD generally strikes during early childhood and usually results in death by age 20. Patients with BMD typically live into their 40s. Patients with Landouzy-Dejerine and Erb's dystrophies usually aren't adversely affected and may live long, healthy lives.

Pathophysiology

The absence or severe reduction of dystrophin protein results in a series of events that lead to myonecrosis with fibrin splitting. Phagocytosis of the muscle cells by inflammatory cells causes scarring and loss of muscle function. As the disease progresses, skeletal muscle becomes almost totally replaced by fat and connective tissue. The skeleton eventually becomes deformed, causing progressive immobility. Cardiac, smooth, and skeletal muscles are affected.

OBSERVING GOWERS' SIGN

Because Duchenne's and Becker's muscular dystrophies weaken pelvic and lower extremity muscles, the patient must use his upper body to maneuver from a prone to an upright position, a maneuver called *Gowers' sign.*

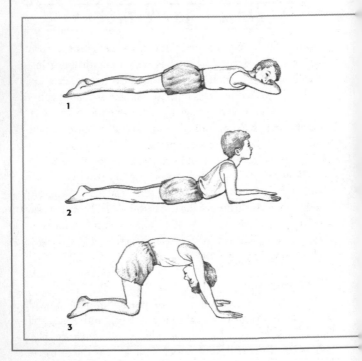

Complications
- Crippling disability
- Contractures
- Pneumonia
- Arrhythmias
- Cardiac hypertrophy

Lying on his stomach with his arms stretched in front of him, the patient raises his head, backs into a crawling position, and then into a half-kneel.

Then stooping, he braces his legs with his hands at the ankles and walks his hands (one after the other) up his legs until he pushes himself upright.

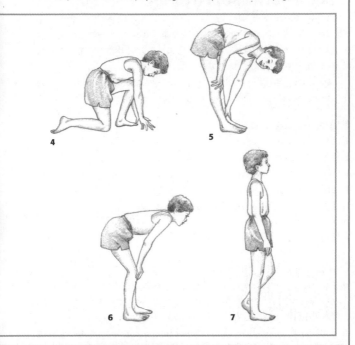

Assessment findings
DMD AND BMD

- Wide stance and waddling gait
- Gowers' sign when rising from a sitting position (see *Observing Gowers' sign*)
- Muscle hypertrophy and atrophy

- Enlarged calves
- Poor posture
- Lordosis with abdominal protrusion
- Scapular "winging" or flaring when raising arms
- Contractures
- Tachypnea and shortness of breath

LANDOUZY-DEJERINE DYSTROPHY

- Pendulous lower lip
- Possible disappearance of nasolabial fold
- Diffuse facial flattening leading to a masklike expression
- Inability to suckle (infants)
- Scapulae with a winglike appearance; inability to raise arms above head (see *Detecting muscular dystrophy*)

ERB'S DYSTROPHY

- Muscle weakness
- Muscle wasting
- Scapulae with a winglike appearance; inability to raise arms above head
- Lordosis with abdominal protrusion
- Waddling gait
- Poor balance

Diagnostic test results

- Electromyography typically demonstrates short, weak bursts of electrical activity or high-frequency, repetitive waxing and waning discharges in affected muscles.
- Muscle biopsy shows variations in the size of muscle fibers and, in later stages, shows fat and connective tissue deposits; dystrophin is absent in DMD and diminished in BMD.
- Serum creatine kinase is markedly elevated in DMD, but only moderately elevated in BMD and Landouzy-Dejerine dystrophy.

DETECTING MUSCULAR DYSTROPHY

In muscular dystrophy, the trapezius muscle typically rises, creating a stepped appearance at the shoulder's point.

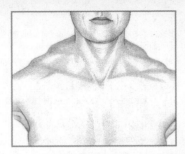

From the posterior view, the scapulae ride over the lateral thoracic region, giving them a winged appearance. In Duchenne's and Becker's dystrophies, this winglike sign appears when the patient raises his arms. In other dystrophies, the sign is obvious without arm raising. (In fact, the patient can't raise his arms.)

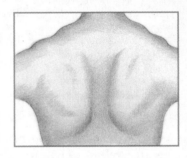

- Immunologic and molecular biological assays available in specialized medical centers facilitate accurate prenatal and postnatal diagnosis of DMD and BMB. These assays are replacing muscle biopsy and elevated serum creatine kinase levels in diagnosing these dystrophies. They can also help to identify carriers.

Treatment

No treatment stops the progressive muscle impairment of muscular dystrophy. However, orthopedic appliances, exercise, physical therapy, and surgery to correct contractures can help preserve the patient's mobility and independence. Prednisone improves muscle strength in patients with DMD.

Nursing interventions
- Encourage coughing, deep-breathing exercises, and diaphragmatic breathing.
- Encourage and assist with active and passive range-of-motion exercises.
- Advise the patient to avoid long periods of bed rest and inactivity.
- Provide trapeze bars, overhead slings, and a wheelchair to assist mobility.
- Encourage adequate fluid intake and provide a low-calorie, high-protein, high-fiber diet.

- Provide emotional support to the patient and his family.
- Provide appropriate education to the patient and his family before discharge. (See *Teaching the patient with muscular dystrophy.*)

MYASTHENIA GRAVIS

Myasthenia gravis (MG) is an autoimmune neuromuscular disease that produces sporadic but progressive weakness and abnormal fatigability of striated (skeletal) muscles. Usually, MG affects muscles innervated by the cranial nerves (face, lips, tongue, neck, and throat), but it can affect any muscle group. It commonly accompanies immune and thyroid disorders such as thymomas. When the disease involves the respiratory system, it may be life-threatening.

MG follows an unpredictable course of recurring exacerbations and periodic remissions. Once a severe and usually fatal disease, newer therapies have improved prognosis and allowed patients to lead relatively normal lives except during exacerbations.

MG occurs at any age, but incidence is highest in females ages 18 to 25 and in males ages 50 to 60. About three times as many females as males develop this disease.

Pathophysiology

For reasons unknown, the patient's blood cells and thymus gland produce antibodies that block, destroy, or weaken the neuroreceptors that transmit nerve impulses, causing a failure in transmission of nerve impulses at the neuromuscular junction. (See *Impaired transmission in myasthenia gravis,* page 224.)

Complications

- Respiratory failure
- Pneumonia
- Aspiration

IMPAIRED TRANSMISSION IN MYASTHENIA GRAVIS

This flowchart and illustration depict how neuromuscular transmission of impulses is impaired in patients with myasthenia gravis.

NORMAL NEUROMUSCULAR TRANSMISSION	NEUROMUSCULAR TRANSMISSION IN MYASTHENIA GRAVIS
Motor nerve impulses travel to motor nerve terminal.	Motor nerve impulses travel to motor nerve terminal.
Acetylcholine (ACh) is released.	ACh is released.
ACh diffuses across synapse.	ACh diffuses across synapse.
ACh receptor sites in motor end plates depolarize muscle fiber.	ACh receptor sites, weakened or destroyed by attached antibodies, block ACh reception.
Depolarization spreads, causing muscle contraction.	Depolarization and muscle contraction don't occur; neuromuscular transmission is blocked.

Axon

Vesicle containing ACh

Neuromuscular junction

ACh receptor site

Muscle

Release site

Junctional fold

Motor end plate

Assessment findings

Depending on the muscles involved and the severity of the disease, assessment findings may vary. Symptoms are milder on awakening and worsen as the day progresses; however, short rest periods temporarily restore muscle function. Symptoms may become more intense during menses and after emotional stress, prolonged exposure to sunlight or cold, or infections. Typical findings may include:

- extreme muscle weakness and fatigue (cardinal signs)
- ptosis and diplopia (most common sign and symptom)
- progressive muscle weakness
- difficulty chewing and swallowing
- impaired speech
- jaw drooping (especially when tired)
- head bobbing
- sleepy, masklike expression
- decreased breath sounds
- unstable or waddling gait.

Diagnostic test results

- Positive Tensilon test confirms the diagnosis of MG.
- Electrodiagnostic testing shows a rapid reduction of more than 10% in the amplitude of evoked response.
- Single-fiber electromyography shows impaired nerve-to-muscle transmission.
- Chest X-rays or computed tomography scan may identify an enlarged thymus gland or thymoma.

Treatment

Measures to relieve symptoms may include anticholinesterase drugs, such as pyridostigmine and neostigmine (less common). These drugs counteract fatigue and muscle weakness and allow approximately 80% of normal muscle function. They become less effective, however, as the disease worsens. Immunosuppressives, such as prednisone or cyclosporine, may also help to relieve symptoms by suppressing production of abnormal antibodies.

If medications prove ineffective, some patients may undergo plasmapheresis—a procedure that removes acetylcholine-receptor antibodies and temporarily reduces the severity of symptoms. I.V. immune globulin is also used for acute exacerbations.

Thymectomy reduces symptoms in 85% of patients with or without thymoma and may even cause complete remission in some individuals. Acute exacerbations that cause severe respiratory distress (myasthenic crisis) necessitate emergency treatment. Tracheotomy or endotracheal intubation, ventilation with a positive-pressure ventilator, and vigorous suctioning to remove secretions usually bring improvement in a few days. Because anticholinesterase drugs aren't effective in myasthenic crisis, they're discontinued until respiratory function begins to improve.

Nursing interventions

- Provide emotional support to the patient and his family
- Assess respiratory and neurologic status per unit protocol and clinical status. Monitor for changes in tidal volume, vital capacity, and inspiratory force.
- Monitor for signs of impending myasthenic crisis (increased muscle weakness, respiratory distress, difficulty talking or chewing).
- Perform orotracheal or nasotracheal suctioning, if appropriate.
- Assist with endotracheal intubation if respiratory failure occurs; monitor ventilation, as ordered.
- Administer medications, as ordered. Be prepared to give atropine in the event of anticholinesterase overdose or toxicity.
- Plan exercise, meals, patient care, and activities at periods of energy peaks.

DISCHARGE TEACHING

TEACHING THE PATIENT WITH MYASTHENIA GRAVIS

Before discharge, teach the patient and his family:
- about the disorder and its implications
- about treatment options, such as surgery and therapy
- about prescribed medications administration, dosages, and possible adverse effects and when to notify the physician
- the importance of good nutrition, including vitamin D and calcium supplementation (long-term steroid use may require caloric restriction)
- how to schedule activities around peak energy periods and the need for frequent rest periods
- the importance of avoiding strenuous exercise, stress, infection, and needless exposure to the sun or cold weather
- the need to check with the primary healthcare provider before using new medications or herbal supplements
- about types of therapy that would be beneficial, such as physical therapy, speech therapy, and occupational therapy
- the signs and symptoms of complications and myasthenia crisis
- the importance of follow-up care
- the benefits of utilizing available community support groups such as the local chapter of the Myasthenia Gravis Foundation of America.

- Provide a diet of semisolid foods, as appropriate, for chewing and swallowing abilities; monitor for signs of aspiration.
- Provide preoperative and postoperative teaching, as indicated.
- Monitor for signs of increased respiratory effort.
- Perform wound care and monitor for signs and symptoms of infection.
- Provide appropriate education to the patient and his family before discharge. (See *Teaching the patient with myasthenia gravis*.)

NONEPILEPTIC SEIZURES

A nonepileptic seizure is one that isn't caused by an electrical disruption of the cerebral cortex. They're usually difficult to differentiate from an epileptic seizure because they may appear the same, although their origins are different. Nonepileptic seizures are classified as physiologic or psychogenic.

A physiologic nonepileptic seizure is caused by a metabolic disturbance that disrupts brain function, such as hypoglycemia or cardiac arrhythmia.

A psychogenic nonepileptic seizure is caused by severe emotional trauma such as rape, or psychological conflict such as divorce.

PAROXYSMAL DISORDERS
EPILEPSY

Epilepsy, also known as *seizure disorder,* is a condition of the brain characterized by a susceptibility to recurrent seizures associated with abnormal electrical discharges of neurons in the brain. Some patients, however, have a seizure related to a particular stimulus, such as a high fever; these patients don't have epilepsy. (See *Nonepileptic seizures.*)

About half the cases of epilepsy are idiopathic; that is, no specific cause can be found and the patient has no other neurologic abnormality. Nonidiopathic epilepsy may be caused by:

- genetic abnormalities, such as tuberous sclerosis and phenylketonuria
- perinatal injuries
- metabolic abnormalities, such as hypocalcemia, hypoglycemia, and pyridoxine deficiency
- brain tumors or other space-occupying lesions
- infections, such as meningitis, encephalitis, or brain abscess
- traumatic injury, especially if the dura mater was penetrated
- ingestion of toxins, such as mercury, lead, or carbon monoxide
- stroke.

Researchers have also detected hereditary EEG abnormalities in some families, and certain seizure disorders appear to have a familial incidence.

Pathophysiology

Some neurons in the brain may depolarize easily or be hyperexcitable; this epileptogenic focus fires more readily than normal when stimulated and spreads electrical current to surrounding cells. In turn, these cells fire and the impulse cascades to one side of the brain (partial seizure), both sides of the brain (generalized seizure), or to the cortical, subcortical, and brain stem area. In response, inhibitory neurons fire, causing the excitatory neurons to slow their firing and eventually stop.

Complications

- Anoxia
- Traumatic injury
- Status epilepticus (see chapter 10 for more information)

Assessment findings

Depending on the type and cause of the seizure, signs and symptoms vary. (See *Differentiating seizures,* pages 230 and 231.)

Physical findings may be normal if the assessment is performed when the patient isn't having a seizure and the cause is idiopathic. If the seizure is associated with an underlying problem, the patient's history and physical examination should reveal signs and symptoms of that problem unless the seizure was caused by a brain tumor, which may produce no other symptoms.

In many cases, the patient's history reveals that seizure occurrence is unpredictable and unrelated to activities. Occasionally, a patient may report precipitating factors or events— for example, that the seizures always take place at a particular time, such as during sleep, or after a particular circumstance, such as lack of sleep or emotional stress. The patient may also

DIFFERENTIATING SEIZURES

The hallmark of epilepsy is recurring seizures, which can be classified as partial or generalized. Some patients may be affected by more than one type.

Partial seizures

Partial seizures arise from a localized area in the brain and cause specific symptoms. In some patients, partial seizure activity spreads to the entire brain, causing a generalized seizure. Partial seizures include simple partial (Jacksonian motor-type and sensory-type), complex partial (psychomotor or temporal lobe), and secondarily generalized partial seizures.

Simple partial (Jacksonian motor-type) seizure

A simple partial (Jacksonian motor-type) seizure begins as a localized motor seizure, which is characterized by a spread of abnormal activity to adjacent areas of the brain. Typically, the patient experiences a stiffening or jerking in one extremity, accompanied by a tingling sensation in the same area. For example, the seizure may start in the thumb and spread to the entire hand and arm. The patient seldom loses consciousness, although the seizure may secondarily progress to a generalized tonic-clonic seizure.

Simple partial (sensory-type) seizure

Perception is distorted in a simple partial (sensory-type) seizure. Symptoms can include hallucinations, flashing lights, tingling sensations, sensing a foul odor, vertigo, or déjà vu.

Complex partial seizure

Symptoms of complex partial seizure vary but usually include purposeless behavior. The patient may experience an aura and exhibit overt signs, including a glassy stare, picking at his clothes, aimless wandering, lip-smacking or chewing motions, and unintelligible speech. A seizure may last for a few seconds or as long as 20 minutes. Afterward, mental confusion may last for several minutes; as a result, an observer may mistakenly suspect psychosis or intoxication with alcohol or drugs. The patient has no memory of his actions during the seizure.

Secondarily generalized partial seizure

This type of seizure can be either simple or complex and can progress to generalized seizures. An aura may precede the progression. Loss of consciousness occurs immediately or within 1 or 2 minutes of the start of the progression.

Generalized seizures

As the term suggests, these seizures cause a generalized electrical abnormality in the brain. They include several distinct types.

Absence (petit mal) seizure

An absence seizure occurs most often in children but may also affect adults.

DIFFERENTIATING SEIZURES *(continued)*

It usually begins with a brief change in level of consciousness, indicated by blinking or rolling of the eyes, a blank stare, and slight mouth movements. The patient retains his posture and continues preseizure activity without difficulty. Typically, a seizure lasts from 1 to 10 seconds. The impairment is so brief that the patient is sometimes unaware of it. If not properly treated, these seizures can recur as often as 100 times a day. An absence seizure can progress to a generalized tonic-clonic seizure.

Myoclonic seizure

A myoclonic seizure–also called *bilateral massive epileptic myoclonus*–is marked by brief, involuntary muscular jerks of the body or extremities, which may occur in a rhythmic manner, and a brief loss of consciousness.

Generalized tonic-clonic (grand mal) seizure

Typically, this seizure begins with a loud cry, precipitated by air rushing from the lungs through the vocal cords. The patient falls to the ground, losing consciousness. The body stiffens (tonic phase) and then alternates between episodes of muscle spasm and relaxation (clonic phase). Tongue biting, incontinence, labored breathing, apnea, and subsequent cyanosis may also occur. The seizure stops in 2 to 5 minutes, when abnormal electrical conduction of the neurons is completed. The patient then regains consciousness but is somewhat confused and may have difficulty talking. If he can talk, he may complain of drowsiness, fatigue, headache, muscle soreness, and arm or leg weakness. He may fall into a deep sleep after the seizure.

Akinetic seizure

An akinetic seizure is characterized by a general loss of postural tone and a temporary loss of consciousness. This type of seizure occurs in young children. Sometimes it's called a *drop attack* because it causes the child to fall.

report nonspecific changes, such as headache, mood changes, lethargy, and myoclonic jerking, occurring up to several hours before the onset of a seizure.

Patients who experience a generalized seizure may describe an aura, which represents the beginning of abnormal electrical discharges within a focal point of the brain. Typical auras may include a pungent smell, GI distress (nausea or indigestion), a dreamy feeling, an unusual taste, or an unusual disturbance such as a flashing light that precedes seizure onset by a few seconds or minutes.

Diagnostic test results

- EEG can identify paroxysmal abnormalities, which may confirm the diagnosis of epilepsy by providing evidence of the continuing tendency to have seizures. A negative EEG doesn't rule out epilepsy because the paroxysmal abnormalities occur intermittently. EEG also helps guide the prognosis and can help to classify the disorder.
- Computed tomography scan and magnetic resonance imaging provide density readings of the brain and may indicate abnormalities in internal structures.

Treatment

Typically, treatment for epilepsy consists of drug therapy specific to the type of seizure. The most commonly prescribed drugs include phenytoin, fosphenytoin, carbamazepine, phenobarbital, valproic acid, and primidone—administered individually for generalized tonic-clonic seizures and complex partial seizures. Valproic acid, clonazepam, and ethosuximide are commonly prescribed for absence (petit mal) seizures. Lamotrigine is also prescribed as adjunct therapy for partial seizures. I.V. fosphenytoin is also an effective treatment.

If drug therapy fails to end seizures, treatment may include surgical removal of a demonstrated focal lesion. Surgery is also performed when epilepsy results from an underlying problem, such as an intracranial tumor, a brain abscess or cyst, and vascular abnormalities.

Vagal nerve stimulation may also be attempted, in which a pacemaker with a stimulator lead is placed on the vagus nerve. The nerve is stimulated for approximately 30 seconds every 5 minutes. This procedure is useful in refractory epilepsy, decreasing seizure frequency and intensity. It may also decrease the need for more medication and increase the quality of life

VAGAL NERVE STIMULATION

The vagal nerve stimulator consists of a pacemaker-like generator and a lead. In a surgical procedure, a small incision is made in the patient's chest and the device is implanted. The surgeon then wraps the lead around the vagus nerve in the neck to connect the device to the nerve.

The device prevents seizures by stimulating the vagus nerve for 30 seconds every 5 minutes around the clock. A magnet over the area can activate the device to give extra, on-demand stimulation if the patient feels a seizure coming on. Adverse effects of the vagal nerve stimulator include voice change, throat discomfort, shortness of breath, and coughing; these are usually felt only when the device is actually stimulating.

for some individuals. (See *Vagal nerve stimulation.*) Although transcranial magnetic stimulators are currently under investigation, their use has proven beneficial for some patients.

Nursing interventions

- Initiate seizure precautions according to your facility's protocol.
- Discuss measures to help prevent recurrent seizures. (See *Preventing seizures,* page 234.)
- Provide emotional support to the patient and his family. Suggest counseling, as appropriate.
- Monitor the patient for signs and symptoms of medication toxicity; check serum drug levels, as ordered.
- Administer medications, as ordered; use a large bore I.V. catheter to infuse phenytoin I.V., administer at a slow rate (not to exceed 50 mg/minute), avoid mixing it with dextrose solutions, and monitor the patient frequently for complications.
- Provide preoperative and postoperative teaching and care, if indicated.

PREVENTING SEIZURES

Teach the patient the following measures to help him control and decrease the occurrence of seizures.
- Take the exact dose of medication at the times prescribed. Missing doses, doubling doses, or taking extra doses can cause a seizure.
- Eat balanced, regular meals. Low blood glucose levels (hypoglycemia) and inadequate vitamin intake can lead to seizures.
- Be alert for odors that may trigger an attack. Advise the patient and his family to inform the physician of any strong odors they notice at the time of a seizure.
- Limit alcohol intake. In fact, the patient should check his physician to find out whether he should drink any alcoholic beverages.
- Get enough sleep. Excessive fatigue can precipitate a seizure.
- Treat a fever early during an illness. If the patient can't reduce a fever, he should notify the physician.
- Learn to control stress. If appropriate, suggest learning relaxation techniques such as deep-breathing exercises.
- Avoid trigger factors, such as flashing lights, hyperventilation, loud noises, heavy musical beats, video games, and television.

DISCHARGE TEACHING

TEACHING THE PATIENT WITH EPILEPSY

Before discharge, teach the patient and his family:
- about the disorder and its implications
- about treatment options, such as surgery and medication
- about prescribed medication administration, dosage, possible adverse effects, and when to notify the physician
- safety measures to follow when the patient is experiencing a seizure
- the importance of eating regular meals and checking with the physician before dieting
- signs and symptoms of complications
- the importance of follow-up care and evaluation of drug blood levels
- the benefits of utilizing available community support groups such as the local chapter of the Epilepsy Foundation.

- Provide appropriate education to the patient and family before discharge. (See *Teaching the patient with epilepsy*.)

HEADACHE

Headache is the most common patient complaint and a leading reason for medical consultations. Within a given year, 90% of men and 95% of women in the United States will experience at least one headache episode. Most headaches are benign in origin, although they may be profoundly disabling. Primary headaches include the chronic recurring types, such as tension, migraine, and cluster headache, not caused by other medical conditions. Secondary headaches are symptoms of another disease or disorder, such as an intracranial lesion, systemic disease, or local disease of the eyes or nasopharynx and may represent a more serious problem. Less than 2% of headaches are secondary headaches.

Pathophysiology

Headache is caused from traction, displacement, inflammation, vascular spasm, or distention of the pain-sensitive structures in the head or neck. Intracranial pain-sensitive structures include venous sinuses; the anterior and middle meningeal arteries; the dura at the base of the skull; the trigeminal (V), glossopharyngeal (IX) and vagus (X) nerves; the proximal portions of the internal carotid artery and its branches near the Circle of Willis; the brainstem periaqueductal gray matter; and the sensory nuclei of the thalamus. Extracranial pain-sensitive structures include the periosteum of the skull; the skin; the subcutaneous tissues, muscles, and arteries; the neck muscles; the second and third cervical nerves; the eyes, ears, teeth, sinuses, and oropharynx; and the mucous membranes of the nasal cavity.

Tension headaches, the most common form of headache, may be episodic or chronic and affect nearly 80% of the population at some point. The exact cause of tension headache is unknown, but both components include a central and peripheral mechanism.

Migraines are the most studied type of headache and are the second most common type of primary headache. Migraines are associated with a hypersensitive reaction to triggers such as stress, food substances (caffeine, alcohol, nicotine, and tyramine), odors, hormones, weather changes, depression, anxiety, and sleep deprivation. Triggers affect branches of the trigeminal nerve, resulting in release of vasoactive amines and substances that lead to inflammation of meningeal arteries and stretching of the trigeminal afferent branches, which can initiate a feedback loop into the trigeminal ganglia and to changes in serotonin levels.

Mutations in mitochondrial deoxyribonucleic acid and calcium channel genes may explain familial cases.

Cluster headaches are the least common type of primary headache and are triggered by alcohol and a history of heavy smoking. They occur with little warning. One to four short-lasting headaches per day during a cluster cycle are common, and the cluster cycle can last for weeks to months followed by a headache-free period that may last from months to years. The pathophysiology of cluster headache is unknown but is associated with elevated histamine levels. There appears to be an alteration in serotonergic nerve transmission but at different loci than in migraine.

Ominous secondary headaches from space occupying lesions and generalized inflammation are caused by increased intracranial pressure (ICP) and irritation of the meninges.

Complications

- Worsening of preexisting hypertension
- Phonophobia
- Emotional lability
- Motor weakness

Assessment findings

Common headache syndromes have considerable overlap in their signs and symptoms. (See *Clinical features of primary headaches,* pages 238 to 240.)

Findings for headaches caused by underlying systemic disease include:

- complaint of "the worst headache of my life," suggesting subarachnoid hemorrhage
- nuchal rigidity and headache, suggesting meningitis or subarachnoid or intraparenchymal hemorrhage
- severe headache with acute onset with such neurological signs as vomiting, seizure, change in level of consciousness, or syncope; headache with fever, neck stiffness, or both; and headache with progressive worsening, suggesting serious pathology
- pain that radiates in the trigeminal nerve distribution, suggesting trigeminal (V) nerve lesion
- pain that originates in the posterior fossa via the glossopharyngeal (IX) and vagus (X) nerves, suggesting an inflammatory disorder
- pain that originates in the posterior fossa and projects to the second and third cervical dermatomes, suggesting cervical disease.

Diagnostic test results

- Skull X-rays may show skull fractures.
- Computed tomography scan may show a tumor or subarachnoid hemorrhage or other intracranial pathology; it may also show sinus pathology.
- Lumbar puncture may identify pathology but it shouldn't be done until the possibility of increased ICP is ruled out by imaging studies.
- EEG may show alterations in the brain's electrical activity.
- Sinus X-rays may show sinusitis.

(Text continues on page 240.)

CLINICAL FEATURES OF PRIMARY HEADACHES

This chart summarizes signs and symptoms of primary headaches.

TYPE	SIGNS AND SYMPTOMS
TENSION HEADACHE	

Muscle-contraction headache
Occurs equally in both genders and in all ages
	• Pain characteristics include at least two of the following:
	  – Pressing/tightening (nonpulsating) quality
	  – Mild or moderate intensity
	  – Bilateral location
	• Gradual onset; may follow stress.
	• Absence of nausea and vomiting
	• Phonophobia or photophobia, but not both at the same time
	• Neck stiffness, shoulder ache, and nausea
	• Depression

COMMON MIGRAINE HEADACHE	

Migraine without aura
Usually occurs on weekends and holidays
	• At least five episodes of an occasional headache lasting 4 to 72 hours, involving two or more of the following:
	  – Nausea with vomiting or phono-phobia and photophobia
	  – Unilateral, throbbing pain wors-ened by movement
	  – Pain that's moderate or severe in nature
	• Fatigue, nausea, vomiting and fluid imbalance that may precede headache by about 1 day

CLASSIC MIGRAINE HEADACHE	
Migraine with aura	• Aura prior to onset of headache

CLINICAL FEATURES OF PRIMARY HEADACHES *(continued)*

TYPE	SIGNS AND SYMPTOMS
CLASSIC MIGRAINE HEADACHE (continued)	
Usually occurs in compulsive personalities and within families	● Visual auras: blinking or brightly colored lights (most common) or halo effect seen around lights or bright objects ● Other aura presentations: episodes of dizziness, confusion, syncope, dysarthria, diplopia, and vomiting Other types of classic migraine: ● Migraine aura without headache: recurrent and periodic headache, in which aura may present without headache (rare); aura may be acute onset, typical, or prolonged

HEMIPLEGIC, OPHTHALMOPLEGIC, RETINAL, AND BASILAR MIGRAINE HEADACHES

Specific types of migraine with aura	● Hemiplegic migraine: aura of hemiplegia and hemiparesis that may persist for several days after headache has subsided; often misdiagnosed as a stroke; possible severe, unilateral pain ● Ophthalmoplegic migraine: extraocular nerve palsies and ptosis (usually involving the third cranial nerve and less frequently the sixth); permanent third nerve injury possible with repeated events ● Retinal migraine: unilateral (monocular) and reversible visual loss ● Basilar migraine: bilateral visual symptoms, unsteadiness, dysarthria, vertigo, limb paraesthesia, and tetraparesis. Possible loss of consciousness that may precede the onset of headache

(continued)

**CLINICAL FEATURES OF
PRIMARY HEADACHES (continued)**

TYPE	SIGNS AND SYMPTOMS

CLUSTER HEADACHE (HISTAMINE CEPHALALGIA, HORTON SYNDROME, AND ERYTHROMELALGIA)

Men and women affected at a ratio of 9:1 More frequent in adults ages 20 to 40.	● Often occurs in middle of the night ● Severe, unilateral pain around the eye, tearing and inflammation of the same eye, and nasal congestion on the affected side ● Typically lasts for 30 to 45 minutes, but may vary from a few minutes to several hours

Treatment

Depending on the diagnosis, pharmaceutical treatment for headache ranges from over-the-counter medications to anti-depressants, selective serotonin reuptake inhibitors, beta-adrenergic blockers, calcium channel blockers, and antiepileptics. Nonpharmaceutical therapies include physical therapy, transcutaneous electrical nerve stimulation, ultrasonography, acupuncture, and improved sleep posture.

Acute tension headaches respond well to aspirin, acetaminophen, and other nonsteroidal anti-inflammatory drugs (NSAIDs), all with or without caffeine, along with reductions in stress and changes in daily living activities designed to reduce the frequency and intensity of episodes. Analgesics with caffeine can stimulate uterine contractions in pregnant women and are therefore contraindicated. Treatment for cluster headaches includes administration of high-flow oxygen for 10 minutes followed by treatment with sumatriptan (subQ), if no response. Other medications include dihydroergotamine (I.M., subQ, or I.V.). Preventive treatments include indomethacin,

PREVENTING HEADACHES

Teach the patient the following measures to help him control and decrease the occurrence of headaches.

● Using the patient's history as a guide, help him understand what precipitates his headaches so that he can avoid such exacerbating factors as hunger, lack of exercise, and erratic sleep schedules.

● Teach the patient how to perform relaxation techniques. Explain that education in relaxation techniques and biofeedback may help him change his attitude toward stress and can help him decrease the frequency of vascular and muscle-contraction headaches.

● Encourage the patient to exercise regularly. Explain that regular exercise promotes relaxation.

● If the patient experiences migraine headaches, instruct him to take the prescribed medication at the onset of migraine symptoms. Also advise him to prevent dehydration by drinking plenty of fluids after nausea and vomiting subside, avoiding long intervals between meals, and awakening at the same time every day. (In some patients, a disruption in normal sleeping patterns can precipitate a headache.)

● Encourage the patient who experiences migraine headaches to keep a journal in which he records activities and events that occurred just before an attack. A record of this information will allow the patient to recognize a pattern that precedes the onset of a migraine, thereby facilitating his ability to avoid precipitating factors.

verapamil, short-term high-dose corticosteroids, and lithium. Due to their short duration, oral medications aren't typically given. (See *Preventing headaches*.)

Medication in the triptan class is the first-line treatment for acute migraine. Medication should be taken within 15 minutes of symptom onset for best relief. Some patients will need an additional dose at 30 minutes to 1 hour. Most patients should be pain free within 2 hours and remain so for 24 hours. Rescue medications after triptan failure include opioids, such as morphine sulfate, diphenhydramine, and prochlorperazine. Other options include ketorolac, dihydroergotamine,

TEACHING THE PATIENT WITH A HEADACHE

Before discharge, teach the patient and his family:
- the causes of headache and its implications
- about treatment options based on the underlying cause
- about prescribed medication administration, dosage, possible adverse effects, and when to notify the physician
- the benefit of keeping a diary of headache occurrence, noting severity, relief, and length of attack
- about trigger recognition and avoidance and recommended lifestyle changes, such as smoking cessation, exercise, and stress reduction
- the importance of establishing a good sleep routine, such as going to bed at same time each night, avoiding stimulants before bedtime, and obtaining 8 hours of uninterrupted sleep
- about foods that may cause or aggravate headaches
- relaxation techniques that may decrease or prevent headaches
- the need for follow-up care, if indicated
- how to contact the National Headache Foundation for further information.

metoclopramide, hydroxyzine, and sodium valproate. For patients with two or more migraines per week, preventive therapy may include tricyclic antidepressants, selective serotonin reuptake inhibitors, NSAIDs, beta-adrenergic blockers, calcium channel blockers, and antiepileptics. However, several trials of different triptan class medications may be needed for long-term success. Each drug should be tried at least three times before moving on to the next medication. Cutaneous allodynia, which occurs with migraine headache, responds poorly to triptans.

Headaches due to subarachnoid hemorrhage, bacterial meningitis, and herniation from intracranial mass lesions are considered life-threatening and require emergency treatment to rectify the underlying cause.

Nursing interventions

- Encourage the use of relaxation techniques.
- Keep the patient's room dark and quiet.
- Administer analgesics, as ordered.
- Place ice packs or a cold cloth on the patient's forehead or eyes.
- Discuss methods to prevent recurring headaches.
- Provide appropriate education to the patient before discharge. (See *Teaching the patient with a headache.*)

Neurologic infections

Neurologic infections can be caused by bacterial or viral infiltration into cerebral tissue. They're an important cause of morbidity and mortality worldwide. Examples of neurologic infection include brain abscess, encephalitis, Guillain-Barré syndrome, and meningitis.

BRAIN ABSCESS

Brain abscess is usually secondary to an existing infection, especially otitis media, sinusitis, dental abscess, and mastoiditis. Other causes include subdural empyema; bacterial endocarditis; human immunodeficiency virus infection; bacteremia; pulmonary or pleural infection; pelvic, abdominal, and skin infections; and cranial trauma, such as a penetrating head wound or compound skull fracture. Brain abscess also occurs in those with congenital heart disease and congenital blood vessel abnormalities of the lungs such as Osler-Weber-Rendu disease.

Pathophysiology
Brain abscess usually begins with localized inflammatory necrosis and edema, septic thrombosis of vessels, and suppurative encephalitis. This is followed by thick encapsulation of accumulated pus and adjacent meningeal infiltration by neutrophils, lymphocytes, and plasma cells.

Complications

- Rupture of abscess into the ventricles or subarachnoid space
- Meningitis
- Epilepsy
- Recurrence of infection
- Death

Assessment findings

Findings may vary according to cause; however, brain abscess generally produces clinical effects similar to those of a brain tumor, including:

- constant intractable headache, worsened by straining
- nausea and vomiting
- confusion
- altered level of consciousness (LOC)
- focal or generalized seizures
- ocular disturbances, such as nystagmus, decreased vision, and unequal pupil size.

Other findings differ with the site of the abscess:

- *temporal lobe abscess:* auditory-receptive dysphasia, central facial weakness, and hemiparesis
- *cerebellar abscess:* dizziness, coarse nystagmus, gaze weakness on lesion side, tremor, and ataxia
- *frontal lobe abscess:* expressive dysphasia, hemiparesis with unilateral motor seizure, drowsiness, inattention, and mental function impairment.

Diagnostic test results

- Complete blood count shows elevated white blood cell count.
- Computed tomography (CT) scan or magnetic resonance imaging (MRI) help locate the site of the abscess.
- Blood culture reveals any bacteria in the bloodstream.
- Chest X-ray may reveal lung infection.
- CT-guided stereotactic biopsy may be performed to drain and culture the abscess.

Treatment

Management of patients with brain abscess has become increasingly challenging because of the proliferation of unusual bacterial, fungal, and parasitic infections, particularly in immunocompromised patients. Therapy consists of antibiotics and antimicrobials, which may be injected directly into the abscess, to combat the underlying infection and surgical excision, aspiration, or drainage of the abscess. (CT scan or MRI can help determine the need for these procedures.) Administration of antibiotics for at least 2 weeks before surgery can reduce the risk of spreading infection.

Other treatments during the acute phase are palliative and supportive and include mechanical ventilation, administration of I.V. fluids with diuretics (urea or mannitol), and glucocorticoids (dexamethasone) to combat increased intracranial pressure (ICP) and cerebral edema. Anticonvulsants, such as phenytoin and phenobarbital, help prevent seizures.

Nursing interventions

- Monitor neurologic status, especially LOC, speech, and sensorimotor and cranial nerve functions. Watch for signs of increased ICP (decreased LOC, vomiting, abnormal pupil response, and depressed respirations), which may lead to cerebral herniation with such signs as fixed and dilated pupils, widened pulse pressure, bradycardia or tachycardia, and absent respirations.
- Assess and record vital signs every hour and as indicated by clinical status.
- Monitor fluid intake and output.

  If surgery is necessary, explain the procedure to the patient and answer his questions. After surgery:
- Continue frequent neurologic assessment. Monitor vital signs and intake and output.
- Watch for signs of meningitis, such as nuchal rigidity, headaches, chills, and sweats.

DISCHARGE TEACHING

TEACHING THE PATIENT WITH A BRAIN ABSCESS

Before discharge, teach the patient and his family:
- about the disorder and its implications
- about treatment options, such as surgery
- about prescribed medication administration, dosage, possible adverse effects, and when to notify the physician
- the signs and symptoms of complications
- how to prevent future brain abscesses
- the importance of follow-up care.

■ Provide appropriate education to the patient and his family before discharge. (See *Teaching the patient with a brain abscess.*)

ENCEPHALITIS

Encephalitis is a severe inflammation of the brain that results from infection with arboviruses specific to rural areas. In urban areas, encephalitis is most commonly caused by enteroviruses (coxsackievirus, poliovirus, and echovirus). Other causes include herpesvirus, mumps virus, adenoviruses, and demyelinating diseases after measles, varicella, rubella, or vaccination. (See *Types of encephalitis,* pages 248 to 251.)

Transmission by means other than arthropod bites may occur through ingestion of infected goat's milk and accidental injection or inhalation of the virus.

Pathophysiology

Virus entry through hematogenous spread or by transmission along the neural and olfactory pathways. Intense lymphocytic infiltration of brain tissues and the leptomeninges causes cerebral edema, degeneration of the brain's ganglion cells, and dif-

(Text continues on page 252.)

TYPES OF ENCEPHALITIS

Four main virus agents cause most cases of encephalitis in the United States: eastern equine encephalitis (EEE), western equine encephalitis (WEE), St. Louis encephalitis (SLE), and La Crosse (LAC) encephalitis, all of which are transmitted by mosquitoes. Another less common cause of encephalitis is the Powassan (POW) virus; it's transmitted by ticks in the northern United States. Most cases of arboviral encephalitis occur from June through September, when arthropods are most active. In milder parts of the country, where arthropods are active late into the year, cases can occur into the winter months.

Vaccines aren't available for these U.S.-based diseases. However, a Japanese encephalitis (JE) vaccine is available for those who will be traveling to Japan, a tick-borne encephalitis vaccine is available for those who will be traveling to Europe, and an equine vaccine is available for EEE, WEE, and Venezuelan equine encephalitis (VEE). Public health measures often require spraying of insecticides to kill larvae and adult mosquitoes as well as controlling standing water, which is a breeding ground for mosquitoes.

Eastern equine encephalitis

● EEE is caused by an alphavirus virus transmitted to humans and equines by the bite of an infected mosquito.

● Incubation is 4 to 10 days.

● Symptoms begin with a sudden onset of fever, general muscle pains, and a headache of increasing severity; it may progress to seizures and coma.

● One-third of those afflicted will die from the disease and of those who recover, many will suffer irreversible brain damage.

● Human cases are usually preceded by outbreaks in horses.

● The virus occurs in natural cycles involving birds in swampy areas nearly every year during the warm months. The virus doesn't escape from these areas, however, and this mosquito doesn't usually bite humans or other mammals.

Western equine encephalitis

● The alphavirus WEE is the causative agent. The virus is closely related to the EEE and VEE viruses.

● The enzootic cycle of WEE involves passerine birds, in which the infection isn't apparent, and culicine mosquitoes, principally *Cx. tarsalis,* a species associated with irrigated agriculture and stream drainages.

● Human WEE cases are usually first seen in June or July.

● Most WEE infections are asymptomatic or present as mild, nonspecific illness. Patients with clinically apparent illness usually have a sudden onset with fever, headache, nausea, vomiting, anorexia, and malaise, followed by altered mental status, weakness, and signs of meningeal irritation.

● Children, especially those younger than age 1, are affected more severely

TYPES OF ENCEPHALITIS *(continued)*

than adults and may be left with permanent sequelae, which is seen in 5% to 30% of young patients.

● Mortality is about 3%.

St. Louis encephalitis

● The leading cause of SLE is flaviviral. It's the most common mosquito-transmitted human pathogen in the United States.

● Mosquitoes become infected by feeding on birds infected with the SLE virus. Infected mosquitoes then transmit the virus to humans and animals during the feeding process. The virus grows both in the infected mosquito and the infected bird, but doesn't make either one sick.

● Less than 1% of SLE viral infections are clinically apparent; the majority are undiagnosed.

● Illness ranges in severity from a simple febrile headache to meningoencephalitis, with an overall case-fatality ratio of 5% to 15%.

● The incubation period is 5 to 15 days.

● Mild infections present with fever and headache. More severe infection is marked by headache, high fever, neck stiffness, stupor, disorientation, coma, tremors, occasional convulsions (especially in infants), and spastic (but rarely flaccid) paralysis.

● The disease is generally milder in children than in adults, but in those children who do have disease, there's a high rate of encephalitis.

● Elderly people are at highest risk for severe disease and death.

● During the summer season, SLE virus is maintained in a mosquito-bird-mosquito cycle, with periodic amplification by peridomestic birds and *Culex* mosquitoes.

La Crosse encephalitis

● The LAC virus, a Bunyavirus, is a zoonotic pathogen cycled between the daytime-biting tree hole mosquito, *Aedes triseriatus,* and vertebrate amplifier hosts (chipmunks, tree squirrels) in deciduous forest habitats. The virus is maintained over the winter by transmission in mosquito eggs. If the female mosquito is infected, she may lay eggs that carry the virus. Vector uses artificial containers (such as tires and buckets) in addition to tree holes.

● LAC encephalitis initially presents as a nonspecific summertime illness with fever, headache, nausea, vomiting, and lethargy.

● Severe disease occurs most commonly in children younger than age 16 and is characterized by seizures, coma, paralysis, and a variety of neurological sequelae after recovery.

● Death occurs in less than 1% of clinical cases.

● Cases are commonly reported as aseptic meningitis or viral encephalitis of unknown etiology.

● During an average year, about 75 cases of LAC encephalitis are reported to the Centers for Disease Control and Prevention.

(continued)

TYPES OF ENCEPHALITIS *(continued)*

Powassan encephalitis
● The POW virus is a flavivirus.
● Recently a Powassan-like virus was isolated from the deer tick, *Ixodes scapularis.* The virus has been recovered from ticks (*Ixodes marxi* and *Dermacentor andersoni*) and from the tissues of a skunk (*Spiligale putorius*).
● It's a rare cause of acute viral encephalitis.
● Patients who recover may have residual neurologic problems.

Venezuelan equine encephalitis
● Like EEE and WEE viruses, VEE is an alphavirus that causes encephalitis in horses and humans. VEE is a significant veterinary and public health problem in Central and South America.
● Infection of humans with the VEE virus is less severe than with EEE and WEE viruses and fatalities are rare.
● Adults usually develop only an influenza-like illness; overt encephalitis is usually confined to children.
● Effective VEE virus vaccines are available for equines.

Japanese encephalitis
● JE virus, which is related to SLE, is a flavivirus. It's widespread throughout Asia.
● Epidemics occur in late summer in temperate regions, but the infection is enzootic and occurs throughout the year in many tropical areas of Asia.
● The virus is maintained in a cycle involving culicine mosquitoes and wa-

terbirds. It's transmitted to humans by Culex mosquitoes, primarily *Cx. tritaeniorhynchus,* which breed in rice fields.
● Mosquitoes become infected by feeding on domestic pigs and wild birds infected with the JE virus. Infected mosquitoes then transmit the virus to humans and animals during the feeding process. The virus is amplified in domestic pigs and wild birds.
● The incubation period is 5 to 14 days.
● Mild infections occur without apparent symptoms other than fever with headache. More severe infection is marked by quick onset, headache, high fever, neck stiffness, stupor, disorientation, coma, tremors, occasional seizures (especially in infants), and spastic (but rarely flaccid) paralysis.
● The illness resolves in 5 to 7 days if there's no central nervous system involvement.
● Mortality is less than 10%, but is higher in children and can exceed 30%. Neurologic sequelae in patients who recover are reported in up to 30% of cases.
● A vaccine is currently available for human use in the United States for individuals who might be traveling to endemic countries.

Tick-borne encephalitis
● Tick-borne encephalitis (TBE) is caused by two closely related flaviviruses. The eastern subtype causes Russian spring-summer encephalitis

TYPES OF ENCEPHALITIS *(continued)*

(RSSE) and is transmitted by *Ixodes persulcatus,* whereas the western subtype is transmitted by *Ixodes ricinus* and causes Central European encephalitis (CEE).

● RSSE is the more severe infection, having a mortality of up to 25% in some outbreaks, whereas mortality in CEE seldom exceeds 5%.

● The incubation period is 7 to 14 days.

● Infection usually presents as a mild, influenza-type illness or as benign, aseptic meningitis, but may result in fatal meningoencephalitis.

● Fever is usually biphasic and there may be severe headache and neck rigidity, with transient paralysis of the limbs, shoulders or, less commonly, the respiratory musculature. Few patients are left with residual paralysis.

● Although the great majority of TBE infections follow exposure to ticks, infection has occurred through the ingestion of infected cows' or goats' milk.

● An inactivated TBE vaccine is currently available in Europe and Russia.

West Nile encephalitis

● West Nile virus (WNV) is a flavivirus belonging to the Japanese encephalitis serocomplex that includes the closely related SLE virus, Kunjin, and Murray Valley encephalitis viruses as well as others.

● WNV can infect a wide range of vertebrates; in humans it usually produces either asymptomatic infection or mild febrile disease, but can cause severe and fatal infection in a small percentage of patients.

● The incubation period is thought to range from 3 to 14 days.

● Symptoms generally last 3 to 6 days.

● Like SLE virus, WNV is transmitted principally by *Culex* species mosquitoes, but can also be transmitted by *Aedes, Anopheles,* and other species.

● The mild form of WNV infection has presented as a febrile illness of sudden onset often accompanied by malaise, anorexia, nausea, vomiting, eye pain, headache, myalgia, rash, and lymphadenopathy.

● A minority of patients with severe disease develop a maculopapular or morbilliform rash involving the neck, trunk, arms, or legs. Some patients experience severe muscle weakness and flaccid paralysis. Neurological presentations include ataxia, cranial nerve abnormalities, myelitis, optic neuritis, polyradiculitis, and seizures. Although not observed in recent outbreaks, myocarditis, pancreatitis, and fulminant hepatitis have been described.

Murray Valley encephalitis

● MVE is endemic in New Guinea and in parts of Australia.

● It's related to the SLE, WN, and JE viruses.

● Infections are common, and the small number of fatalities have mostly been seen in children.

fuse nerve cell destruction. Resultant parenchymal damage may range from mild to severe.

Complications
- Bronchial pneumonia
- Urinary tract infection
- Coma
- Epilepsy
- Parkinsonism
- Mental deterioration

Assessment findings
Findings for encephalitis include:
- fever, headache, and vomiting
- altered levels of consciousness (LOC), from lethargy or drowsiness to stupor
- seizures, which may be the only presenting sign of encephalitis.
- confusion, disorientation, or hallucinations
- tremors, cranial nerve palsies, exaggerated deep tendon reflexes, absent superficial reflexes, and paresis or paralysis of the extremities
- stiff neck.

If the cerebral hemispheres are involved, assessment findings may include:
- aphasia
- involuntary movements
- ataxia
- sensory defects such as disturbances of taste and smell
- poor memory retention.

Diagnostic test results
- Blood analysis or, rarely, cerebrospinal fluid (CSF) analysis identifies the virus and confirms the diagnosis.
- Serologic studies in herpes encephalitis may show rising titers of complement-fixing antibodies. Serologic studies may also be diagnostic in other types of encephalitis.

- Lumbar puncture reveals elevated CSF in all forms of encephalitis. White blood cell count and protein levels in CSF are slightly elevated, but glucose level remains normal.
- EEG reveals abnormalities such as generalized slowing of waveforms.
- Computed tomography scan or magnetic resonance imaging may reveal temporal lobe lesions that indicate herpesvirus and may rule out cerebral hematoma.

Treatment

The antiviral agent acyclovir is effective only against herpes encephalitis. Antibiotics may be prescribed if the infection is caused by bacteria.

Treatment of all other forms of encephalitis is supportive. Drug therapy includes reduction of intracranial pressure (ICP) with I.V. mannitol and corticosteroids (to reduce cerebral inflammation and resulting edema); phenytoin or another anticonvulsant, usually given I.V.; sedatives for restlessness; and aspirin or acetaminophen to relieve headache and reduce fever. Ribavirin and interferon alpha-2b were have shown some effect on West Nile encephalitis.

Other supportive measures include adequate fluid and electrolyte administration to prevent dehydration and appropriate antibiotics for associated infections, such as pneumonia or sinusitis; maintenance of the patient's airway; administration of oxygen to maintain arterial blood gas levels; and maintenance of nutrition, especially during periods of coma. Isolation is unnecessary.

Nursing interventions

- Monitor neurologic status. Observe LOC and signs of increased ICP. Watch for cranial nerve involvement (ptosis, strabismus, diplopia), abnormal steep patterns, and behavior changes.
- Administer fluid to prevent dehydration but avoid fluid overload, which may increase cerebral edema. Measure and record intake and output accurately.

TEACHING THE PATIENT WITH ENCEPHALITIS

Before discharge, teach the patient and his family:
- about the disorder and its implications
- about prescribed medication administration, dosage, possible adverse effects, and when to notify the physician
- the importance of good nutrition and fluid intake
- about rehabilitation if neurologic deficits occur
- the signs and symptoms of complications
- the importance of follow-up care
- how to contact the National Institute of Neurological Disorders and Stroke for more information.

- Position the patient to prevent joint stiffness and neck pain and reposition every 2 hours. Assist with range-of-motion exercises.
- Provide adequate nutrition. Give the patient small, frequent meals, or administer with nasogastric tube or parenteral feedings.
- Administer medications, as ordered.
- Provide good mouth care.
- Maintain a quiet environment.
- Initiate seizure precautions, if indicated.
- Provide emotional support and reassure the patient and his family.
- Provide appropriate education to the patient and his family before discharge. (See *Teaching the patient with encephalitis*.)

GUILLAIN-BARRÉ SYNDROME

Guillain-Barré syndrome is an acute, rapidly progressive, and potentially fatal form of polyneuritis that causes segmented demyelination of peripheral nerves. It's thought to be a cell-mediated immunologic attack on peripheral nerves in response to a virus. When infection precedes onset of Guillain-Barré syndrome, signs of infection subside before neurologic symptoms appear. Other possible precipitating factors include surgery, vaccination (such as flu, tetanus), Hodgkin's or other malignant disease, drugs, and lupus erythematosus.

The clinical course of Guillain-Barré syndrome has three phases. The acute phase begins when the first definitive symptom develops; it ends 1 to 3 weeks later, when no further deterioration is noted. The plateau phase lasts for several days to 2 weeks and is followed by the recovery phase, which is believed to coincide with remyelination and axonal process regrowth. The recovery phase extends over 4 to 6 months; however, patients with severe disease may take up to 2 to 3 years to recover, and recovery may not be complete. The disorder is also known as *infectious polyneuritis, Landry-Guillain-Barré syndrome,* or *acute idiopathic polyneuritis.*

Pathophysiology

The major pathologic effect is segmental demyelination of the peripheral nerves, which prevents normal transmission of electrical impulses along the sensorimotor nerve roots. (See *Understanding sensorimotor nerve degeneration,* page 256.)

Complications

- Thrombophlebitis
- Pulmonary embolism
- Myocardial infarction
- Pressure ulcers
- Contractures
- Muscle wasting
- Aspiration
- Respiratory tract infections
- Life-threatening respiratory and cardiac compromise

Assessment findings

Findings for Guillain-Barré syndrome include:

UNDERSTANDING SENSORIMOTOR NERVE DEGENERATION

Guillain-Barré syndrome attacks the peripheral nerves, impairing their ability to correctly transmit messages to the brain.

The myelin sheath degenerates for unknown reasons. This sheath covers the nerve axons and conducts electrical impulses along the nerve pathways. Degeneration brings inflammation, swelling, and patchy demyelination. As this disorder destroys myelin, the nodes of Ranvier (at the junction of the myelin sheaths) widen. This delays and impairs impulse transmission along the dorsal and anterior nerve roots.

Because the dorsal nerve roots handle sensory function, the patient may experience tingling and numbness. Similarly, because the anterior nerve roots are responsible for motor function, impairment causes varying weakness, immobility, and paralysis.

- history of a minor febrile illness (usually an upper respiratory tract infection or, less commonly, GI infection) 1 to 4 weeks before current symptoms
- tingling and numbness (paresthesia) in the feet and then hands
- back pain or a severe "charley horse"
- muscle weakness (major neurologic sign) and sensory loss, initially in the legs but may have progressed to the arms
- difficulty talking, chewing, and swallowing
- loss of position sense and diminished or absent deep tendon reflexes.

Diagnostic test results

- Cerebrospinal fluid (CSF) analysis may show a normal white blood cell count, an elevated protein count and, in severe disease, increased CSF pressure.
- Electromyography may demonstrate repeated firing of the same motor unit instead of widespread sectional stimulation.

- Electrophysiologic testing may reveal marked slowing of nerve conduction velocities.
- Antiganglioside antibody testing may help establish disease subclassification.

Treatment

Treatment is primarily supportive and may require endotracheal intubation or tracheotomy if the patient has difficulty clearing secretions and mechanical ventilation if the patient has respiratory failure.

Continuous electrocardiogram monitoring is necessary to identify and treat cardiac arrhythmias. Atropine may be administered to treat bradycardia. Marked hypotension may require volume replacement.

Plasmapheresis produces a temporary reduction in circulating antibodies and is most effective when performed during the first few weeks of the disease. The patient may receive three to five plasma exchanges. I.V. immune globulin is given to reduce the severity and duration of symptoms.

Nursing interventions

- Monitor vital signs and neurological status. (See *Testing for thoracic sensation*, page 258.)
- Monitor respiratory status and pulse oximetry. Assist with intubation, if indicated.

RED FLAG Because neuromuscular disease results in primary hypoventilation with hypoxemia and hypercapnia, watch for partial pressure of arterial oxygen below 70 mm Hg, which signals respiratory failure. Be alert for confusion and tachypnea, which are signs of rising partial pressure of arterial carbon dioxide.

- Reposition every 2 hours. Provide skin care and assess for skin breakdown.
- Perform passive range-of-motion (ROM) exercises and assist with active ROM exercises for as long as the patient can participate.

TESTING FOR THORACIC SENSATION

When Guillain-Barré syndrome progresses rapidly, test for ascending sensory loss by touching the patient or pressing his skin lightly with a pin every hour. Move systematically from the iliac crest (T12) to the scapula, occasionally substituting the blunt end of the pin to test the patient's ability to discriminate between sharp and dull.

Mark the level of diminished sensation to measure any change. If diminished sensation ascends to T8 or higher, the patient's intercostal muscle function (and consequently respiratory function) will probably be impaired. As Guillain-Barré syndrome subsides, sensory and motor weakness descends to the lower thoracic segments, heralding a return of intercostal and extremity muscle function.

SEGMENTAL DISTRIBUTION OF SPINAL NERVES TO BACK

T6
T7
T8
T9
T10
T11
T12

Key: T = thoracic segments

- Elevate the head of the bed for eating. Assess gag reflex before allowing the patient to eat. Watch for signs of aspiration. Administer tube feedings if the patient can't safely swallow or is intubated.
- Initiate prophylactic measures to prevent deep vein thrombophlebitis. Apply sequential compresion stockings. Inspect the patient's legs regularly for signs of thrombophlebitis (localized pain, tenderness, erythema, edema, Homans' sign). Administer anticoagulants, as ordered.
- Monitor intake and output. Insert an indwelling urinary catheter, as indicated.

DISCHARGE TEACHING

TEACHING THE PATIENT WITH GUILLIAN-BARRÉ SYNDROME

Before discharge, teach the patient and his family:
● about the disorder and its implications
● the patient's treatment plan
● about prescribed medication administration, dosage, possible adverse effects, and when to notify the physician
● about the importance of good nutrition and what types of food may be best for the patient to handle and swallow
● range-of-motion exercises to improve the muscle tonicity and control spasms
● about activity recommendations and how to prevent skin breakdown
● how to establish a bowel and bladder program
● rehabilitation available for recovery
● the signs and symptoms of complications
● the importance of follow-up care
● the benefits of utilizing available community support groups such as the local chapter of the Guillain-Barré Syndrome Foundation International.

■ Provide emotional support to the patient and his family. Listen to their concerns and answer all questions.
■ Administer medications, as ordered. Analgesics may be prescribed to relieve muscle stiffness and spasm.
■ Provide appropriate education to the patient and his family before discharge. (See *Teaching the patient with Guillain-Barré syndrome*.)

MENINGITIS

Meningitis is inflammation of the brain and the spinal cord meninges. Inflammation may involve all three meningeal membranes: the dura mater, arachnoid membrane, and pia mater.

Meningitis can be caused by bacteria, viruses, protozoa, or fungi. However, it most commonly results from bacterial infection, usually due to *Neisseria meningitides, Haemophilus influenzae, Streptococcus pneumoniae,* or *Escherichia coli.* Occasionally, the causative organism can't be determined.

In most patients, the infection that causes meningitis is secondary to another bacterial infection, such as bacteremia (especially from pneumonia, empyema, osteomyelitis, and endocarditis), sinusitis, otitis media, encephalitis, myelitis, or brain abscess. Meningitis can also follow a skull fracture, a penetrating head wound, lumbar puncture, or ventricular shunting procedures.

Meningitis caused by a virus is called aseptic viral meningitis. (See *Understanding aseptic viral meningitis.*)

Pathophysiology

With meningitis, an invading organism triggers an inflammatory response in the meninges. In an attempt to ward off the invasion, neutrophils gather in the area and produce an exudate in the subarachnoid space, causing the cerebrospinal fluid (CSF) to thicken. In turn, this thickened CSF flows less readily around the brain and spinal cord, and it can block the arachnoid villi, obstructing absorption of CSF and causing hydrocephalus. The exudate also exacerbates the inflammatory response, increasing the pressure in the brain; it may extend to the cranial and peripheral nerves, triggering additional inflammation; and it irritates the meninges, disrupting their cell membranes and causing edema.

Complications

- Visual impairment
- Optic neuritis
- Cranial nerve palsies
- Deafness
- Personality change
- Headache
- Paresis or paralysis
- Endocarditis

UNDERSTANDING ASEPTIC VIRAL MENINGITIS

Aseptic viral meningitis is a benign syndrome characterized by headache, fever, vomiting, and meningeal symptoms. It results from viral infections, including enteroviruses (most common), arboviruses, herpes simplex virus, mumps virus, or lymphocytic choriomeningitis virus.

Assessment findings

The history of a patient with aseptic viral meningitis usually shows sudden onset of signs and symptoms with a fever up to 104° F (40° C), alterations in consciousness (drowsiness, confusion, and stupor), and neck or spine stiffness when bending forward; this stiffness is initially slight. The patient's history may also reveal a recent illness.

Other signs and symptoms may include headaches, nausea, vomiting, abdominal pain, poorly defined chest pain, and sore throat.

The patient's history and the physician's knowledge of seasonal epidemics are essential in differentiating among the many forms of aseptic viral meningitis. Negative bacteriologic cultures and cerebrospinal fluid (CSF) analysis showing pleocytosis and increased protein suggest the diagnosis. Isolation of the virus from CSF confirms it.

Supportive treatment

Management of aseptic meningitis involves bed rest, maintenance of fluid and electrolyte balance, analgesics for pain, and exercises to combat residual weakness. Isolation isn't necessary. Careful handling of body fluids and excretions and good hand-washing technique prevent the spread of the disease.

- Coma
- Vasculitis
- Cerebral infarction

IN CHILDREN

- Sensory hearing loss
- Epilepsy
- Mental retardation
- Hydrocephalus
- Subdural effusions

TWO TELLTALE SIGNS OF MENINGITIS

Brudzinski's sign
Place the patient in a dorsal recumbent position, put your hands behind her neck, and bend it forward. Pain and resistance may indicate meningeal inflammation, neck injury, or arthritis. If the patient also flexes her hips and knees in response to this manipulation, chances are she has meningitis.

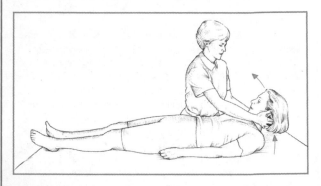

Assessment findings
Findings for meningitis include:
- classic triad of fever, headache, and nuchal rigidity
- malaise
- photophobia
- chills
- vomiting
- twitching and seizures
- altered level of consciousness (LOC), such as confusion and delirium
- opisthotonus
- petechial, purpuric, or ecchymotic rash on the lower part of the body

Kernig's sign

Place the patient in a supine position. Flex her leg at the hip and knee and then straighten the knee. Pain or resistance points to meningitis.

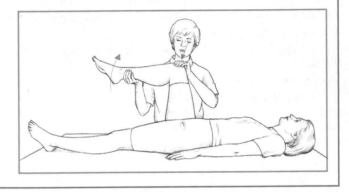

- positive Brudzinski's and Kernig's signs and exaggerated and symmetrical deep tendon reflexes (See *Two telltale signs of meningitis.*)
- diplopia and other vision problems.

Diagnostic test results

- Computed tomography scan can rule out cerebral hematoma, hemorrhage, or tumor and should be done before a lumbar puncture is performed.
- Lumbar puncture shows cloudy or milky white CSF, high levels of protein, positive Gram stain and culture that usually identifies the infecting organism unless it's a virus, and depressed CSF glucose concentration.

- Chest X-rays may reveal pneumonitis or lung abscess, tubercular lesions, or granulomas secondary to fungal infection.
- Sinus and skull films may help identify the presence of cranial osteomyelitis, paranasal sinusitis, or skull fracture.
- White blood cell count usually indicates leukocytosis.

Treatment

Treatment for bacterial meningitis includes appropriate antibiotic therapy and vigorous supportive care; for viral meningitis, treatment is primarily supportive.

Usually, I.V. antibiotics are given for a minimum of 4 days followed by oral antibiotics; overall length of treatment is dependent on causative organism and resistance.

Typical agents include ampicillin, cefotaxime, ceftriaxone, and nafcillin. Other drugs include mannitol to decrease cerebral edema, an anticonvulsant (usually given I.V.) or a sedative to reduce restlessness, and aspirin or acetaminophen to relieve headache and fever.

Supportive measures consist of bed rest, hypothermia, and fluid therapy to prevent dehydration. Isolation is necessary for first 24 hours if nasal cultures are positive. Other treatment includes appropriate therapy for any coexisting conditions, such as endocarditis or pneumonia.

Nursing interventions

- Monitor neurologic status and vital signs continually.

RED FLAG Watch for signs of deterioration. Be especially alert for increased temperature, deteriorating LOC, onset of seizures, and altered respirations, all of which may signal an impending crisis.

- Obtain arterial blood gas measurements, as ordered, and administer oxygen, as required, to maintain partial pressure of oxygen at desired levels. If necessary, maintain the patient on mechanical ventilation and care for his endotracheal tube or tracheostomy.

TEACHING THE PATIENT WITH MENINGITIS

Before discharge, teach the patient and his family:
- about the disorder and its implications
- about treatment plan
- about prescribed medication administration, dosage, possible adverse effects, and when to notify the physician
- the importance of good nutrition and fluid intake
- about activity recommendations and how to prevent skin breakdown
- rehabilitation available for recovery
- the signs and symptoms of complications
- the importance of follow-up care
- the benefits of utilizing available community support groups such as the local chapter of the National Meningitis Association.

- Monitor fluid balance. Maintain adequate fluid intake to avoid dehydration but avoid fluid overload because of the danger of cerebral edema. Measure central venous pressure and intake and output accurately.
- Administer prescribed medications and note their effects. Watch for adverse reactions.
- Position the patient carefully to prevent joint stiffness and neck pain. Reposition him every 2 hours. Assist with range-of-motion exercises.
- Provide skin care and assess for skin breakdown.
- Provide adequate nutrition with small, frequent meals or nasogastric tube or parenteral feedings.
- Provide mouth care regularly.
- Maintain a quiet environment. Darken the room to decrease photophobia.
- Provide reassurance and emotional support. Answer all questions.
- Provide appropriate education to the patient and his family before discharge. (See *Teaching the patient with meningitis.*)

Neurovascular and neurodegenerative disorders

Neurovascular disorders impair cerebral blood flow and may cause permanent physical deficits. Examples of neurovascular disorders include cerebral aneurysm and stroke. Neurodegenerative disorders are neurologic disorders that cause progressive deterioration of cerebral and motor function. Alzheimer's disease, Creutzfeldt-Jakob disease, Huntington's disease, multiple sclerosis, and Parkinson's disease are neurodegenerative disorders.

CEREBRAL ANEURYSM

Cerebral aneurysm is a localized dilation of a cerebral artery that results from a weakness in the arterial wall. The most common form is the saccular (berry) aneurysm, a saclike outpouching in a cerebral artery. (See *Comparing types of aneurysms.*) Cerebral aneurysms commonly rupture, causing subarachnoid hemorrhage.

Most cerebral aneurysms occur at bifurcations of major arteries in the circle of Willis and its branches. An aneurysm can produce neurologic symptoms by exerting pressure on the surrounding structures such as the cranial nerves. (See *Common sites of cerebral aneurysm,* page 268.)

Cerebral aneurysm results from a congenital defect of the vessel wall, head trauma, hypertensive vascular disease, ad-

COMPARING TYPES OF ANEURYSMS

Saccular (berry) aneurysm

- Most common type
- Secondary to congenital weakness of media
- Usually occurs at major vessel bifurcations
- Occurs at the circle of Willis
- Has a neck or stem
- Has a sac that may be partly filled with a blood clot

Giant aneurysm

- Similar to saccular aneurysm, but larger—3 cm or more in diameter
- Behaves like a space-occupying lesion, producing cerebral tissue compression and cranial nerve damage
- Associated with hypertension

Fusiform (spindle-shaped) aneurysm

- Occurs with atherosclerotic disease
- Characterized by irregular vessel dilation
- Develops on internal carotid or basilar arteries
- Rarely ruptures
- Produces brain and cranial nerve compression or cerebrospinal fluid obstruction

Dissecting aneurysm

- Caused by arteriosclerosis, head injury, syphilis, or trauma during angiography
- Develops when blood is forced between layers of arterial walls, stripping intima from the underlying muscle layer

Traumatic aneurysm

- Develops in the carotid system
- Associated with fractures and intimal damage
- May thrombose spontaneously

Charcot-Bouchard aneurysm

- Microscopic
- Associated with hypertension
- Involves basal ganglia or brain stem

Mycotic (infectious) aneurysm

- Rare
- Associated with septic emboli that occur secondary to bacterial endocarditis
- Develops when emboli lodge in arterial lumen, causing arteritis and weakening and dilation of arterial wall

vancing age, infection, or atherosclerosis, which can weaken the vessel wall. Cerebral aneurysm is more common in women than in men; however, the opposite is true in children and adolescents, with a male to female ratio of 2:1. Additionally, cerebral aneurysm rupture is most prevalent in the 35- to 60-year-old age-group, with 50 being the mean age of occurrence.

COMMON SITES OF CEREBRAL ANEURYSM

Cerebral aneurysms usually arise at arterial bifurcations in the circle of Willis and its branches. This illustration shows the most common aneurysm sites around this circle.

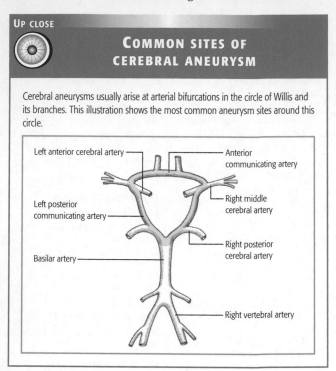

The prognosis is usually guarded, but it depends on the patient's age and neurologic condition, presence of other diseases, and the extent and location of the aneurysm. About half the patients who suffer subarachnoid hemorrhages die immediately. However, with new and better treatment, the prognosis is improving.

Pathophysiology

Blood flow exerts pressure against a congenitally weak arterial wall, stretching it like an overblown balloon and making it likely to rupture. Such a rupture is followed by a subarachnoid hemorrhage, in which blood spills into the space normally occupied by cerebrospinal fluid (CSF). Sometimes blood spills into the brain tissue, where a large clot can cause potentially fatal increased intracranial pressure (ICP) and brain tissue damage.

Complications
- Rupture
- Subarachnoid hemorrhage
- Brain tissue infarction
- Cerebral vasospasm
- Death
- Rebleeding
- Hydrocephalus

Assessment findings
Most cerebral aneurysms produce no symptoms until rupture occurs and include the following:
- sudden onset of an unusually severe headache
- nausea and vomiting
- altered level of consciousness (LOC)
- history of a period of activity, such as exercise, labor and delivery, or sexual intercourse, before the rupture.

Other findings vary with the location of the aneurysm and the extent and severity of hemorrhage and may include:
- pain above or behind an eye
- possible photophobia
- nuchal rigidity
- back and leg pain
- fever
- restlessness and irritability
- seizures
- blurred vision
- ptosis and vision disturbances (aneurysm adjacent to the oculomotor nerve)
- hemiparesis, unilateral sensory deficits, dysphagia, vision deficits, and altered LOC (bleeding into the brain tissue).

COMPLICATIONS OF A RUPTURED ANEURYSM

If your patient survives a ruptured cerebral aneurysm, monitor her closely for rebleeding, cerebral vasospasm, and acute hydrocephalus, which are life-threatening complications. This table lists the signs and symptoms of each complication and tells when it's most likely to occur and how it should be treated.

COMPLICATION	SIGNS AND SYMPTOMS	ONSET	TREATMENT
Rebleeding	Deterioration of neurologic status, decrease in level of consciousness (LOC), intensifying headache	7 to 10 days after rupture	● Sedation, rest ● Avoidance of Valsalva's maneuver
Cerebral vasospasm	Decrease in LOC, motor weakness or paralysis, vision deficits, changes in vital signs (particularly respiratory patterns)	Several hours to days after rupture	● Intravascular volume expanders ● Induced hypertensive therapy ● Calcium channel blockers
Hydrocephalus	Mental changes, gait disturbances, general mental and physical deterioration	Can occur several hours to days later as a result	● Cerebrospinal fluid drainage via intraventricular catheter

Additional findings may result from complications. (See *Complications of a ruptured aneurysm.*)

To better describe the condition of patients with ruptured cerebral aneurysm, the following grading system was developed.

■ *Grade I (minimal bleeding):* The patient is alert, with no neurologic deficit; she may have a mild headache and nuchal rigidity.

- *Grade II (mild bleeding):* The patient is alert, with a mild to severe headache, nuchal rigidity and, possibly, third-nerve palsy.
- *Grade III (moderate bleeding):* The patient is confused or drowsy, with nuchal rigidity and, possibly, a mild focal deficit.
- *Grade IV (severe bleeding):* The patient is stuporous, with nuchal rigidity, early decerebrate rigidity and, possibly, mild to severe hemiparesis.
- *Grade V (moribund [usually fatal]):* If not fatal, the patient is in a deep coma or is decerebrate.

Diagnostic test results

- Angiography confirms the aneurysm's location and displays the vessels' condition.
- Lumbar puncture may detect blood in the CSF, but this procedure is contraindicated if the patient shows signs of increased ICP.
- Computed tomography scanning locates the clot and identifies hydrocephalus, areas of infarction, and the extent of blood spillage in the cisterns around the brain.
- Magnetic resonance imaging and magnetic resonance angiography show the extent of bleeding and the vessels' condition.

Treatment

Initial treatment includes supportive measures, such as oxygenation and ventilation. Surgical repair includes clipping, ligating, or wrapping the aneurysm neck and usually takes place as soon as the patient is stable enough, generally 7 to 10 days after the initial bleed. (See *Aneurysm clip,* page 272.) Although surgery has been the standard of treatment for ruptured and nonruptured cerebral aneurysms, new interventional procedures, using such devices as coils, balloons, and stents, are proving successful.

ANEURYSM CLIP

Clipping is a method of surgical repair for a cerebral aneurysm. The neurosurgeon grasps the clip, opens the jaw, and then slides the clip over the hemorrhaging blood vessel. He then closes the clip over the blood vessel, and the applied pressure stems the hemorrhaging without compromising vessel integrity.

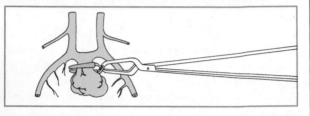

After surgical repair, treatment is based on the extent of damage from the initial bleed and the degree of success in treating the resulting complications. Surgery won't improve the patient's neurologic condition unless it removes a hematoma or reduces the compression effect.

When surgical correction poses too much risk (in very elderly patients and those with heart, lung, or other serious diseases), when the aneurysm is in a particularly dangerous location, or when vasospasm necessitates a delay in surgery, the patient may receive conservative treatment, including:

- bed rest in a quiet, darkened room (may last for 4 to 6 weeks)
- avoidance of coffee, other stimulants, and aspirin
- codeine or another analgesic, as needed
- hydralazine (Apresoline) or another antihypertensive, if needed
- a vasoconstrictor to maintain blood pressure at the optimum level (20 to 40 mm Hg above normal), if needed
- corticosteroids to reduce meningeal irritation
- phenytoin (Dilantin) or another anticonvulsant

- phenobarbital (Luminal) or another sedative to relax the patient
- nimodipine (Nimotop), a calcium channel blocker, to decrease cerebral vessel vasospasm
- albumin for volume expansion, to decrease vasospasm
- aminocaproic acid (Amicar), a fibrinolytic inhibitor, to minimize the risk of rebleeding by delaying blood clot lysis. (However, this drug's effectiveness has been disputed.)

Nursing interventions

- Maintain a patent airway and provide oxygen and ventilation, as needed.
- Monitor the patient's neurologic status.
- Suction the patient cautiously (less than 20 seconds) to avoid increased ICP.
- Monitor vital signs and pulse oximetry readings.
- Provide frequent nose and mouth care.
- Initiate aneurysm precautions: a quiet room, bed rest in the dark (with the head of the bed flat or elevated less than 30 degrees, as ordered), limited visitors, avoidance of such stimulants as coffee, avoidance of Valsalva's maneuver and other strenuous activity, and restricted fluid intake.
- Monitor for signs of rebleeding, intracranial clot, vasospasm, or other complications.
- Administer medications, as ordered, and monitor effects.
- Provide emotional support to the patient and his family. Encourage them to talk about their concerns. Listen carefully and answer their questions honestly and completely.
- Reposition the patient every 2 hours and assess skin condition. Provide skin care.
- Assist with active range-of-motion (ROM) exercises; if the patient is paralyzed, perform passive ROM exercises.
- Administer I.V. fluids and monitor intake and output. Maintain fluid volume to decrease the risk of vasospasm.
- Assess swallowing ability and assist with meals, as appropriate; administer enteral feedings, if ordered.

TEACHING THE PATIENT WITH A CEREBRAL ANEURYSM

Before discharge, be sure to cover with the patient and his family:
● the disorder and its implications
● treatment options, such as surgery and therapy
● medication administration, dosage, and possible adverse effects, and when to notify the physician
● the importance of good nutrition and what types of food may be best based on swallowing ability
● range-of-motion exercises to improve muscle tone and strength
● types of therapy that would be beneficial, such as physical therapy, speech therapy, and occupational therapy
● signs and symptoms of complications
● the importance of follow-up care
● the benefit of utilizing available community support groups such as the local chapter of the Brain Aneurysm Foundation.

■ Initiate seizure precautions, if indicated.
■ Monitor head dressings and provide wound care.
■ Monitor ICP and cerebral perfusion pressures, and provide measures to maintain adequate readings.
■ Monitor for postoperative complications, including sudden hemiplegia, psychological changes (disorientation, amnesia, Korsakoff's syndrome, personality impairment), fluid and electrolyte disturbances, and GI bleeding.
■ Provide appropriate education to the patient and his family before discharge. (See *Teaching the patient with a cerebral aneurysm.*)

STROKE

Also known as *brain attack* or *cerebrovascular accident,* stroke is a sudden impairment of cerebral circulation in one or more blood vessels supplying the brain. Stroke interrupts or diminishes oxygen supply and commonly causes serious damage or necrosis in brain tissues. The sooner circulation returns to normal after stroke, the better chances are for complete recovery. About half of those who survive stroke suffer a disability and experience a recurrence within weeks, months, or years.

Causes of stroke include cerebral thrombosis, embolism, and hemorrhage. (See *Types of stroke,* page 276.)

Thrombosis is the most common cause of stroke in middle-age and elderly people. *Embolism,* the second most common cause of stroke, is especially prevalent among patients with a history of rheumatic heart disease, endocarditis, posttraumatic valvular disease, or myocardial fibrillation and other cardiac arrhythmias. It may also occur after open-heart surgery. *Hemorrhage,* the third most common cause of stroke, results from chronic hypertension or aneurysms.

Strokes are classified according to their course of progression. The least severe is the transient ischemic attack (TIA), which results from a temporary interruption of blood flow, most often in the carotid and vertebrobasilar arteries. (See *Transient ischemic attack: A warning sign of stroke,* page 277.)

A progressive stroke, or stroke-in-evolution (thrombus-in-evolution), begins with a minor neurologic deficit and worsens over the course of 2 days. In a complete stroke, neurologic deficits are at the maximum at the onset.

Risk factors for stroke include:
- atrial fibrillation
- TIA
- atherosclerosis
- hypertension
- renal disease
- carotid stenosis
- diabetes mellitus
- cardiac or myocardial enlargement
- sickle cell anemia
- hypercoagulable states
- hyperlipidemia

TYPES OF STROKE

Strokes are typically classified as ischemic or hemorrhagic, depending on the underlying cause. This chart describes the major types of stroke.

TYPE OF STROKE	DESCRIPTION
ISCHEMIC	
Thrombotic	● Most common type of stroke ● Commonly the result of atherosclerosis; also associated with hypertension, smoking, or diabetes (disease process similar to myocardial infarction [MI]) ● Thrombus in extracranial or intracranial vessel blocks blood flow to the cerebral cortex ● Carotid artery most commonly affected extracranial vessel ● Common intracranial sites include bifurcation of carotid arteries, distal intracranial portion of vertebral arteries, and proximal basilar arteries ● May occur during sleep or shortly after awakening, during surgery, or after an MI
Embolic	● Second most common type of stroke ● Embolus from heart or extracranial arteries floats into cerebral bloodstream and lodges in middle cerebral artery or branches ● Embolus commonly originates during atrial fibrillation ● Typically occurs during activity ● Develops rapidly
Lacunar	● Subtype of thrombotic stroke ● Hypertension creates cavities deep in white matter of the brain, affecting the internal capsule, basal ganglia, thalamus, and pons ● Lipid coating lining of the small penetrating arteries thickens and weakens wall, causing microaneurysms and dissections
HEMORRHAGIC	
	● Third most common type of stroke ● Typically caused by hypertension or aneurysm rupture ● Blood supply to area from the ruptured artery diminished and surrounding tissue compressed by accumulated blood

TRANSIENT ISCHEMIC ATTACK: A WARNING SIGN OF STROKE

A transient ischemic attack (TIA) is an episode of neurologic deficit lasting less than 1 hour without permanent neurologic defects. It's usually considered a warning sign of an impending stroke and may be recurrent. TIAs are reported in 50% to 80% of patients who had a cerebral infarction from such thrombosis. The age of onset varies. Incidence increases dramatically after age 50 and is highest among blacks and males.

With a TIA, microemboli released from a thrombus may temporarily interrupt blood flow, especially in the small distal branches of the brain's arterial tree. Small spasms in those arterioles may impair blood flow and also precede a TIA. Predisposing factors are the same as those for thrombotic strokes.

Clinical features
The most distinctive characteristics of a TIA are the transient duration of neurologic deficits and the complete return of normal function. The signs and symptoms of a TIA correlate with the location of the affected artery. They include double vision, speech deficits (slurring or thickness), unilateral blindness, staggering or uncoordinated gait, unilateral weakness or numbness, falling because of weakness in the legs, and dizziness.

Treatment
During an active TIA, treatment aims to prevent a completed stroke and consists of aspirin, antiplatelet drugs, or anticoagulants to minimize the risk of thrombosis. After or between attacks, preventive treatment includes carotid endarterectomy or cerebral microvascular bypass.

- individual history of stroke
- family history of stroke
- advanced age
- smoking
- use of hormonal contraceptives
- lack of exercise.

Pathophysiology
Stroke that results from thrombosis causes ischemia, congestion, and edema in the brain tissue supplied by the affected

HOW STROKE AFFECTS THE BODY

Stroke affects not only the brain and nervous system but other major body systems as well, which are outlined here. In addition, the patient with an acute stroke requires multidisciplinary care.

Nervous system

Pathophysiologic processes vary depending on the type of stroke.

Ischemic stroke

● An *ischemic stroke,* which can be *thrombotic* or *embolic,* causes ischemia. Some of the neurons served by the occluded vessel die from lack of oxygen and nutrients.
● Neuron death results in cerebral infarction, in which tissue injury triggers an inflammatory response that increases intracranial pressure (ICP).
● Injury to surrounding cells disrupts metabolism and leads to changes in ionic transport, localized acidosis, and free radical formation.
● Calcium, sodium, and water accumulate in the injured cells, and excitatory neurotransmitters are released.
● Consequent continued cellular injury and swelling set up a cycle of further damage.

Hemorrhagic stroke

● Impaired cerebral perfusion causes infarction, and the blood itself acts as a space-occupying mass, exerting pressure on brain tissues.
● The brain's regulatory mechanisms attempt to maintain equilibrium by increasing blood pressure to maintain cerebral perfusion pressure.

● The increased ICP forces cerebrospinal fluid out, thus restoring the balance. If the hemorrhage is small, the patient may live with only minimal neurologic deficits. If the bleeding is heavy, ICP increases rapidly and perfusion stops. Even if the pressure returns to normal, many brain cells die.
● Initially, the ruptured cerebral blood vessels may constrict to limit the blood loss.
● This vasospasm further compromises blood flow, leading to more ischemia and cellular damage.
● If a clot forms in the vessel, decreased blood flow promotes ischemia.
● If the blood enters the subarachnoid space, meningeal irritation occurs.
● Blood cells that pass through the vessel wall into the surrounding tissue may break down and block the arachnoid villi, causing hydrocephalus.

Cardiovascular system

● Cerebral ischemia and infarction can ultimately affect the autonomic nervous system, which can alter blood vessel constriction and dilation, heart rate, blood pressure, and cardiac contractility.
● Cardiovascular effects are increasingly problematic if the patient has an underlying disorder, such as heart disease or hypertension.

HOW STROKE AFFECTS THE BODY *(continued)*

Musculoskeletal system

● Cerebral infarction can lead to a disturbance in impulse transmission via the cranial and peripheral nerves, altering motor and sensory function.

● Changes in sensation or mobility can lead to pressure areas, especially with prolonged bed rest or limited activity. In addition, the ability of the blood vessels to constrict and dilate as necessary may be altered, increasing the risk of impaired blood flow to the area. Subsequently, pressure ulcers may develop.

Respiratory system

● If infarction resulting from increased ICP and decreased perfusion involves the respiratory center in the medulla, respiration—including the depth and rate—can be affected because nerve impulse transmission via the phrenic nerves to the diaphragm and intercostal nerves to the intercostal muscles is interrupted.

● If the pons (the location for apneustic and pneumotaxic centers) is affected, breathing patterns become altered and impulse transmission via the cranial nerves (CN) may be interrupted.

● If the glossopharyngeal (CN IX) and vagus nerves (CN X) are affected, swallowing may be impaired and aspiration may occur.

Collaborative management

Typically, emergency services personnel are involved in confirming the signs and symptoms of an acute stroke, completing the primary survey, and transporting the patient to the health care facility. A speech therapist may assist the patient with defects in swallowing as well as speaking. A physical therapist helps the patient relearn basic activities of daily living, such as dressing, bathing, and cooking. The patient and his family may benefit from pastoral or spiritual counseling and support groups. Social services ensures continuity of care after discharge to the patient's home or to a rehabilitation facility and assists with follow-up care and financial and emotional concerns.

vessel; edema may produce more clinical effects than thrombosis itself, but these effects subside along with the edema. (See *How stroke affects the body*.)

An embolism usually develops rapidly—in 10 to 20 seconds—and without warning. When an embolus reaches the cerebral vasculature, it cuts off cerebral circulation by lodging in a narrow portion of an artery, most commonly the middle cerebral artery, causing necrosis and edema. If the embolus is septic and infection extends beyond the vessel wall, encephalitis or an abscess may develop.

Hemorrhage diminishes blood supply to the area served by the ruptured artery. In addition, blood accumulates deep within the brain, further compressing neural tissue and causing even greater damage.

Complications
- Sensory impairment
- Motor impairment
- Altered level of consciousness (LOC)
- Aspiration
- Contractures
- Complications of immobility
- Deep vein thrombosis (DVT)
- Pulmonary emboli
- Depression
- Malnutrition

Assessment findings
Clinical features of stroke vary with the artery affected and, consequently, the portion of the brain it supplies; the severity of the damage; and the extent of collateral circulation that develops to help the brain compensate for a decreased blood supply. The examination may reveal:
- history of one or more risk factors for stroke
- sudden loss of voluntary muscle control or onset of hemiparesis or hemiplegia
- sudden onset of speech disturbance or communication problem
- sudden change in LOC
- sudden change in mental status
- headache
- seizure
- urinary incontinence

- decreased deep tendon reflexes (Reflexes return to normal after the initial phase, along with an increase in muscle tone and, in some cases, muscle spasticity on the affected side.)
- hemianopsia on the affected side of the body and, in patients with left-sided hemiplegia, problems with visuospatial relations
- sensory losses, ranging from slight impairment of touch to the inability to perceive the position and motion of body parts; the patient may also have difficulty interpreting visual, tactile, and auditory stimuli. (See *Understanding neurologic deficits in stroke,* page 282.)

Diagnostic test results

- Computed tomography (CT) scan and CT angiography show immediate evidence of hemorrhagic stroke, but may not show evidence of thrombotic infarction for 48 to 72 hours.
- Magnetic resonance imaging may identify ischemic or infarcted areas and cerebral swelling.
- An electrocardiogram may identify a cardiac arrhythmia.
- Carotid duplex may detect carotid artery stenosis.
- Angiography outlines blood vessels and pinpoints occlusion or the rupture site.
- EEG helps localize the damaged area.

Treatment

Initial supportive measures include airway maintenance, oxygenation, and ventilation. Tissue plasminogen activator is recommended if the diagnosis of stroke is established within 3 hours of the onset of symptoms and the patient fits the criteria for administration. (See *Treating ischemic stroke,* pages 284 and 285.) Depending on the cause and extent of the stroke, the patient may undergo a craniotomy to remove a hematoma, endarterectomy to remove atherosclerotic plaques from the inner arterial wall, or extracranial-intracranial bypass to circumvent

UNDERSTANDING NEUROLOGIC DEFICITS IN STROKE

Stroke can leave one patient with midhand weakness and another with complete unilateral paralysis. In both patients, the functional loss reflects damage to the brain area normally perfused by the occluded or ruptured artery. But the damage doesn't stop there. Resulting hypoxia and ischemia produce edema that affects distal parts of the brain, causing further neurologic deficits.

Most strokes occur in the anterior cerebral circulation and cause symptoms from damage in the middle cerebral artery, internal carotid artery, or anterior cerebral artery. Strokes can also occur in the posterior circulation. These originate in the vertebral arteries and result in signs and symptoms caused by damage to the vertebral or basilar artery and posterior cerebral artery, resulting in higher mortality. Described here are the signs and symptoms that accompany stroke at the following sites.

Middle cerebral artery
The patient may experience aphasia, dysphasia, reading difficulty (dyslexia), writing inability (dysgraphia), visual field cuts, and hemiparesis on the affected side (more severe in the face and arm than in the leg).

Internal carotid artery
The patient may complain of headache. Expect to find weakness, paralysis, numbness, sensory changes, and vision disturbances such as blurring on the affected side. You may also detect altered level of consciousness, bruits over the carotid artery, aphasia, dysphasia, and ptosis.

Anterior cerebral artery
You may note confusion, weakness, and numbness (especially of the arm) on the affected side, paralysis of the contralateral foot and leg with accompanying footdrop, incontinence, loss of coordination, impaired motor and sensory functions, and personality changes (flat affect, distractibility).

Vertebral or basilar artery
The patient may complain of numbness around the lips and mouth and dizziness. You may note weakness on the affected side, poor coordination, dysphagia, slurred speech, amnesia, ataxia, and vision deficits, such as color blindness, lack of depth perception, and diplopia.

Posterior cerebral artery
The patient may experience visual field cuts, sensory impairment, dyslexia, coma, and cortical blindness from ischemia in the occipital area. Usually, paralysis is absent.

an artery blocked by occlusion or stenosis. Ventricular shunts may also be necessary to drain cerebrospinal fluid.

Medications useful in stroke include the following:

- Antihypertensives may be given to control blood pressure.
- Anticoagulants, such as heparin or warfarin (Coumadin), may be used as well as aspirin and other antiplatelet drugs.
- Antiplatelet drugs may be more appropriate for a TIA and ischemic strokes as secondary stroke risk reduction.
- Anticonvulsants may be used to treat or prevent seizures.
- Stool softeners may be used to prevent straining, which increases intracranial pressure.
- Corticosteroids may be indicated to minimize associated cerebral edema.
- Analgesics may be used to relieve the headache that typically follows hemorrhagic stroke.

Other treatment initiatives include physical rehabilitation, dietary and drug regimens to help decrease risk factors, possible surgery, prevention of DVT, and care measures to help the patient adapt to specific deficits, such as swallowing difficulties, speech impairment, and paralysis. Counseling may be indicated for depression.

Nursing interventions

- Maintain a patent airway, adequate oxygenation, and ventilation assistance, if necessary.
- Monitor the patient's neurologic and respiratory status.
- Monitor vital signs, pulse oximetry, and cardiac rhythm.
- Reposition the patient every 2 hours, assess his skin condition, and provide skin care.
- Assess swallowing abilities, assist with meals and monitor for signs of aspiration, and administer enteral feedings, if indicated.
- Administer I.V. fluids, as ordered; monitor intake and output.
- Encourage active range-of-motion (ROM) exercises; provide passive ROM exercises, if indicated.

(Text continues on page 286.)

TREATING ISCHEMIC STROKE

In an ischemic stroke, a thrombus occludes a cerebral vessel or one of its branches and blocks blood flow to the brain. The thrombus may either have formed in that vessel or have lodged there after traveling through the circulation from another site such as the heart. Prompt treatment with a thrombolytic or an anticoagulant helps to minimize the effects of the occlusion. This flowchart shows how these drugs disrupt an ischemic stroke, thus minimizing the effects of cerebral ischemia and infarction. Keep in mind that thrombolytics can only be used within 3 hours after onset of the patient's symptoms.

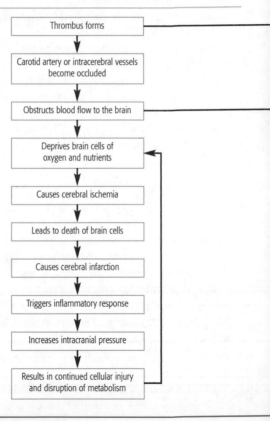

Thrombus forms

↓

Carotid artery or intracerebral vessels become occluded

↓

Obstructs blood flow to the brain

↓

Deprives brain cells of oxygen and nutrients

↓

Causes cerebral ischemia

↓

Leads to death of brain cells

↓

Causes cerebral infarction

↓

Triggers inflammatory response

↓

Increases intracranial pressure

↓

Results in continued cellular injury and disruption of metabolism

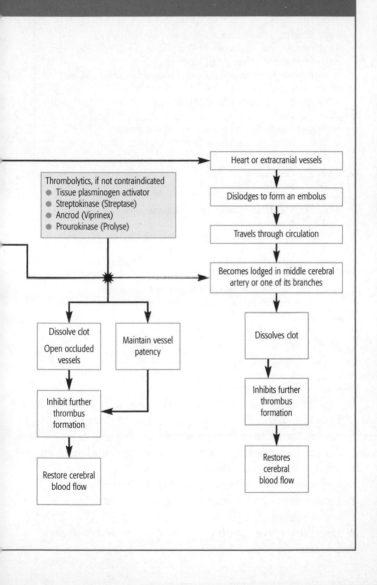

Heart or extracranial vessels

↓

Dislodges to form an embolus

↓

Travels through circulation

↓

Becomes lodged in middle cerebral artery or one of its branches

↓

Dissolves clot

↓

Inhibits further thrombus formation

↓

Restores cerebral blood flow

Thrombolytics, if not contraindicated
- Tissue plasminogen activator
- Streptokinase (Streptase)
- Ancrod (Viprinex)
- Prourokinase (Prolyse)

Dissolve clot

Open occluded vessels

Maintain vessel patency

↓

Inhibit further thrombus formation

↓

Restore cerebral blood flow

TEACHING THE PATIENT ABOUT STROKE

Before discharge, be sure to cover with the patient and his family:
- the disorder and its implications
- treatment options, such as surgery and therapy
- medication administration, dosage, and possible adverse effects, and when to notify the physician
- the importance of good nutrition and what types of food may be best based on swallowing ability
- range-of-motion exercises to improve muscle tone and strength
- types of therapy that would be beneficial, such as physical therapy, speech therapy, and occupational therapy
- available counseling and home health care
- signs and symptoms of complications
- the importance of follow-up care
- the benefit of utilizing available community support groups such as the local chapter of the American Stroke Association.

To reduce the risk of another stroke, teach the patient and his family:
- the need to eliminate risk factors such as smoking
- the importance of maintaining an ideal weight and following a low-cholesterol, low-salt diet
- the need to control such diseases as diabetes and hypertension
- the importance of increasing activity, avoiding prolonged bed rest, and minimizing stress
- early recognition of signs and symptoms of impending stroke and seeking prompt treatment.

- Initiate DVT prophylaxis.
- Provide an alternate method of communication, if indicated.
- Refer the patient to physical therapy, speech therapy, and occupational therapy, as appropriate.
- Provide emotional support to the patient and his family. Encourage them to talk about their concerns. Listen carefully, and answer their questions honestly and completely.
- Protect the patient from injury; initiate fall precautions, as appropriate.
- If surgery is necessary, provide preoperative and postoperative care.

- Provide appropriate education to the patient and his family before discharge. (See *Teaching the patient about stroke*.)

NEURODEGENERATIVE DISORDERS
ALZHEIMER'S DISEASE

Alzheimer's disease is a progressive degenerative disorder of the cerebral cortex (especially the frontal lobe) that impairs memory, thinking, and behavior and accounts for more than half of all cases of dementia. An estimated 5% of people older than age 65 have a severe form of this disease, and 12% suffer from mild to moderate dementia. Because Alzheimer's disease causes progressive dementia, the prognosis is poor.

The cause of Alzheimer's disease is unknown, but several factors are thought to be closely connected to this disease. These include neurochemical factors, such as deficiencies of the neurotransmitters acetylcholine, somatostatin, substance P, and norepinephrine; environmental factors, such as aluminum and manganese; trauma; genetic immunologic factors; and viral factors such as slow-growing central nervous system viruses.

Genetic studies revealed an autosomal dominant form of Alzheimer's disease associated with early onset and early death; this form accounts for about 100,000 deaths per year. A family history of Alzheimer's disease and the presence of Down syndrome are two established risk factors.

Pathophysiology
The brain tissue of patients with this dementia has three distinguishing features: neurofibrillary tangles, beta-amyloid plaques, and granulovascular degeneration.

Additional structural changes include cortical atrophy, ventricular dilation, deposits of amyloid (a glycoprotein) around the cortical blood vessels, and reduced brain volume. There's also a selective loss of cholinergic neurons in the pathways to the frontal lobes and hippocampus—areas that are more important for memory and cognitive functions. Post-mortem examination of the brain reveals diffuse atrophy of the cerebral cortex; a weight of less than 1,000 g is common. Normal brain weight is about 1,380 g.

Complications
- Injury
- Pneumonia and other infections
- Malnutrition
- Constipation
- Aspiration

Assessment findings
- History of memory loss, forgetfulness, and difficulty learning and remembering new information
- General deterioration in personal hygiene and appearance and an inability to concentrate
- Difficulty with abstract thinking and activities that require judgment
- Progressive difficulty in communicating
- Decreased motor function
- Repetitive actions
- Restlessness
- Personality changes, such as irritability, depression, paranoia, hostility, and combativeness; nocturnal awakening; and disorientation
- Labile emotions or mood swings
- Misperception of environment and misidentification of objects and people
- Impaired sense of smell (usually an early symptom)
- Positive snout reflex
- Urinary or fecal incontinence
- Seizures (see *Stages of Alzheimer's disease,* pages 290 and 291)

Diagnostic test results

Alzheimer's disease is diagnosed by exclusion. Various tests, such as those described here, are performed to rule out other disorders. However, the diagnosis can't be confirmed until death, when pathologic findings are identified at autopsy.

- Positron emission tomography measures the metabolic activity of the cerebral cortex and may help rule out other disease.
- Magnetic resonance imaging (MRI) may show atrophy in the hippocampus and enlarged ventricles. MRI also evaluates the condition of the brain and rules out intracranial lesions as the source of dementia.
- Computed tomography scanning (in some patients) shows progressive brain atrophy in excess of that which occurs in normal aging.
- EEG evaluates the brain's electrical activity and may show slowing of the brain waves in the late stages of the disease. This test also helps identify tumors, abscesses, and other intracranial lesions that might be causing the patient's symptoms.
- Cerebrospinal fluid analysis may help determine if the patient's signs and symptoms stem from a chronic neurologic infection. Cerebral blood flow studies may detect abnormalities in blood flow to the brain.
- Neuropsychologic testing consists of a battery of tests designed to assess cognitive ability and reasoning. These tests can help differentiate Alzheimer's disease from other types of dementia.

Treatment

Because there's no cure for Alzheimer's disease, treatment focuses on attempting to slow disease progression; identifying and treating the underlying disorder that may be contributing to the patient's confusion, such as hypoxia; managing behavioral problems; implementing modifications of the home environment; and eliciting family support.

STAGES OF ALZHEIMER'S DISEASE

Alzheimer's disease progresses in three stages. The symptoms of each stage are outlined here.

MILD OR EARLY STAGE		MODERATE OR
FUNCTIONS/TESTS	**SYMPTOMS**	**FUNCTIONS/TESTS**
Language	Anomia, empty speech	Language
Memory	Defective	Memory
Visuospatial skills	Impaired	Visuospatial skills
Calculation	Impaired	Personality
Personality	Indifferent, occasionally irritable, sad, or depressed	Motor system
Klüver-Bucy syndrome	Absent	EEG
Motor system	Normal	CT scan/MRI
EEG	Normal	
Computed tomography (CT) scan/magnetic resonance imaging (MRI)	Normal	

Some medications have proven helpful. Anticholinesterase agents, such as donepezil (Aricept), rivastigmine (Exelon), and galantamine (Reminyl) slow progression of the disease and improve cognitive function. Memantine (Namenda), a N-methyl-D-aspartate receptor agonist, provides symptomatic improvement of cognitive and psychomotor functioning.

Nursing interventions

- Provide emotional support to the patient and his family. Encourage them to talk about their concerns. Listen carefully,

MIDDLE STAGE	SEVERE OR LATE STAGE	
SYMPTOMS	**FUNCTIONS/TESTS**	**SYMPTOMS**
Fluent aphasia	Intellectual function	Severely impaired
Severely impaired	Language	Palilalia, echolalia, or mutism
Severely impaired		
Indifferent or irritable; suspicious and angry	Motor system	Limb rigidity
	Sphincter control	Incontinence
Restlessness, pacing	EEG	Diffuse slowing
Slowing of background rhythms	CT scan/MRI	Diffuse atrophy
Atrophy		

and answer their questions honestly and completely. (See *The progression of Alzheimer's disease*, pages 292 and 293.)

- Use a soft tone and a slow, calm manner when dealing with the patient.
- Allow sufficient time for response because thought processes are slow, impairing the patient's ability to communicate verbally.
- Administer medications, as ordered, and monitor their effects.
- Monitor swallowing ability; assist with meals and assess for signs of aspiration.

THE PROGRESSION OF ALZHEIMER'S DISEASE

Counsel family members to expect progressive deterioration in the patient with Alzheimer's disease. To help them plan future patient care, discuss the stages of this neurodegenerative disease.

Bear in mind that family members may refuse to believe that the disease is advancing. Be sensitive to their concerns and, if necessary, review the information again when they're more receptive.

Forgetfulness

The patient becomes forgetful, especially of recent events. He frequently loses everyday objects such as keys. Aware of his loss of function, he may compensate by relinquishing tasks that might reveal his forgetfulness. Because his behavior isn't disruptive and may be attributed to stress, fatigue, or normal aging, he usually doesn't consult a physician at this stage.

Confusion

The patient has increasing difficulty with activities that require planning, decision making, and judgment, such as managing personal finances, driving a car, and performing his job. He does retain skills such as personal grooming. Social withdrawal occurs when the patient feels overwhelmed by a changing environment and his inability to cope with multiple stimuli. Travel is difficult and tiring. As he becomes aware of his progressive loss of function, he may become severely depressed.

Safety becomes a concern when the patient forgets to turn off appliances or recognize unsafe situations such as boiling water. At this point, the family may need to consider day care or a supervised residential facility.

Decline in activities of daily living

The patient at this stage loses his ability to perform such daily activities as eating or washing without direct supervision. Weight loss may occur. He withdraws from the family and increasingly depends on the primary caregiver. Communication becomes difficult as his understanding of written and spoken language declines. Agitation, wandering, pacing, and nighttime awakening are linked to his inability to cope with a multisensory environment. He may mistake his mirror image for a real person (pseudohallucination). Caregivers must be constantly vigilant, which may lead to physical and emotional exhaustion. They may also become angry and feel a sense of loss.

Total deterioration

In the final stage of Alzheimer's disease, the patient no longer recognizes himself, his body parts, or other family members. He becomes bedridden,

THE PROGRESSION OF ALZHEIMER'S DISEASE
(continued)

and his activity consists of small, purposeless movements. Verbal communication stops, although he may scream spontaneously. Complications of immobility may include pressure ulcers, urinary tract infections, pneumonia, and contractures.

DISCHARGE TEACHING

TEACHING THE PATIENT WITH ALZHEIMER'S DISEASE

Before discharge, be sure to cover with the patient and his family:
- the disorder and its implications
- medication administration, dosage, and possible adverse effects, and when to notify the physician
- the importance of good nutrition and selecting foods may be best based on swallowing ability
- exercise and activity schedule to maintain muscle strength and function
- establishing a routine that will help maintain independence and avoid confusion
- environmental and personal safety issues
- the importance of wearing a medical identification bracelet
- types of therapy that would be beneficial, such as physical therapy, speech therapy, and occupational therapy
- available counseling and home health care
- signs and symptoms of complications
- the importance of follow-up care
- the benefit of utilizing available community support groups such as the local chapter of the Alzheimer's Association.

- Monitor nutritional and fluid intake.
- Provide safety measures to protect the patient from injury.
- Encourage exercise and active range-of-motion exercises.

- Encourage participation in care; help the patient maintain independence as much as possible but assist with hygiene and dressing, as necessary.
- Assist with toileting habits, as needed, to prevent incontinence and constipation.
- Provide appropriate education to the patient and his family before discharge. (See *Teaching the patient with Alzheimer's disease,* page 293.)

CREUTZFELDT-JAKOB DISEASE

Creutzfeldt-Jakob disease (CJD) is a rare, rapidly progressive viral disease that attacks the central nervous system, causing dementia and neurologic signs and symptoms, such as myoclonic jerking, ataxia, aphasia, vision disturbances, and paralysis. CJD is always fatal. A new variant of CJD—vCJD— emerged in Europe in 1996. (See *Understanding vCJD.*)

CJD generally affects adults ages 40 to 65 and occurs in more than 50 countries. Males and females are affected equally. In people younger than age 30, incidence is 5 in 1,000,000; in all other age-groups, incidence is 1 in 100,000,000. Most cases are sporadic; 5% to 15% are familial, with an autosomal dominant pattern of inheritance. Although CJD isn't transmitted by normal casual contact, human-to-human transmission can occur during certain medical procedures, such as corneal and cadaveric dura mater grafts. Isolated cases have been attributed to treatment during childhood with human growth hormone and to improperly decontaminated neurosurgical instruments and brain electrodes.

Pathophysiology

CJD is caused by the abnormal accumulation or metabolism of prion proteins (isoform). These modified proteins are resistant to proteolyte digestion and aggregate in the brain to produce rodlike particles. The accumulation of these modified cellular

UNDERSTANDING vCJD

Like conventional Creutzfeldt-Jakob disease (CJD), the variant form (vCJD) is also a rare, fatal neurodegenerative disorder. Most reported cases have occurred in the United Kingdom. vCJD is most likely caused by ingestion of beef products from cattle infected with bovine spongiform encephalopathy (BSE), a fatal brain disease also known as *mad cow disease.*

vCJD affects patients at a much younger age (younger than 55 years) than CJD does, and the duration of the illness is much longer (14 months).

Regulations have been established in Europe to control outbreaks of BSE in cattle and prevent contaminated meat from entering the food supply. The Centers for Disease Control and Prevention and the World Health Organization continue to investigate vCJD and its relationship to BSE.

proteins result in neuronal degeneration and spongiform changes in brain tissue.

Complications
- Severe, progressive dementia
- Complications of immobility
- Death

Assessment findings
- Difficulty in performing rapid alternating movements and point-to-point movements (typically evident early in the disease)
- Mental impairment that progressively deteriorates: slowness in thinking, difficulty concentrating, impaired judgment, and memory loss
- Involuntary movements: muscle twitching, trembling, and peculiar body movements
- Vision disturbances
- Gait disturbances
- Hallucinations

TEACHING THE PATIENT WITH CJD

Before discharge, be sure to cover with the patient and his family:
● the disorder and its implications
● medication administration, dosage, and possible adverse effects, and when to notify the physician
● the importance of good nutrition and what types of food may be best based on swallowing ability
● range-of-motion exercises to improve muscle tone and strength
● types of therapy that would be beneficial, such as physical, speech, and occupational therapy
● signs and symptoms of complications
● the importance of follow-up care
● establishing end-of-life care
● the benefit of utilizing available community support groups such as the local chapter of the Creutzfeldt-Jakob Disease Foundation, Inc.

Diagnostic test results

Neurologic examination is the most effective tool in diagnosing CJD.

Definitive diagnosis usually isn't obtained until an autopsy is done and brain tissue is examined; however, the following tests may prove useful:

- EEG may assess the patient for typical changes in brain wave activity.
- Computed tomography scan, magnetic resonance imaging of the brain, and lumbar puncture may rule out other disorders that cause dementia.

Treatment

Because CJD can't be cured, nor can its progress be slowed, treatment focuses on palliative care to make the patient comfortable and ease symptoms. Such medications as sedatives and antipsychotics may be needed to control aggressive behaviors.

Providing a safe environment, controlling aggressive or agitated behavior, and meeting the patient's physiologic needs may require monitoring and assistance in the home or in an institutionalized setting. Family counseling may help in coping with the changes required for home care.

Behavior modification may be helpful, in some cases, for controlling unacceptable or dangerous behaviors. Reality orientation, with repeated reinforcement of environmental and other cues, may help reduce disorientation.

Nursing interventions

- Provide supportive and palliative care.
- Provide emotional support to the patient and his family. Encourage them to talk about their concerns. Listen carefully, and answer their questions honestly and completely.
- Contact social services and hospice, as appropriate, to assist the family with their needs.
- Use caution when handling body fluids and other materials to prevent disease transmission.
- Encourage the patient and his family to seek legal advice to decide and establish advance directives, assign power of attorney, and set up other provisions for end-of-life care.
- Provide appropriate education to the patient and his family before discharge. (See *Teaching the patient with CJD.*)

HUNTINGTON'S DISEASE

With Huntington's disease (also called *Huntington's chorea, hereditary chorea, chronic progressive chorea,* or *adult chorea*), degeneration in the cerebral cortex and basal ganglia causes chronic progressive chorea (dancelike movements) and mental deterioration, ending in dementia.

Huntington's disease usually strikes people from ages 25 to 55 (the average age is 35), but 2% of cases occur·in children, and 5% occur as late as age 60. Death usually results 10 to 15 years after onset from heart failure or pneumonia. The exact cause of Huntington's disease is unknown. Because it's transmitted as an autosomal dominant trait, either sex can transmit and inherit it. If the gene is inherited, the person will eventually develop the disease. If the gene is not inherited, it can't be passed on to subsequent generations. Genetic studies have identified a marker for the gene linked to Huntington's disease, and testing is available for people with a family history of the disease.

Pathophysiology

Huntington's disease involves a disturbance in neurotransmitter substances, primarily gamma aminobutyric acid (GABA) and dopamine. In the basal ganglia, frontal cortex, and cerebellum, GABA neurons are destroyed and replaced by glial cells. The subsequent deficiency of GABA results in a relative excess of dopamine and abnormal neurotransmission along the affected pathways.

Complications

- Choking
- Aspiration
- Pneumonia
- Heart failure
- Infections

Assessment findings

Assessment findings vary depending on disease progression, but may include:

- family history
- clumsy, irritable, or impatient behavior and fits of anger and periods of suicidal depression, apathy, or elation (early stages)
- judgment and memory impairment
- hallucinations, delusions, and paranoid thinking
- gradual loss of intellectual ability
- choreic movements that progress from mild fidgeting to grimacing, tongue smacking, dysarthria (indistinct speech),

athetoid movements (especially of the hands) related to emotional state, and torticollis; in later stages, constant writhing and twitching, unintelligible speech, chewing and swallowing difficulties, immobility, and appearing emaciated and exhausted
- ravenous appetite, especially for sweets
- loss of bladder and bowel control (later stages).

Diagnostic test results

Diagnosis is largely based on a characteristic clinical history that includes progressive chorea and dementia, onset in early middle age (35 to 40), and confirmation of a genetic link. Other tests include the following:
- Positron emission tomography and deoxyribonucleic acid analysis may detect Huntington's disease.
- Magnetic resonance imaging shows characteristic butterfly dilation of the brain's lateral ventricles.
- Computed tomography scanning shows brain atrophy.

Treatment

Because there's no known cure for Huntington's disease, treatment is supportive, protective, and specific to the patient's symptoms. Antipsychotics, such as haloperidol (Haldol), a dopamine blocker, and benzodiazepines, such as clonazepam (Klonopin), help control choreic movements and reduce abnormal behaviors (hallucinations, agitation, and psychotic delusions); however, antipsychotics may also cause tardive dyskinesia, so they should be reserved for severe disabling chorea while using the lowest possible dose. Reserpine (Harmonyl), amantadine (Symmetrel), and other drugs have been used for chorea with less chance of causing tardive dyskinesia; however, these medications pose other adverse effects, which limits their usefulness.

Psychotherapy to decrease anxiety and stress may also be helpful. The patient may also require institutionalization because of mental deterioration.

TEACHING THE PATIENT WITH HUNTINGTON'S DISEASE

Before discharge, be sure to cover with the patient and his family:
- the disorder and its implications
- medication administration, dosage, and possible adverse effects, and when to notify the physician
- the importance of good nutrition and what types of food may be best based on swallowing ability
- range-of-motion exercises to improve muscle tone and strength
- available counseling and home health care
- types of therapy that would be beneficial, such as physical therapy and speech therapy
- signs and symptoms of complications
- the importance of follow-up care
- genetic counseling
- establishing end-of-life care
- the benefit of utilizing available community support groups such as the local chapter of Huntington's Disease Society of America.

Nursing interventions

- Provide emotional support to the patient and his family. Encourage them to talk about their concerns. Listen carefully, and answer their questions honestly and completely.
- Assess self-care deficits and assist with care, as needed.
- Administer medications, as ordered. Monitor for desired effects and adverse reactions.
- Support independence as much as possible.
- Provide alternate methods of communication, if needed.
- Provide safety measures and assess for the possibility of self-injury.
- Reposition the patient every 2 hours, assess his skin condition, and provide appropriate skin care.
- Encourage physical activity as much as possible.
- Follow standard precautions.

- Monitor vital signs, temperature, and white blood cell count for signs of infection.
- Assist with meals and assess for signs of aspiration.
- Provide appropriate education to the patient and his family before discharge. (See *Teaching the patient with Huntington's disease*.)

MULTIPLE SCLEROSIS

Multiple sclerosis (MS) is a chronic disease caused by progressive demyelination of the white matter of the brain and spinal cord. Demyelination is the destruction of the covering of the nerve cells, which results in plaque formation. These sporadic patches of demyelination in the central nervous system (CNS) cause widespread and varied neurologic dysfunction. The exact cause of MS is unknown, but may result from a slow-acting viral infection that may precede an autoimmune response of the nervous system or an allergic response. Other possible factors include trauma, anoxia, toxins, nutritional deficiencies, vascular lesions, and anorexia nervosa, all of which may help destroy axons and the myelin sheath. Emotional stress, overwork, fatigue, pregnancy, cold or hot weather, hot baths, fever, menstruation, and acute respiratory tract infections may precede symptom onset. Genetic factors may also be involved.

MS is a major cause of chronic disability in young adults ages 20 to 40 and is characterized by exacerbations and remissions. MS may progress rapidly, causing death within months or disability by early adulthood. The prognosis varies; about 70% of patients lead active, productive lives with prolonged remissions.

The incidence of MS is highest in females and among people in northern urban areas, higher socioeconomic groups, and in those living in a cold, damp climate.

Pathophysiology

With MS, sporadic patches of axon demyelination and nerve fiber loss occur throughout the CNS, producing widely dis-

UP CLOSE

WHEN MYELIN BREAKS DOWN

Myelin plays a key role in speeding electrical impulses to the brain for interpretation. A lipoprotein complex formed of glial cells or oligodendrocytes, the myelin sheath protects the neuron's long nerve fiber (the axon) much like the insulation on an electrical wire. Its high electrical resistance and low capacitance allow the myelin sheath to permit sufficient conduction of nerve impulses from one node of Ranvier to the next.

Myelin is susceptible to injury by hypoxemia, toxic chemicals, vascular insufficiency, and autoimmune responses. When injury occurs, the myelin sheath becomes inflamed and the membrane layers break down into smaller components that become well-circumscribed plaques (filled with microglial elements, macroglia, and lymphocytes). This process is called *demyelination.*

The damaged myelin sheath impairs normal conduction, causing partial loss or dispersion of the action potential and consequent neurologic dysfunction.

New evidence of nerve fiber loss may explain the invisible neurologic deficits experienced by many patients with multiple sclerosis. The axons control the presence or absence of function. Loss of myelin doesn't correlate with loss of function.

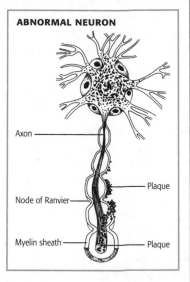

ABNORMAL NEURON

Axon

Plaque

Node of Ranvier

Myelin sheath

Plaque

---

seminated and varied neurologic dysfunction. (See *When myelin breaks down.*) New evidence of nerve fiber loss may provide an explanation for the invisible neurologic deficits experienced by many patients with MS. Indeed, immune system B-cells exhibit energy production in nerve fiber cells during an MS attack, causing them to degenerate and die. Axons determine the presence or absence of function; however, loss of myelin doesn't correlate with loss of function.

Complications

- Injury
- Urinary tract infection
- Constipation
- Joint contractures
- Pressure ulcers
- Rectal distention
- Pneumonia
- Depression

Assessment findings

Clinical findings in MS correspond to the extent and site of myelin destruction, extent of remyelination, and adequacy of subsequent restored synaptic transmission. Symptoms may be transient or may last for hours or weeks. Clinical effects may be so mild that the patient is unaware of them or so intense that they're disabling. (See *Describing MS,* page 304.) Look for the following characteristics in your assessment:

- ocular disturbances—optic neuritis, diplopia, ophthalmoplegia, blurred vision, and nystagmus
- psuedobulbar affect—difficulty controlling emotions
- muscle dysfunction—weakness, paralysis ranging from monoplegia to quadriplegia, spasticity, hyperreflexia, intention tremor, and gait ataxia
- urinary disturbances—incontinence, frequency, urgency, and frequent urinary infections
- bowel disturbances—involuntary evacuation or constipation
- fatigue—usually the most disabling symptom
- neurologic problems—poorly articulated speech, scanning speech, or dysarthria disturbances
- Lhermitte's sign—an electrical sensation that travels down the back or legs, which is precipitated by flexion of the neck.

DESCRIBING MS

Multiple sclerosis (MS) may be described in various terms.

● *Relapsing-remitting:* Clear relapses (or acute attacks or exacerbations) with full recovery and lasting disability. Between the attacks there's no worsening of the disease.

● *Primary progressive:* Steady progression or worsening of the disease from the onset with minor recovery or plateaus. This form is uncommon and may involve different brain and spinal cord damage than other forms.

● *Secondary progressive:* Begins as a pattern of clear-cut relapses and recovery but becomes steadily progressive and worsens between acute attacks.

● *Progressive relapsing:* Steadily progressive from the onset but also has clear, acute attacks. This form is rare. In addition, differential diagnosis must rule out spinal cord compression, foramen magnum tumor (which may mimic the exacerbations and remission of MS), multiple small strokes, syphilis or another infection, thyroid disease, and chronic fatigue syndrome.

Diagnostic test results

- EEG shows abnormalities in one-third of patients.
- Cerebrospinal fluid (CSF) analysis reveals elevated immunoglobulin (Ig) G levels but normal total protein levels. Elevated IgG levels are significant only when serum gamma globulin levels are normal, and they reflect hyperactivity of the immune system due to chronic demyelination.
- Laboratory studies may reveal a slightly increased white blood cell count.
- Evoked potential studies demonstrate slowed conduction of nerve impulses in 80% of patients with MS.
- Magnetic resonance imaging is the most sensitive method of detecting MS lesions. More than 90% of patients with MS show multifocal white matter lesions when this test is performed. It's also used to evaluate disease progression.
- Computed tomography scanning may disclose lesions within the brain's white matter.

- Electrophoresis may detect oligoclonal bands of Ig in CSF. They're present in most patients and can be found even when the percentage of gamma globulin in CSF is normal.

Treatment

Treatment aims to shorten exacerbations and relieve neurologic deficits. Those with relapsing-remitting courses are placed on immune modulating therapy with interferon beta-1A (Avonex) or glatiramer (Copaxoner). Natalizumab (Tysabri) has been recently approved as monotherapy for relapsing-remitting MS. Steroids are used to reduce the associated edema of the myelin sheath during exacerbations.

Other drugs that may be administered include baclofen (Baclofen), tizanidine (Zanaflex), or diazepam (Valium) to relieve spasticity; cholinergic agents to relieve urine retention and minimize frequency and urgency; amantadine (Symmetrel) to relieve fatigue; and antidepressants to help with mood or behavioral symptoms. During acute exacerbations, supportive measures include bed rest, comfort measures such as massages, prevention of fatigue, prevention of pressure ulcers, bowel and bladder training (if necessary), and administration of antibiotics for bladder infections. Physical therapy, speech therapy, occupational therapy, and support groups and counseling are also useful. Planned exercise programs help with maintaining muscle tone. Counseling may be needed for coping with depression.

Associated signs and symptoms are treated with medications, supportive measures, and aggressive management to prevent deterioration. (See *Treating signs and symptoms of MS*, page 306.)

Nursing interventions

- Provide emotional support to the patient and her family. Encourage them to talk about their concerns. Listen carefully, and answer their questions honestly and completely.

TREATING SIGNS AND SYMPTOMS OF MS

Signs and symptoms of multiple sclerosis (MS) include spasticity, fatigue, bladder and bowel problems, sensory symptoms, and cognitive and motor dysfunction. Each symptom is treated with many medications and supportive measures.

● *Spasticity* occurs when opposing muscle groups relax and contract at the same time. Stretching and range-of-motion exercises, coupled with correct positioning, are helpful in relaxing muscles and maintaining function. Drug therapy for spasticity includes baclofen (Lioresal) and tizanidine (Zanaflex). For severe spasticity, Botox injections, intrathecal injections, nerve blocks, and surgery may be necessary.

● *Fatigue* in MS is characterized by an overwhelming feeling of exhaustion that can occur at any time of the day without warning. The cause is unknown. Changes in environmental conditions, such as heat and humidity, can aggravate fatigue. Amantadine (Symmetrel) and methylphenidate (Ritalin) are beneficial, as are antidepressants, to manage fatigue.

● *Bladder problems* may arise from failure to store urine, failure to empty the bladder or, more commonly, a combination of both. Treatment ranges from simple strategies, such as drinking increased fluids, to the placement of an indwelling urinary catheter and suprapubic tubes. Intermittent self-catheterization programs are ben-

eficial. In addition, anticholinergic medications may be helpful.

● *Bowel problems,* such as constipation and involuntary evacuation of stool, can be managed by increasing fiber. Bulking agents, such as psyllium (Metamucil), assist in relief and prevention of bowel problems. Other bowel-training strategies, such as daily suppositories and rectal stimulation, may be necessary.

● *Sensory symptoms,* such as pain, numbness, burning, and tingling sensations, can be well managed by low-dose tricyclic antidepressants, phenytoin (Dilantin), or carbamazepine (Tegretol).

● *Cognitive dysfunction* occurs in 50% of patients with MS. Cognitive problems tend to be minor; short-term memory loss is the most frequently experienced symptom. For more severe issues, a neuropsychological consultation could be beneficial.

● *Motor dysfunction,* such as problems with balance, strength, and muscle coordination, may be present in MS. Adaptive devices and physical therapy intervention help to maintain mobility.

● *Other symptoms,* such as tremors, may be treated with beta-adrenergic blockers, sedatives, or diuretics. Dysarthria requires speech therapy consultation. Vertigo may be managed with antihistamines, vision therapy, or exercise. Vision changes may require vision therapy or adaptive lenses.

TEACHING THE PATIENT WITH MS

Before discharge, be sure to cover with the patient and her family:
- the disorder and its implications
- medication administration, dosage, and possible adverse effects, and when to notify the physician
- avoidance of stress, infections, and fatigue
- the importance of good nutrition and fluid intake
- range-of-motion exercises to improve muscle tone and strength
- available counseling and home health care
- types of therapy that would be beneficial, such as physical therapy and occupational therapy
- signs and symptoms of complications
- the importance of follow-up care
- the benefit of utilizing available community support groups such as the local chapter of National Multiple Sclerosis Society.

- Encourage active range-of-motion exercises and participation in physical therapy. Assist with exercises to maintain muscle tone and joint mobility, decrease spasticity, improve coordination, and boost morale. Provide rest periods between exercises.
- Help establish a daily routine to maintain optimal functioning.
- Assist with elimination needs. Evaluate the need for bowel and bladder training.
- Encourage adequate fluid intake.
- Administer medications and monitor for adverse reactions.
- Provide appropriate education to the patient and her family before discharge. (See *Teaching the patient with MS*.)

PARKINSON'S DISEASE

Named for the English physician who first accurately described the disease in 1817, Parkinson's disease is a chronic progressive disorder that's characterized by progressive muscle rigidity, akinesia, and involuntary tremors. Deterioration commonly progresses, culminating in death, which usually results from aspiration pneumonia or some other infection.

Parkinson's disease is also called *parkinsonism, paralysis agitans,* or *shaking palsy.* It's one of the most common crippling diseases in the United States, occurring in 2 of every 1,000 people older than age 50 and affecting more males than females. However, due to advances in the treatment of complications, patients are experiencing increased longevity.

Pathophysiology

Studies of the extrapyramidal brain nuclei (corpus striatum, globus pallidus, and substantia nigra) have established that a dopamine deficiency prevents affected brain cells from performing their normal inhibitory function within the central nervous system. The presence of fibrous tissue deposits, known as *Lewy bodies,* are present in the substantia nigra; however, it isn't yet known the role (if any) that Lewy bodies play in the development and progression of the disease.

Some cases of Parkinson's disease are caused by external factors, such as medication, and environmental toxins, such as manganese dust and carbon monoxide. (See *Understanding Parkinson's disease.*)

Complications

- Injury
- Aspiration
- Urinary tract infection
- Complications of immobility
- Depression

Assessment findings

- Insidious tremor, commonly known as *unilateral pill-roll tremor,* that begins in the fingers
- Dysphagia
- Muscle cramps of the legs, neck, and trunk

> ## UNDERSTANDING
> ## PARKINSON'S DISEASE
>
> Research into the pathogenesis of Parkinson's disease focuses on damage to the substantia nigra due to oxidative stress. Types of damage include:
> - alterations in brain iron content
> - impaired mitochondrial function
> - alterations in antioxidant and protective systems
> - reduced glutathione
> - damage to lipids, proteins, and deoxyribonucleic acid.

- Increased perspiration
- Insomnia
- Dysarthria and speaking in a high-pitched monotone
- Drooling
- Masklike facial expression
- Difficulty walking; gait commonly lacks normal parallel motion and may be retropulsive or propulsive
- Akinesia that causes loss of posture control, oculogyric crises (eyes fixed upward, with involuntary tonic movements) or blepharospasm (eyelids closed) and delay in initiating movement to perform a purposeful action
- Muscle rigidity that may be uniform (lead-pipe rigidity) or jerky (cogwheel rigidity)
- Cognitive changes, dementia
- Depression, emotional changes
- Urinary problems, constipation

Diagnostic test results
A conclusive diagnosis of Parkinson's disease is possible only after ruling out other causes of tremor, involutional depression, cerebral arteriosclerosis and, in patients younger than age 30, intracranial tremors, Wilson's disease, or phenothiazine (antipsychotic) or other drug toxicity.

- Urinalysis may reveal decreased dopamine levels.
- Computed tomography scanning or magnetic resonance imaging may rule out other disorders.

Treatment

No cure exists for Parkinson's disease; therefore, treatment focuses on relieving symptoms and maintaining the patient's ability to function as long as possible. Treatment may include drugs, physical therapy and, in severe disease unresponsive to drugs, deep brain stimulation, stereotaxic neurosurgery, or fetal cell transplantation. In this treatment, fetal brain tissue is injected into the patient's brain. If the injected cells grow within the recipient's brain, they allow the brain to process dopamine, thereby either halting or reversing disease progression. Neurotransplantation techniques, including the use of nerve cells from other parts of the patient's body, have been attempted with mixed results.

Standard treatment for Parkinson's disease is dopamine replacement therapy in combination with a peripheral decarboxylase inhibitor—levodopa-carbidopa (Sinemet).

Other drug therapy usually includes such enzyme-inhibiting agents as selegiline (Atapryl) and rasagiline (Azilect), which allow for conservation of dopamine and enhance the therapeutic effect of levodopa. The patient may receive bromocriptine (Parlodel) as an additive to reduce the levodopa dose. If levodopa is ineffective or if the patient can't tolerate it, alternative drug therapy includes anticholinergics (such as trihexyphenidyl [Artane] or benztropine [Cogentin]), antivirals (such as amantadine [Symmetrel]), and antihistamines (such as diphenhydramine [Benedryl]), all of which help to decrease tremors, rigidity, and akinesia.

When drug therapy fails, neurosurgery may be warranted to help control symptoms. Traditional procedures, such as thalamotomy and pallidotomy, have been replaced with more advanced treatments, such as deep brain stimulation (neurostimulation)—which targets the thalamus, subthalamus, or globus pallidus—to improve dyskinesia and motor function.

TEACHING THE PATIENT WITH PARKINSON'S DISEASE

Before discharge, be sure to cover with the patient and his family:
- the disorder and its implications
- treatment options, such as therapy and surgery
- medication administration, dosage, and possible adverse effects, and when to notify the physician
- avoidance of stress, infections, and fatigue
- the importance of good nutrition and fluid intake
- range-of-motion exercises to improve muscle tone and strength
- environmental safety measures
- available counseling and home health care
- types of therapy that would be beneficial, such as physical and occupational therapy
- signs and symptoms of complications
- the importance of follow-up care
- the benefit of utilizing available community support groups such as the local chapter of the National Parkinson Foundation.

As a complement to drug treatment and neurosurgery, physical therapy helps to maintain the patient's normal muscle tone and function. Appropriate physical therapy includes active and passive range-of-motion (ROM) exercises, routine daily activities, walking, and baths and massage to help relax muscles.

Tricyclic antidepressants may help alleviate the depression that commonly accompanies the disease.

Nursing interventions

- Provide emotional support to the patient and his family. Encourage them to talk about their concerns. Listen carefully, and answer their questions honestly and completely.
- Encourage active ROM exercises and participation in physical therapy. Assist with exercises to maintain muscle tone and joint mobility, decrease spasticity, improve coordina-

tion, and boost morale. Provide rest periods between exercises.

- Protect the patient from injury.
- Assist with meals and assess for signs of aspiration.
- Help establish a daily routine to maintain optimal functioning.
- Assist with elimination needs. Evaluate the need for bowel and bladder training.
- Encourage adequate fluid intake.
- Administer medications and monitor for adverse reactions.
- Provide preoperative and postoperative care, as appropriate.
- Provide appropriate education to the patient and his family before discharge. (See *Teaching the patient with Parkinson's disease,* page 311.)

Nerve and pain disorders

With nerve and pain disorders, damage that causes impairment is the focus of the patient's problem and may cause significant distress or dysfunction. Nerve disorders include Bell's palsy, extraocular motor nerve palsies, peripheral neuritis, and trigeminal neuralgia. Pain disorders include complex regional pain syndrome.

NERVE DISORDERS
BELL'S PALSY

With Bell's palsy, impulses from the seventh cranial nerve—the nerve responsible for motor innervation of the facial muscles—are blocked.

Although the exact cause of Bell's palsy is unknown, possible causes include ischemia, viral disease such as herpes simplex or herpes zoster, local traumatic injury, or autoimmune disease.

Bell's palsy can affect all age-groups; however, it occurs most commonly in people ages 20 to 60. Onset is rapid. In 80% to 90% of patients, the disorder subsides spontaneously, with complete recovery in 1 to 8 weeks. If recovery is partial, contractures may develop on the paralyzed side of the face. The disorder may recur on the same or the opposite side of the face.

NEUROLOGIC DYSFUNCTION IN BELL'S PALSY

This illustration shows how motor conduction of the seventh cranial nerve (facial) is blocked in Bell's palsy, causing a unilateral facial weakness.

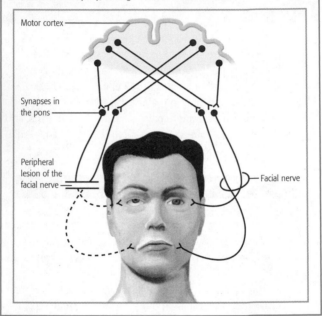

Pathophysiology

Bell's palsy reflects an inflammatory reaction around the seventh cranial nerve, usually at the internal auditory meatus where the nerve leaves bony tissue. This inflammatory reaction produces a conduction block that inhibits appropriate neural stimulation to the muscle by the motor fibers of the facial nerve, resulting in the characteristic unilateral or bilateral facial weakness. (See *Neurologic dysfunction in Bell's palsy*.)

FACIAL PARALYSIS IN BELL'S PALSY

Unilateral facial paralysis typifies Bell's palsy. The paralysis produces a distorted appearance and an inability to wrinkle the forehead, close the eyelid, smile, show the teeth, or puff out the cheek on the affected side.

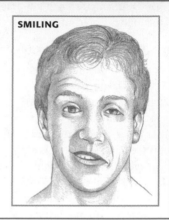

SMILING

Complications
- Corneal ulceration
- Blindness
- Impaired nutrition
- Psychosocial problems

Assessment findings
- Pain on the affected side
- Difficulty eating on the affected side
- Difficulty speaking clearly
- Drooping mouth and drooling
- Distorted taste perception over the affected anterior portion of the tongue
- Inability to raise the eyebrow, smile, show teeth, or puff out the cheek on the affected side
- Difficulty closing the eye on the affected side; if attempted, the eye rolls upward (Bell's phenomenon) and shows excessive tearing (see *Facial paralysis in Bell's palsy*)

Diagnostic test results

- Diagnosis is based on clinical presentation.
- Electromyography helps predict the level of expected recovery by distinguishing temporary conduction defects from a pathologic interruption of nerve fibers.

Treatment

Appropriate treatment consists of administration of corticosteroids to reduce facial nerve edema and improve nerve conduction and blood flow. Corticosteroid therapy is especially helpful when started within a week of the symptom's onset. After 2 weeks of corticosteroid therapy, electrotherapy may help prevent facial muscle atrophy.

Analgesics help to control facial pain and discomfort. Moist heat applied to the affected side may also provide some comfort. Lubricants or an eye ointment may be needed to protect the eye; patching during sleep may also be necessary.

If the patient fails to recover from facial paralysis, surgery that involves exploration of the facial nerve may be necessary.

Nursing interventions

- Provide psychological support to the patient. Reassure him that he hasn't had a stroke. Tell him that spontaneous recovery usually occurs within 8 weeks. This should help decrease his anxiety and help him adjust to the temporary change in his body image.
- Administer medications and monitor for adverse reactions.
- Monitor serum glucose levels during corticosteroid therapy.
- Apply moist heat to the affected side of the face, as ordered.
- Massage the patient's face with a gentle upward motion two to three times daily for 5 to 10 minutes; teach massage to the patient.
- Apply a facial sling, if necessary, to improve lip alignment.
- Provide frequent and complete mouth care, taking special care to remove residual food that collects between the cheeks and gums.

DISCHARGE TEACHING

TEACHING THE PATIENT WITH BELL'S PALSY

Before discharge, be sure to cover with the patient and his family:
● the disorder and its implications
● medication administration, dosage, and possible adverse effects, and when to notify the physician
● about protecting his affected eye by covering it with an eye patch, especially when outdoors
● facial exercises
● the importance of maintaining good nutrition
● signs and symptoms of complications
● the importance of follow-up care
● the benefit of utilizing available community support groups such as the local chapter of the Bell's Palsy Research Foundation.

■ Provide a soft, nutritionally balanced diet, eliminating hot foods and fluids.
■ Provide preoperative and postoperative care, as appropriate.
■ Provide appropriate education to the patient and his family before discharge. (See *Teaching the patient with Bell's palsy*.)

EXTRAOCULAR MOTOR NERVE PALSIES

In patients with extraocular motor nerve palsies, dysfunction affects cranial nerves (CNs) III, IV, and VI. These nerves are responsible for innervating eye movements. The most common causes of extraocular motor nerve palsies include diabetic neuropathy, trauma, and pressure from an aneurysm or a brain tumor. Other causes vary depending on the cranial nerve involved. (See *Causes of extraocular motor nerve palsies,* page 318.)

Pathophysiology

Nerve palsies occur with inflammation of the nerve and affect their function. The extraocular nerves perform several func-

CAUSES OF EXTRAOCULAR MOTOR NERVE PALSIES

Causes of extraocular nerve palsies may include the following:
- Oculomotor (cranial nerve [CN] III) palsy or acute ophthalmoplegia, may result from brain stem ischemia or other cerebrovascular disorders, poisoning (lead, carbon monoxide, botulism), alcohol abuse, infections (measles, encephalitis), trauma to the extraocular muscles, myasthenia gravis, or tumors in the cavernous sinus area.
- Trochlear (CN IV) palsy may result from closed head trauma (for example, a blow-out fracture) or sinus surgery.
- Abducens (CN VI) palsy may result from increased intracranial pressure, brain abscess, stroke, meningitis, arterial brain occlusions, infections of the petrous bone (rare), lateral sinus thrombosis, myasthenia gravis, and thyrotropic exophthalmos.

tions. The superior branch of the oculomotor nerve (CN III) innervates the levator superior muscle of the upper eyelid and the superior rectus muscle of the eye; the inferior branch innervates the interior rectus, medial rectus, and inferior oblique muscles. It also supplies the intrinsic pupillary and ciliary muscles, which control lens shape and accommodation. The trochlear nerve (CN IV) innervates the superior oblique muscles, which control downward rotation, intorsion, and abduction of the eye. The abducens nerve (CN VI) innervates the lateral rectus muscles, which control inward movement of the eye.

Complications

- Diplopia
- Ptosis
- Strabismus
- Nystagmus
- Ocular torticollis

Assessment findings

- Recent onset of diplopia (varies in different fields of gaze based on the eye muscles affected)
- Torticollis (from repeatedly turning the head to compensate for visual field defects)
  With CN III palsy:
- Ptosis
- Extropia (eye positioned outward)
- Pupillary dilation and unresponsiveness to light and accommodation
- Inability to move the eye
  With CN IV palsy:
- Inability to move the eye downward or upward
  With CN VI palsy:
- Estropia (inward deviation of the eye)

Diagnostic test results

- Diagnosis is based on neuro-ophthalmologic examination.
- Blood studies may detect diabetes.
- Computed tomography scanning, magnetic resonance imaging, or skull X-rays may be done to rule out intracranial tumors.
- Angiography may be done to evaluate possible vascular abnormalities.
- Culture and sensitivity tests may rule out infection.

Treatment

Appropriate treatment varies depending on the cause. For example, neurosurgery may be necessary for a brain tumor or an aneurysm. For infection, massive doses of antibiotics may be appropriate. After treating the primary condition, the patient may need to perform exercises that stretch the neck muscles to correct acquired torticollis (wry neck). Other care and treatments depend on residual symptoms.

TEACHING THE PATIENT WITH EXTRAOCULAR MOTOR NERVE PALSIES

Before discharge, be sure to cover with the patient:
● the disorder and its implications
● medication administration, dosage, and possible adverse effects, and when to notify the physician
● exercises to improve neck movement
● signs and symptoms of complications
● the importance of follow-up care
● the benefit of utilizing available community support groups.

Nursing interventions

■ Provide emotional support to help minimize the patient's anxiety about the cause of the motor nerve palsy.
■ Provide treatment appropriate for the specific cause of the palsy.
■ Encourage neck exercises if torticollis is present.
■ Provide appropriate education to the patient before discharge. (See *Teaching the patient with extraocular motor nerve palsies.*)

PERIPHERAL NEURITIS

Peripheral neuritis, also called *multiple neuritis, peripheral neuropathy,* and *polyneuritis*, is the inflammatory degeneration of peripheral nerves that primarily supply the distal muscles of the extremities. It results in muscle weakness with sensory loss and atrophy and decreased or absent deep tendon reflexes. Because onset is usually insidious, patients may compensate by overusing unaffected muscles. If the cause can be identified and eliminated, the prognosis is good.

Although the exact cause of peripheral neuritis is unknown, it's thought to be mediated by inflammation, ischemia, and demyelination of the larger peripheral nerves, as a result of diabetes, alcohol use, and Guillain-Barré syndrome.

Drugs that may cause peripheral neuritis include thalidomide (Talomid); metronidazole (Flagyl); phenytoin (Dilantin); amitriptyline (Elavil); dapsone (DDS); nitrofurantoin (Macrodantin); cholesterol-lowering drugs, such as lovastatin (Mevacor), indapamide (Lozol) and gemfibrozil (Lopid); thallium; and chemotherapy (cisplatin [Platinol], vincristine [Oncovin]).

Pathophysiology

Peripheral neuritis is damage to nerves that run from the spinal cord to the rest of the body, which impairs function of the sensory, motor, and autonomic nerves.

- *Sensory changes:* Damage to sensory fibers results in changes in sensation, such as burning, nerve pain, tingling or numbness, or an inability to determine joint position. Changes in sensation commonly begin in the feet and progress toward the center of the body with subsequent involvement of other areas as the condition worsens.
- *Motor changes:* Damage to the motor fibers interferes with muscle control and can cause weakness, cramping, loss of muscle bulk, and loss of dexterity. Other muscle-related symptoms include lack of muscle control, difficulty or inability to move a part of the body, muscle atrophy, muscle twitching, difficulty breathing or swallowing, or falling.
- *Autonomic changes:* Damage to autonomic nerves can cause blurred vision, decreased ability to sweat, dizziness that occurs when standing up or fainting associated with a decrease in blood pressure, heat intolerance with exertion, nausea or vomiting after meals, abdominal bloating, feeling full after eating a small amount, diarrhea, constipation, unintentional weight loss (more than 5% of body weight), urinary incontinence, feeling of incomplete bladder emptying, difficulty beginning to urinate, and male impotence.

Complications

- Chronic pain
- Depression
- Drug dependence

Assessment findings

Symptoms vary according to which type of nerve is affected (sensory, motor, or autonomic) and may include:

- altered sensations or paresthesias
- impaired balance when standing or walking
- difficulty maintaining a grip on objects
- muscle weakness.

Diagnostic test results

- Patient history and physical examination delineate characteristic distribution of motor and sensory deficits.
- Electromyography may show a delayed action potential if the condition impairs motor nerve function.
- Nerve biopsy and nerve conduction tests can confirm the diagnosis.

Treatment

Effective treatment of peripheral neuritis consists of supportive measures to relieve pain; adequate bed rest; physical, vocational, and occupational therapy; and orthopedic interventions to promote independence. Most importantly, however, the underlying cause must be identified and treated. For instance, it's essential to identify and remove the toxic agent, correct nutritional and vitamin deficiencies (the patient needs a high-calorie diet rich in vitamins, especially B-complex), and counsel the patient to avoid alcohol.

Over-the-counter analgesics or prescription pain medications may be needed to control nerve pain. Anticonvulsants (phenytoin [Dilantin], carbamazepine [Tegretol], and gabapentin [Neurotin]) or tricyclic antidepressants may be used to reduce the stabbing pains that some patients experience. Whenever possible, medication use should be minimized to avoid adverse effects.

Duloxetine (Cymbalta) may be prescribed specifically for the treatment of diabetic neuropathy, but shouldn't be given to patients with end-stage renal disease, hepatic impairment, uncontrolled hypertension, and those who have substantial alcohol intake or are on thioridazine (Mellaril) because of the potential risk of cardiac arrhythmias.

Fludrocortisone (Florinef) or similar medications may be beneficial in reducing postural hypotension for some patients. Metoclopramide (Reglan) may be helpful for patients with reduced gastric motility.

For patients with bladder dysfunction, manual expression of urine (pressing over the bladder with the hands), intermittent catheterization, or medications, such as bethanechol (Urecholine), may be necessary.

Other types of therapy may include acupuncture, plasmapheresis and I.V. gamma globulin, electrical nerve stimulation, and biofeedback.

Nursing interventions

- Encourage participation in physical therapy. Provide range-of-motion exercises, if necessary. Teach use of assistive devices, if appropriate.
- Assess affected areas frequently for bruises, open skin areas, or other injuries and provide appropriate care.
- Provide safety measures to prevent injury.
- Reposition the patient every 2 hours or teach him to change position frequently if nerve damage prevents adequate sensation of pressure.
- Provide small, frequent meals, if appropriate.
- Assist the patient with bladder dysfunction with manual expression of urine and intermittent catheterization, as necessary.

TEACHING THE PATIENT WITH PERIPHERAL NEURITIS

Before discharge, be sure to cover with the patient and his family:
- the disorder and its implications
- medication administration, dosage, and possible adverse effects, and when to notify the physician
- protecting the affected area by avoiding pressure and performing appropriate exercises
- available therapies, such as physical therapy, occupational therapy, and use of a transcutaneous electrical stimulation unit
- signs and symptoms of complications
- the importance of follow-up care
- the benefit of utilizing available community support groups such as the local chapter of the Neuropathy Association.

■ Provide appropriate education to the patient and his family before discharge. (See *Teaching the patient with peripheral neuritis.*)

TRIGEMINAL NEURALGIA

Trigeminal neuralgia, also known as *tic douloureux,* is a disorder of one or more branches of the fifth cranial nerve. This nerve affects chewing movements and sensations of the face, scalp, and teeth. On stimulation of a trigger zone, the patient experiences paroxysmal attacks of excruciating facial pain, most likely produced by an interaction or short-circuiting of touch and pain fibers. (See *Trigeminal nerve function and distribution.*)

The disease occurs mostly in people older than age 40 (about 25% more females than men) and on the right side of the face more commonly than the left. Trigeminal neuralgia can subside spontaneously, with remissions lasting from several months to years.

TRIGEMINAL NERVE FUNCTION AND DISTRIBUTION

Function
- Motor: chewing movements
- Sensory: sensations of face, scalp, and teeth (mouth and nasal chamber)

Distribution
I   ophthalmic
II maxillary
III mandibular

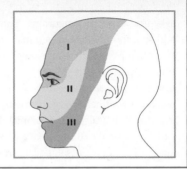

Pathophysiology

Seven forms of trigeminal neuralgia have been described based on the pathophysiologic cause: typical trigeminal neuralgia, atypical trigeminal neuralgia, pre-trigeminal neuralgia, multiple sclerosis (MS)-related trigeminal neuralgia, secondary trigeminal neuralgia, posttraumatic trigeminal neuralgia (trigeminal neuropathy), and failed trigeminal neuralgia.

- *Typical trigeminal neuralgia* (also known as *classical, idiopathic,* and *essential trigeminal neuralgia*): This is the most common form of trigeminal neuralgia. Nearly all cases of typical trigeminal neuralgia are caused by blood vessels compressing the trigeminal nerve root as it enters the brain stem. The superior cerebellar artery is the vessel usually responsible for neurovascular compression, although other arteries or veins may be involved.

- *Atypical trigeminal neuralgia:* This is characterized by a unilateral, prominent, constant, and severe aching, boring, or burning pain superimposed upon otherwise typical trigeminal neuralgia symptoms. Vascular compression is thought to be the most common cause of atypical trigeminal neuralgia; however, some believe that the more severe symptoms are caused by compression on a specific part of the trigeminal nerve (the portio minor), while others theorize that atypical trigeminal neuralgia represents a more severe form or progression of typical trigeminal neuralgia.

- *Pre-trigeminal neuralgia:* Days to years before the first attack of typical trigeminal neuralgia, some patients experience odd sensations in the trigeminal distributions, such as pain, described as a toothache; or discomfort, described as "pins and needles" or paresthesia.

- *MS-related trigeminal neuralgia:* The characteristics of MS-related trigeminal neuralgia are identical to those for typical trigeminal neuralgia. Approximately 2% to 4% of patients with trigeminal neuralgia have evidence of MS and approximately 1% of patients suffering from MS develop trigeminal neuralgia. Those with MS-related trigeminal neuralgia tend to be younger when they experience their first attack of pain, and the pain progresses over a shorter period than in those with typical trigeminal neuralgia. Furthermore, bilateral trigeminal neuralgia is more commonly seen in people with MS.

- *Secondary trigeminal neuralgia:* Trigeminal neuralgia pain caused by a lesion, such as a tumor, is referred to as *secondary trigeminal neuralgia*. A tumor that severely compresses or distorts the trigeminal nerve may cause facial numbness, weakness of chewing muscles, or constant aching pain.

- *Posttraumatic trigeminal neuralgia:* Posttraumatic trigeminal neuralgia may develop following craniofacial trauma (such as from a motor vehicle accident), dental trauma, sinus trauma, or after destructive procedures (rhizotomies) used to treat trigeminal neuralgia. Following trigeminal nerve injury, numbness may become associated with bothersome sensations or pain, sometimes called *phantom pain* or *deafferentation pain*. These pain conditions are caused by irreparable damage to the trigeminal nerve and secondary hyperactivity of the trigeminal nerve nucleus. The pain is usually constant and aching or burning, but may be worsened by exposure to triggers, such as wind and cold. Such deafferentation pain can start immediately or days to years after injury to the trigeminal nerve. In the most extreme form, called *anesthesia dolorosa*, there's continuous, severe pain in areas of complete numbness.

- *Failed trigeminal neuralgia:* Unfortunately, in a very small proportion of trigeminal neuralgia sufferers, all medications, microvascular decompression, and destructive rhizotomy procedures prove ineffective in controlling trigeminal neuralgia pain. This condition is called *failed trigeminal neuralgia.* Such individuals typically suffer from additional post-traumatic trigeminal neuralgia as a result of the destructive interventions previously undertaken.

Complications
- Intractable pain
- Lack of self-care
- Depression

Assessment findings
- Localized searing or burning pain that occurs in lightning-like jabs and lasts from 1 to 2 minutes (Pain is usually initiated by a light touch to a hypersensitive area, such as the tip of the nose, cheeks, or gums. Pain may also follow a draft of air, exposure to heat or cold, eating, smiling, talking, or drinking hot or cold beverages.)
- Constant, dull ache
- Splinting of the affected area

Diagnostic test results
- Patient history and physical examination guide the use of diagnostic tests.
- Skull X-rays, computed tomography scan, and magnetic resonance imaging are performed to rule out sinus or tooth infections and tumors. If the patient has trigeminal neuralgia, these test results are normal.

Treatment

The primary oral medication used to treat trigeminal neuralgia is carbamazepine (Tegretol), an antiseizure drug. Initial relief is readily achieved in most patients. Clinicians commonly consider its use as a means to confirm the diagnosis of trigeminal neuralgia. The drug is introduced slowly and increased to a level where the patient is either pain-free or adverse effects occur. Extended-release carbamazepine is also available as Carbatrol and Tegretol XR.

A newer medication, oxcarbazepine (Trileptal), has been used more frequently as a first-line drug for trigeminal neuralgia. Although it's structurally related to carbamazepine, it may be preferable due to its mild adverse effects. Other medications used in the treatment of trigeminal neuralgia include baclofen (Lioresal), gabapentin (Neurontin), clonazepam (Klonopin), sodium valproate (Depakote), lamotrigine (Lamictal), and topiramate (Topamax). Analgesics and opioids aren't effective in addressing the pain of trigeminal neuralgia.

Surgery is indicated for those patients who can't tolerate medications or who exhibit serious adverse reactions. Procedures range from nerve blocks injections and percutaneous surgery (through the cheek) to open skull surgery and pinpoint radiation. Each procedure has certain advantages and disadvantages. Ease of the procedure, effectiveness, long-term results, recurrences, and possible complications must all be carefully weighed. There isn't one medical or surgical treatment that's effective for all patients. The choice between a procedure performed on an outpatient basis (such as radiofrequency coagulation or glycerol injection) or one requiring several days in the hospital (microvascular decompression) depends on patient preference, physical well-being, previous surgeries, presence of MS, and area of trigeminal nerve involvement. (Some procedures are particularly indicated when the upper/ophthalmic branch is involved.)

TEACHING THE PATIENT WITH TRIGEMINAL NEURALGIA

Before discharge, be sure to cover with the patient and her family:
- the disorder and its implications
- treatment options, such as surgery and medication
- medication administration, dosage, and possible adverse effects, and when to notify the physician
- avoidance of pain triggers
- the importance of maintaining adequate nutrition
- signs and symptoms of complications
- the importance of follow-up care
- the benefit of utilizing available community support groups such as the local chapter of the Neuropathy Association.

Nursing interventions

- Provide emotional support to the patient and her family. Encourage them to talk about their concerns. Listen carefully, and answer their questions honestly and completely.
- Observe and record the characteristics of each attack, including the patient's protective mechanisms.
- Provide small, frequent meals at room temperature to maintain adequate nutrition.
- Assist the patient in identifying factors that precipitate an attack, and urge the patient to avoid stimulation (air, heat, cold) of trigger zones (lips, cheeks, gums).
- Administer medications, as ordered, and monitor for adverse effects.
- Provide appropriate preoperative and postoperative care, as appropriate.
- Provide appropriate education to the patient and her family before discharge. (See *Teaching the patient with trigeminal neuralgia*.)

PAIN DISORDERS

COMPLEX REGIONAL PAIN SYNDROME

Complex regional pain syndrome (CRPS), also known as *reflex sympathetic dystrophy (CRPS1)* or *causalgia (CRPS2)*, is a chronic pain disorder that results from abnormal healing after an injury—either minor or major—to a bone, muscle, or nerve. The development of symptoms is commonly disproportionate to the severity of the injury and seems to result from abnormal functioning of the sympathetic nervous system (the part of the nervous system that controls the diameter of blood vessels). One or more extremities or other body parts may be affected. With early diagnosis, prognosis improves. (See *Stages of CRPS,* pages 332 and 333.)

Pathophysiology

The exact cause of CRPS is unknown. Impaired communication between the damaged nerves of the sympathetic nervous system and the brain may impede normal signals for sensations, temperature, and blood flow. This impedance leads to problems in the nerves, blood vessels, skin, bones, and muscles. Infection or injury to an arm or leg may initiate CRPS. It can also occur after a myocardial infarction or stroke. The condition may occasionally appear without obvious injury to the affected limb. The syndrome also occurs in patients who have had surgery and in patients with diseases that can cause chronic pain, such as cancer and arthritis. (See *Theories of pain,* pages 334 and 335.)

Complications
- Chronic pain
- Depression
- Drug dependence

Assessment findings

- Severe and constant pain
- Altered blood flow to the affected area
- Discoloration, sweating, or swelling of the affected area (may also be warm or cool to the touch)
- Skin, hair, and nail changes
- Impaired mobility and muscle wasting (if adequate treatment is delayed)

Diagnostic test results

- Diagnosis is based on the patient's history and clinical findings.
- Bone X-rays may aid in ruling out other conditions, such as osteomyelitis and stress fractures, which cause similar signs and symptoms. Additional tests may include bone scans, nerve conduction studies, and thermography (a test that indicates temperature changes and lack of blood supply in the painful area of the affected limb).

Treatment

Treatment typically consists of a combination of therapies, including administration of anti-inflammatory, antidepressant, vasodilator, and analgesic agents used singly or in varying combinations, depending on the patient and the severity of symptoms. Corticosteroids may be prescribed for some patients; others may be given bone loss medications, such as risedronate (Actonel). Physical therapy to the injured area, application of heat and cold, the use of a transcutaneous electrical nerve stimulator unit, biofeedback, and psychological support are helpful for some patients.

Treatment may also include techniques for interrupting the hyperactivity of the sympathetic nervous system such as nerve or regional blocks. Surgical sympathectomy—a radical procedure in which nerves are cut to destroy the pain—may be done in severe cases; however, this method is rarely used because other sensations may be destroyed in the process.

STAGES OF CRPS

Complex regional pain syndrome (CRPS) is divided into three stages. The stages aren't always distinct and not all of the signs may be present.

STAGE	DURATION	PAIN, SWELLING, AND IMMOBILITY
I *(ACUTE)*	● Symptoms beginning with-in hours, days, or weeks of the injury, lasting several weeks	● Gradual or abrupt onset of severe aching, throbbing, and burning pain at site of injury ● Pain may be accompanied by sensitivity to touch, swelling, muscle spasm, stiffness, and limited mobility
II *(SUBACUTE OR DYSTROPHIC)*	● Lasts 3 to 6 months	● Continuous burning, aching, or throbbing pain that's more severe than stage I ● Swelling spreads and changes from soft to brawny and firm ● Loss of range of motion, muscle wasting
III *(CHRONIC OR ATROPHIC)*	● Lasts more than 6 months	● Pain spreads proximately and may be intractable, but sometimes lessens and stabilizes ● More distinct dystrophic changes and irreversible tissue damage ● Muscle atrophy and contractures

Nursing interventions

■ Administer medications, monitor their effects, and observe for adverse reactions.

■ Assist with range-of-motion exercises. Provide rest periods, as needed.

■ Provide emotional support to the patient and his family. Encourage them to talk about their concerns. Listen carefully, and answer their questions honestly and completely.

■ Consult a pain care specialist to provide additional options for the patient and help manage discomfort.

SKIN	HAIR AND NAILS	OSTEOPOROSIS
● Warm, red, dry skin at onset; changes to bluish and becomes cold and sweaty	● Accelerated hair and nail growth	● Early osteoporosis symptoms
● Cool, pale, bluish, sweaty	● Altered hair growth; cracked, grooved, or ridged nails	● More apparent osteoporosis
● Thin, shiny	● Increasingly brittle and ridged nails	● Marked diffuse osteoporosis

■ Provide appropriate education to the patient and his family before discharge. (See *Teaching the patient with complex regional pain syndrome*, page 336.)

THEORIES OF PAIN

Over the years numerous theories have attempted to explain the sensation of pain and describe how it occurs. This chart highlights some major theories about pain.

THEORY	MAJOR ASSUMPTIONS	COMMENT
Specificity	● Four types of cutaneous sensation (touch, warmth, cold, pain); each results from stimulation of specific skin receptor sites and neural pathways. ● Specific pain neurons transmit pain sensation along specific pain fibers. ● At synapses in the substantia gelatinosa, pain impulses cross to the opposite side of the cord and ascend the specific pain pathways of the spinothalamic tract to the thalamus and the pain receptor areas of the cerebral cortex.	● Focuses on the direct relationship between the pain stimulus and perception; doesn't account for adaptation to pain and the psychosocial factors modulating it.
Intensity	● Pain results from excessive stimulation of sensory receptors. Disorders or processes causing pain create an intense summation of nonnoxious stimuli.	● Doesn't explain existence of intense stimuli not perceived as pain.
Pattern	● Nonspecific receptors transmit specific patterns (characterized by the length of the pain sensation, the amount of involved tissue, and the summation of impulses) from the skin to the spinal cord, leading to pain perception.	● Includes some components of the intensity theory; pain possibly a response to intense stimulation of the sensory receptors regardless of receptor type or pathway.
Neuromatrix	● A pattern theory. Sensations imprinted in the brain. Sensory inputs may trigger a pattern of sensation from the neuromatrix (a proposed network of neurons looping between the thalamus and the cortex, and the cortex and the limbic system). ● Sensation pattern is possible without the sensory trigger.	● Explains existence of phantom pain.

THEORIES OF PAIN *(continued)*

THEORY	MAJOR ASSUMPTIONS	COMMENT
Gate control	● Pain is transmitted from skin via the small diameter A delta and C fibers to cells of the substantia gelatinosa in the dorsal horn, where interconnections between other sensory pathways exist. Stimulation of the large-diameter fast, myelinated A beta and A alpha fibers closes gate, which restricts transmission of the impulse to the central nervous system (CNS) and diminishes pain perception. ● Large fiber stimulation is possible through massage, scratching or rubbing the skin, or through electrical stimulation. Concurrent firing of pain and touch paths reduces transmission and perception of the pain impulses but not of touch impulses. ● An increase in small-fiber activity inhibits the substantia gelatinosa cells, "opening the gate" and increasing pain transmission and perception. ● Substantia gelatinosa acts as a gate-control system to inhibit the flow of nerve impulses from peripheral fibers to the CNS. ● Central T cells act as a CNS control to stimulate selective brain processes that influence the gate-control system. Inhibition of T cells closes the gate, and pain impulses aren't transmitted to the brain. ● T-cell activation of neural mechanisms in the brain is responsible for pain perception and response; transmitters partly regulate the release of substance P, the peptide that conveys pain information. Pain modulation is also partly controlled by the neurotransmitters, enkephalin and serotonin. ● Persistent pain initiates a gradual decline in the fraction of impulses that pass through the various gates. ● Descending efferent impulses from the brain may be responsible for closing, partially opening, or completely opening the gate.	● Provides the basis for use of massage and electrical stimulation in pain management; being used to develop additional theories and models.

DISCHARGE TEACHING

TEACHING THE PATIENT WITH COMPLEX REGIONAL PAIN SYNDROME

Before discharge, be sure to cover with the patient and his family:
● the disorder and its implications
● medication administration, dosage, and possible adverse effects, and when to notify the physician
● the importance of maintaining good nutrition and obtaining adequate rest
● appropriate exercises and therapy
● pain reduction measures and relaxation techniques
● available counseling options
● signs and symptoms of complications
● the importance of follow-up care
● the benefit of utilizing available community support groups such as the local chapter of the Reflex Sympathetic Dystrophy Syndrome Association.

Neurologic emergencies and neurologic malignancies

Neurologic emergencies include acceleration-deceleration injury, myelitis, Reye's syndrome, skull fracture, spinal cord injury and traumatic brain injury. Neurologic malignancies include malignant brain tumors and spinal neoplasms.

NEUROLOGIC EMERGENCIES

ACCELERATION-DECELERATION INJURY

An acceleration-deceleration injury results from a sharp hyper-extension and flexion of the neck that damage muscles, ligaments, disks, and nerve tissue. It commonly results from a motor vehicle accident and is also known as *whiplash*. It may also occur from a fall or sports activity. While this type of injury usually has an excellent prognosis, it's a neck injury and carries the risk of paralysis occurring as a complication. Symptoms usually subside with symptomatic treatment. One million cases of whiplash occur each year in the United States. The average age of these patients is the late 40s.

Pathophysiology

Any unexpected force that causes the head to jerk back and then forward may cause the neck bones to snap out of position, causing injury. Irritated nerves can interfere with blood flow and transmission of nerve impulses. Pinched nerves can affect certain body part functions. Usually pain is the result of the injury, with some limitation in neck movement.

Complications

- Temporomandibular joint disorder
- Nerve damage

Assessment findings

- Mechanism of injury identifies acceleration-deceleration action
- Pain initially minimal but increases 12 to 72 hours after the accident
- Dizziness
- Headache
- Back pain
- Shoulder pain
- Vision disturbances
- Tinnitus
- Neck muscle asymmetry
- Reduced neck mobility
- Gait disturbances
- Rigidity or numbness in the arms
- Tenderness at the exact location of the injury
- Decreased active and passive range of motion

Diagnostic test results

- Full cervical spine X-rays rule out cervical fracture.

Treatment

- Until X-rays rule out cervical fracture, treatment focuses on protecting the cervical spine through immobilization. After cervical spine injury has been ruled out, initial treatment includes limited activity during the first 72 hours after the injury, use of a soft cervical collar, and application of ice packs. (See *Using a cervical collar.*) Oral analgesics provide pain relief, and oral corticosteroids help reduce inflammation and relieve chronic discomfort. To restore flexibility,

USING A CERVICAL COLLAR

Cervical collars are used to support an injured or weakened cervical spine and to maintain alignment during healing. The soft cervical color, made of spongy foam, provides gentler support and reminds the patient to avoid cervical spine motion.

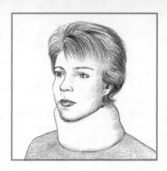

physical therapy, including mobilization exercises, is started 72 hours after the injury. It's combined with the application of moist heat and a gradually decreased use of the soft collar.

- If the patient experiences persistent ligamentous or articular pain, he may benefit from cervical traction and diathermy treatment. Surgical stabilization may be necessary with severe cervical acceleration-deceleration injury.

Nursing interventions

- Maintain spinal immobilization until cervical X-rays are evaluated.
- Protect the patient's spine during all care.
- Give prescribed drugs.
- Apply a soft cervical collar.
- Monitor pain level, administer analgesics as ordered, and evaluate response to medications.
- Observe for signs and symptoms of complications.
- Assess the patient's neurologic status per facility protocol and clinical status.

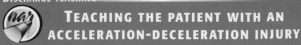

■ Provide appropriate education to the patient before discharge. (See *Teaching the patient with an acceleration-deceleration injury.*)

MYELITIS AND ACUTE TRANSVERSE MYELITIS

Myelitis, or inflammation of the spinal cord, can result from several diseases. Poliomyelitis affects the cord's gray matter and produces motor dysfunction; leukomyelitis affects only the white matter and produces sensory dysfunction.

The prognosis depends on the severity of cord damage and prevention of complications. If spinal cord necrosis occurs, the prognosis for a complete recovery is poor. Even without necrosis, residual neurologic deficits usually persist after recovery. Patients who develop spastic reflexes early in the course of the illness are more likely to recover than those who don't.

Acute transverse myelitis has many causes. It commonly follows acute infectious diseases, such as measles or pneumonia (the inflammation occurs after the infection has subsided), and primary infections of the spinal cord itself, such as syphilis or acute disseminated encephalomyelitis. Acute transverse myelitis may also accompany demyelinating diseases, such as acute multiple sclerosis, and inflammatory and necrotizing disorders of the spinal cord such as hematomyelia.

Such toxic agents as carbon monoxide, lead, and arsenic can cause a type of myelitis in which acute inflammation (followed by hemorrhage and possible necrosis) destroys the entire circumference (myelin, axis cylinders, and neurons) of the spinal cord. Other forms of myelitis may result from poliovirus, herpes zoster, herpesvirus B, or rabies virus; disorders that cause meningeal inflammation, such as syphilis, abscesses, tuberculosis, and other suppurative conditions; smallpox or polio vaccination; parasitic and fungal infections; and chronic adhesive arachnoiditis.

Peak incidence occurs from ages 10 to 19 and then again from ages 30 to 39. About 33,000 Americans have some type of disability from this disorder, with approximately 1,400 new cases diagnosed each year.

Pathophysiology

Myelitis is an inflammation of the spinal cord. Only the cord's gray matter may be affected, producing motor dysfunction, or the white matter may be affected, producing sensory dysfunction. These types of myelitis can attack any level of the spinal cord, causing partial destruction or scattered lesions. Acute transverse myelitis, which affects the entire thickness of the spinal cord, produces motor and sensory dysfunction. It's rapid in onset and is the most devastating form of myelitis.

Complications

- Shock
- Motor impairment
- Sensory impairment

Assessment findings

- Sensory or motor dysfunction, depending on the site of damage to the spinal cord
- Rapid onset with motor and sensory dysfunctions below the level of spinal cord damage appearing in 1 to 2 days
- Flaccid paralysis of the legs (sometimes beginning in just one leg) with loss of sensory and sphincter functions; may follow pain in the legs or trunk
- Absent reflexes in early stages but possibly reappearing in later stages
- Extent of damage dependent on level of the spinal cord affected; transverse myelitis seldom involving the arms; with severe spinal cord damage, shock possible (hypotension and hypothermia)

Diagnostic test results

- Neurologic examination confirms paraplegia or neurologic deficit below the level of the spinal cord lesion and absent (or, in later stages) hyperactive reflexes.
- Cerebrospinal fluid may be normal or show increased lymphocytes or elevated protein levels.
- Magnetic resonance imaging rules out spinal cord tumor.
- Culture specimens identify the cause of any underlying infection.

Treatment

No definitive treatment exists for acute transverse myelitis. Rather, the condition requires appropriate treatment of the underlying infection. Steroid therapy is a possible treatment modality; however, more research is needed to determine its benefits.

Nursing interventions

- Monitor vital signs. Watch carefully for signs of spinal shock (hypotension and excessive sweating).

DISCHARGE TEACHING

TEACHING THE PATIENT WITH MYELITIS

Before discharge, be sure to cover with the patient and his family:
- the disorder and its implications
- medication administration, dosage, and possible adverse effects, and when to notify the physician
- when to report changes in mental status, level of consciousness, or motor ability
- types of therapy that may be beneficial, such as physical therapy, occupational therapy, or counseling
- the importance of maintaining adequate nutrition
- bowel and bladder training
- exercises to maintain or improve muscle tone and function
- signs and symptoms of complications
- the importance of follow-up care
- the benefit of utilizing available community support groups such as the local chapter of the Transverse Myelitis Association.

- Assist with range-of-motion exercises and proper body alignment.
- Reposition the patient every 2 hours, assess his skin condition, and provide appropriate skin care.
- Monitor intake and output.
- Initiate rehabilitation immediately. Assist the patient with physical therapy, bowel and bladder training, and lifestyle changes that his condition requires.
- Provide appropriate education to the patient and his family before discharge. (See *Teaching the patient with myelitis.*)

NEUROLOGIC MALIGNANCIES

BRAIN TUMOR, MALIGNANT

A malignant brain tumor is an abnormal growth of cancerous cells within the intracranial space. The tumor may affect brain tissue, the meninges, the pituitary gland, and blood vessels. In adults, the most common tumor types are gliomas and meningiomas, which usually occur above the covering of the cerebellum, or supratentorial tumors. In children, the most common tumor types are astrocytomas, medulloblastomas, ependymomas, and brain stem gliomas. The exact cause unknown, but risk factors include preexisting cancer, radiation or chemical exposure, and head trauma.

Malignant brain tumors are slightly more common in males than in females and have an overall incidence of 4.5 per 100,000 people. They can occur at any age. In adults, incidence is highest between ages 40 and 60. Most tumors in children occur before age 1 or between ages 2 and 12.

 AGE AWARE Brain tumors are one of the most common causes of cancer death in children.

Pathophysiology
Tumors are classified based on histology or grade of cell malignancy. Central nervous system changes are caused by cancer cells invading and destroying tissues and by compression of the brain, cranial nerves, and cerebral vessels; cerebral edema; and increased intracranial pressure (ICP).

Complications
- Radiation encephalopathy
- Cerebral edema
- Seizures
- Neurologic deficits
- Hydrocephalus
- Brain herniation

LIFE-THREATENING COMPLICATIONS FROM INCREASED ICP
- Coma
- Respiratory or cardiac arrest
- Brain herniation

Assessment findings

- Headache
- Nausea and vomiting
- Signs and symptoms of increased ICP
  - Vision disturbances
  - Weakness, paralysis
  - Aphasia, dysphagia
  - Ataxia, incoordination
  - Seizures (see *Brain tumors: Site-specific signs and symptoms,* pages 346 and 347, and *Assessment findings in malignant brain tumors,* pages 348 to 353)

Diagnostic test results

- Skull X-rays confirm tumor.
- Brain scan confirms tumor.
- Computed tomography scan confirms tumor.
- Magnetic resonance imaging evaluates tumor location, size, and vascularity and cerebral edema.
- Cerebral angiography confirms tumor.
- Positron emission tomography confirms tumor.
- Tissue biopsy confirms the type of tumor.
- Lumbar puncture may show increased cerebrospinal fluid (CSF) pressure, which reflects ICP, increased protein levels, decreased glucose levels and, occasionally, tumor cells in CSF.

Treatment

Specific treatments vary with the tumor's histologic type, radiosensitivity, and location. Such treatments may include surgery, radiation therapy, chemotherapy, and decompression of increased ICP (with diuretics, corticosteroids, or possibly, ventriculoatrial or ventriculoperitoneal shunting of the CSF).

Treatment of a glioma usually consists of resection by craniotomy. Radiation therapy and chemotherapy follow resection. The combination of carmustine (BiCNU), lomustine

(Text continues on page 352.)

BRAIN TUMORS: SITE-SPECIFIC SIGNS AND SYMPTOMS

A brain tumor usually produces signs and symptoms specific to its location. Recognizing the effects helps identify the tumor site and guide treatment before and after surgery and can help you spot life-threatening complications, such as increasing intracranial pressure and imminent brain herniation. A brain tumor may cause all, some, or none of the effects shown here.

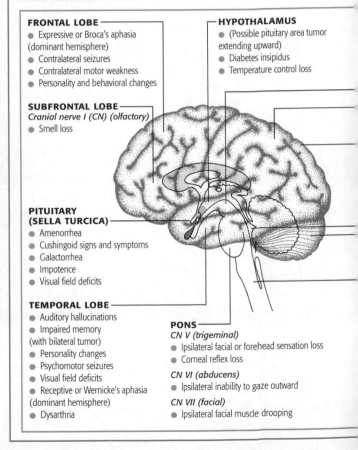

FRONTAL LOBE
- Expressive or Broca's aphasia (dominant hemisphere)
- Contralateral seizures
- Contralateral motor weakness
- Personality and behavioral changes

SUBFRONTAL LOBE
Cranial nerve I (CN) (olfactory)
- Smell loss

PITUITARY (SELLA TURCICA)
- Amenorrhea
- Cushingoid signs and symptoms
- Galactorrhea
- Impotence
- Visual field deficits

TEMPORAL LOBE
- Auditory hallucinations
- Impaired memory (with bilateral tumor)
- Personality changes
- Psychomotor seizures
- Visual field deficits
- Receptive or Wernicke's aphasia (dominant hemisphere)
- Dysarthria

HYPOTHALAMUS
- (Possible pituitary area tumor extending upward)
- Diabetes insipidus
- Temperature control loss

PONS
CN V (trigeminal)
- Ipsilateral facial or forehead sensation loss
- Corneal reflex loss

CN VI (abducens)
- Ipsilateral inability to gaze outward

CN VII (facial)
- Ipsilateral facial muscle drooping

MIDBRAIN
CN III (oculomotor)
- Ptosis
- Diplopia
- Dilated pupil
- Inability to gaze up, down, or in-ward (all ipsilateral)

PARIETAL LOBE
- Dyslexia (left side)
- Position sense loss
- Perceptual problems
- Contralateral sensory disturbances
- Visual field deficits

OCCIPITAL LOBE
- Visual agnosia
(inability to name objects)
- Visual field deficits

CEREBELLOPONTINE ANGLE
CN VII (facial)
- Ipsilateral facial muscle drooping

CN VIII (acoustic)
- Tinnitus
- Hearing loss

MEDULLA
CN IX (glossopharyngeal)
- Difficulty swallowing
CN X (vagus)
- Gag and cough reflex loss
- Difficulty swallowing
- Hoarseness
- Projectile vomiting
CN XI (spinal accessory)
- Inability to shrug shoulders or turn head toward tumor side
CN XII (hypoglossal)
- Tongue protrusion
(deviating toward tumor side)
- Respiratory pattern changes

CEREBELLUM
- Disturbed gait
- Impaired balance
- Incoordination

ASSESSMENT FINDINGS IN MALIGNANT BRAIN TUMORS

TUMOR AND CHARACTERISTICS

GLIOBLASTOMA MULTIFORME (SPONGIOBLASTOMA MULTIFORME)
- Most common; accounts for 60% of all gliomas
- Peak incidence between ages 50 and 60; more common in males than in females
- Unencapsulated, highly malignant; grows rapidly and infiltrates the brain extensively; may become enormous before diagnosed
- Usually occurs in cerebral hemispheres, especially frontal and temporal lobes (rarely in brain stem and cerebellum)
- Occupies more than one lobe of affected hemisphere; may spread to opposite hemisphere by corpus callosum or metastasize into cerebrospinal fluid (CSF), producing tumors in distant parts of the central nervous system (CNS)

ASTROCYTOMA
- Second most common malignant glioma, accounting for 10% of all gliomas
- Occurs at any age; incidence higher in males than in females
- Usually occurs in central and subcortical white matter; may originate in any part of CNS
- Cerebellar astrocytomas usually confined to one hemisphere

OLIGODENDROGLIOMA
- Third most common glioma; accounts for less than 5% of all gliomas
- Occurs in middle adult years; more common in females than in males
- Slow growing

ASSESSMENT FINDINGS

GENERAL
- Increased intracranial pressure (ICP) (nausea, vomiting, headache, papilledema)
- Mental and behavioral changes; speech and sensory disturbances
- Altered vital signs (increased systolic pressure, widened pulse pressure, respiratory changes)
- In children, irritability and projectile vomiting

LOCALIZING
- Midline: headache (bifrontal or bioccipital) that's worse in morning; intensified by coughing, straining, or sudden head movements
- Temporal lobe: psychomotor seizures
- Central region: focal seizures
- Optic and oculomotor nerves: vision deficits
- Frontal lobe: abnormal reflexes and motor responses

GENERAL
- Headache and mental activity changes
- Decreased motor strength and coordination
- Seizures and scanning speech
- Altered vital signs

LOCALIZING
- Third ventricle: changes in mental activity and level of consciousness, nausea, pupillary dilation and sluggish light reflex; paresis or ataxia in later stages of disease
- Brain stem and pons: ipsilateral trigeminal, abducens, and facial nerve palsies in early stages; cerebellar ataxia, tremors, and other cranial nerve deficits as disease progresses
- Third or fourth ventricle or aqueduct of Sylvius: secondary hydrocephalus
- Thalamus or hypothalamus: various endocrine, metabolic, autonomic, and behavioral changes

GENERAL
- Mental and behavioral changes
- Decreased visual acuity and other vision disturbances
- Increased ICP

LOCALIZING
- Temporal lobe: hallucinations and psychomotor seizures
- Central region: seizures (confined to one muscle group or unilateral)

(continued)

ASSESSMENT FINDINGS IN
MALIGNANT BRAIN TUMORS (continued)

TUMOR AND CHARACTERISTICS

OLIGODENDROGLIOMA (continued)

EPENDYMOMA
- Rare glioma
- Most common in children and young adults
- Usually located in fourth and lateral ventricles

MEDULLOBLASTOMA
- Rare glioma
- Most common in children and young adults
- Incidence highest in children ages 4 to 6
- Affects males more than females
- Frequently metastasizes by way of CSF

MENINGIOMA
- Most common nongliomatous brain tumor, constituting 15% of primary brain tumors
- Usually occurs in people in their 50s; rare in children; more common in females than in males (ratio 3:2)
- Arises from the meninges
- Common locations: parasagittal area, sphenoidal ridge, anterior part of base of skull, cerebellopontine angle, and spinal canal
- Benign, well-circumscribed, highly vascular tumor that compresses underlying brain tissue by invading overlying skull

ASSESSMENT FINDINGS

● Midbrain or third ventricle: pyramidal tract symptoms (dizziness, ataxia, paresthesia of face)
● Brain stem and cerebrum: nystagmus, hearing loss, dizziness, ataxia, paresthesia of face, cranial nerve palsies, hemiparesis, suboccipital tenderness, loss of balance

GENERAL
● Increased ICP and obstructive hydrocephalus, depending on tumor size
● Other assessment findings similar to those of oligodendroglioma

GENERAL
● Increased ICP
LOCALIZING
● Brain and cerebrum: papilledema, nystagmus, hearing loss, perception of flashing lights, dizziness, ataxia, paresthesia of face, cranial nerve palsies (V, VI, VII, IX, X, primarily sensory), hemiparesis, suboccipital tenderness; compression of supratentorial area produces other general and focal symptoms

GENERAL
● Headache
● Seizures (in two-thirds of patients)
● Vomiting
● Changes in mental activity
● Other assessment findings similar to those of schwannomas
LOCALIZING
● Skull changes (bony bulge) over tumor
● Sphenoidal ridge, indenting optic nerve: unilateral
● Vision changes and papilledema
● Prefrontal parasagittal: personality and behavioral changes
● Motor cortex: contralateral motor changes
● Anterior fossa compressing both optic nerves and frontal lobes: headaches and bilateral vision loss
● Pressure on cranial nerves, causing varying symptoms

(continued)

ASSESSMENT FINDINGS IN
MALIGNANT BRAIN TUMORS *(continued)*

TUMOR AND CHARACTERISTICS

SCHWANNOMA (ACOUSTIC NEUROMA, NEURILEMOMA, CEREBELLOPONTINE ANGLE TUMOR)

- Accounts for about 10% of all intracranial tumors
- Onset of symptoms between ages 30 and 60; higher incidence in females than in males
- Affects the craniospinal nerve sheath, usually cranial nerve VIII; also, V and VII, and to a lesser extent, VI and X on the same side as tumor
- Benign, but usually classified as malignant because of its growth patterns; slow-growing; may be present for years before symptoms occur

(CeeNU), or procarbazine (Matulane) with radiation therapy is more effective than radiation alone.

For low-grade cystic cerebellar astrocytomas, surgical resection permits long-term survival. For other astrocytomas, treatment consists of repeated surgery, radiation therapy, and shunting of fluid from obstructed CSF pathways. Radiation therapy works best in radiosensitive astrocytomas; some astrocytomas are radioresistant.

Treatment of oligodendrogliomas and ependymomas include surgical resection and radiation therapy. Medulloblastomas call for surgical resection and, possibly, intrathecal infusion of methotrexate (Rheumatrex) or another antineoplastic drug. Meningiomas require surgical resection, including the dura mater and bone.

For schwannomas, microsurgical technique allows complete resection of the tumor and preservation of the facial

ASSESSMENT FINDINGS

GENERAL
- Unilateral hearing loss with or without tinnitus
- Stiff neck and suboccipital discomfort
- Secondary hydrocephalus
- Ataxia and uncoordinated movements of one or both arms due to pressure on brain stem and cerebellum

LOCALIZING
- V: early signs including facial hypoesthesia and paresthesia on the side of hearing loss; unilateral loss of corneal reflex
- VI: diplopia
- VII: paresis progressing to paralysis (Bell's palsy)
- X: weakness of palate, tongue, and nerve muscles on same side as tumor

nerve. Although schwannomas are moderately radioresistant, treatment still calls for postoperative radiation therapy.

Chemotherapy for malignant brain tumors includes the nitrosoureas that help break down the blood-brain barrier and allow other chemotherapeutic drugs to go through as well. Intrathecal and intra-arterial administration of drugs maximizes drug action.

Palliative measures for gliomas, astrocytomas, oligodendrogliomas, and ependymomas include dexamethasone (Decadron) for cerebral edema; osmotic diuretics, such as urea and mannitol, to reduce brain swelling; analgesics to control pain; and antacids and histamine-2 receptor antagonists for stress ulcers. These tumors and schwannomas may also require anticonvulsants, such as phenytoin (Dilantin) to prevent seizures.

Before discharge, be sure to cover with the patient and his family:
● the disorder and its implications
● medication administration, dosage, and possible adverse effects, and when to notify the physician
● the importance of good nutrition
● signs of infection or bleeding that may result from chemotherapy
● adverse effects of chemotherapy and other treatments and actions that may alleviate them
● physical and cognitive limitations that may occur
● seizure precautions
● early signs of tumor recurrence
● wound care
● types of therapy that would be beneficial, such as physical therapy, speech therapy, and occupational therapy
● signs and symptoms of complications, espically increased intracranial pressure and infection
● information regarding end-of-life care, such as advance directives and hospice
● the importance of follow-up care
● the benefit of available community support groups such as the local chapter of the National Brain Tumor Foundation.

Nursing interventions

■ Maintain a patent airway.
■ Document the occurrence, nature, and duration of seizure activity.
■ Take steps to protect the patient's safety.
■ Give prescribed drugs and note any adverse reactions.
■ Monitor for changes in the patient's neurologic status and observe for signs of increased ICP.
■ Monitor vital signs and pulse oximetry. Note changes in respiratory status and temperature.
■ After supratentorial craniotomy, elevate the head of the bed about 30 degrees.

- After infratentorial craniotomy, keep the patient flat for 48 hours.
- Monitor ICP and cerebral perfusion pressures, and provide measures to maintain adequate readings.
- Monitor head dressings and provide wound care.
- As appropriate, instruct the patient to avoid Valsalva's maneuver and isometric muscle contractions when moving or sitting up in bed.
- Consult with occupational, speech, and physical therapists.
- Provide emotional support to the patient and his family. Encourage them to talk about their concerns. Listen carefully and answer their questions honestly and completely.
- Provide appropraite education to the patient and his family before discharge. (See *Teaching the patient with a malignant brain tumor.*)

REYE'S SYNDROME

Reye's syndrome is an acute childhood illness that causes fatty infiltration of the liver with concurrent hyperammonemia, encephalopathy, and increased intracranial pressure (ICP). Reye's syndrome affects children from infancy to adolescence and occurs equally in boys and girls. It affects whites older than age 1 more often than it does blacks.

Reye's syndrome almost always follows within 1 to 3 days of an acute viral infection, such as an upper respiratory tract infection, type B influenza, or varicella (chickenpox).

The prognosis depends on the severity of central nervous system depression. Previously, mortality was as high as 90%. Today, however, increased awareness of Reye's syndrome, early detection, and prompt, aggressive treatment have reduced mortality to about 5%. Death is usually a result of cerebral edema or respiratory arrest. Most comatose patients who survive have some residual brain damage, such as developmental and neuropsychological difficulties.

The cause of Reye's syndrome is unknown, but viral and toxic agents, especially salicylates, have been implicated. Studies have demonstrated a link between aspirin administration during a viral infection and onset of Reye's syndrome. For this reason, use of aspirin in children younger than age 15 is prohibited. Incidence of Reye's syndrome has decreased dramatically because parents know to give their children acetaminophen (Tylenol) instead of aspirin for flulike symptoms or fever.

Pathophysiology
Damaged hepatic mitochondria disrupt the urea cycle, which normally changes ammonia to urea for its excretion. This disruption results in hyperammonemia, hypoglycemia, and an increase in serum short-chain fatty acids, leading to encephalopathy. As the ammonia level increases, the brain, a secondary site of urea metabolism, swells markedly. At the same time, fatty infiltration occurs in renal tubular cells, neuronal tissue, and muscle tissue, including the heart.

Complications
- Increased ICP
- Brain damage
- Coma

Assessment findings
The severity of signs and symptoms varies with the degree of encephalopathy and cerebral edema, but may include:
- history of recent viral infection
- intractable vomiting
- progressive changes in level of consciousness, from drowsiness and lethargy to stupor and coma
- low-grade fever or normal temperature
- slight tachycardia, rapid respirations
- diaphoresis
- agitated, confused, or combative behavior
- hyperreflexia.

Diagnostic test results

- Serum ammonia levels are elevated, serum glucose levels are normal or low (in 15% of cases), and serum fatty acid and lactate levels are increased.
- Liver function studies indicate aspartate aminotransferase and alanine aminotransferase at twice the normal levels.
- Coagulation studies demonstrate increased prothrombin time and partial thromboplastin time.
- Liver biopsy reveals fatty droplets uniformly distributed throughout liver cells.
- Cerebrospinal fluid analysis shows a white blood cell count of less than 10/μl.

Treatment

Treatment must be started as soon as Reye's syndrome is diagnosed because the disease progresses rapidly. Initially, therapy consists of I.V. administration of glucose to prevent the onset of coma. Other treatments include airway maintenance, adequate oxygenation, and control of cerebral edema. (See *Reye's syndrome: Stages and treatment*, pages 358 and 359.)

Nursing interventions

- Provide emotional and psychological support to the child, as appropriate, and his family. Listen to their concerns, and stay with them during periods of acute stress.
- Monitor the patient's vital signs and neurologic status.
- Assist with endotracheal intubation and mechanical ventilation, as indicated.
- Elevate the head of the bed 30 degrees (if the patient's blood pressure tolerates it) to increase venous outflow and decrease ICP.
- Monitor ICP and report changes.
- Monitor the patient's cardiovascular status with a pulmonary artery catheter or central venous line.

(Text continues on page 360.)

REYE'S SYNDROME: STAGES AND TREATMENT

Each stage of Reye's syndrome produces its own set of signs and symptoms that require appropriate medical treatment and nursing interventions, as outlined here.

SIGNS AND SYMPTOMS	TREATMENT
STAGE I Vomiting, lethargy, hepatic dysfunction	● Give glucose I.V. to help reduce the risk of coma. ● Give I.V. fluids at two-thirds of maintenance dose and an osmotic diuretic or furosemide (Lasix) to decrease intracranial pressure (ICP) and cerebral edema. ● Give vitamin K to decrease hypoprothrombinemia; if unsuccessful, give fresh frozen plasma.
STAGE II Hyperventilation, delirium, hepatic dysfunction, hyperactive reflexes	● Continue baseline treatment.
STAGE III Coma, hyperventilation, decorticate rigidity, hepatic dysfunction	● Continue baseline treatment and supportive care. ● Monitor ICP with a subarachnoid screw or other invasive device. ● Perform endotracheal intubation, and institute ventilation to control $Paco_2$ levels. Administering a paralyzing agent, such as vecuronium (Norcuron) I.V., may help maintain ventilation. ● Administer mannitol (Osmitrol) I.V., thiopental (Sodium Pentalhol) I.V., or glycerol by NG tube to help control ICP.
STAGE IV Deepening coma; decerebrate rigidity; large, fixed pupils; minimal hepatic dysfunction	● Continue baseline treatment and supportive care. ● If all previous measures fail, some pediatric centers use barbiturate coma, decompressive craniotomy, hypothermia, or exchange transfusion.
STAGE V Seizures, loss of deep tendon reflexes, flaccidity, respiratory arrest, ammonia level greater than 300 mg/dl	● Continue baseline and supportive care. The prognosis is poor at this stage; usually the child doesn't recover.

NURSING INTERVENTIONS

● Obtain serum ammonia, blood glucose, and plasma osmolality values every 4 to 8 hours to monitor patient progress.
● Monitor fluid intake and output to prevent fluid overload. Maintain urine output at 1 ml/kg/hour, plasma osmolality at 290 mOsm/kg, and blood glucose level at 150 mg/dl. (Goal: Keep glucose levels high, osmolality normal to high, and ammonia levels low.) Restrict protein intake.

● Institute seizure precautions.
● Watch closely for signs of coma that require invasive supportive therapy such as intubation.
● Keep head of bed at 30 degrees.

● Continue seizure precautions.
● Monitor ICP (should be < 20 mm Hg before suctioning).
● When ventilating the patient, maintain $Paco_2$ between 20 and 30 mm Hg and partial pressure of arterial oxygen between 80 and 100 mm Hg.
● Insert a pulmonary artery catheter or central venous pressure catheter to monitor cardio-vascular status.
● Provide good skin and mouth care, and perform range-of-motion exercises.

● Check the patient for loss of reflexes and signs of flaccidity.
● Give the family the extra support they need, considering their child's poor prognosis.

● Help the family face the patient's impending death.

DISCHARGE TEACHING

TEACHING THE PATIENT WITH REYE'S SYNDROME

Before discharge, be sure to cover with the child and his parents:
- the disorder and its implications
- medication administration, dosage, and possible adverse effects, and when to notify the physician
- using nonsalicylate analgesics and antipyretics such as acetaminophen (Tylenol)
- when to report changes in mental status, level of consciousness, or motor ability
- types of therapy that may be beneficial, such as physical therapy, occupational therapy, or counseling
- the importance of maintaining adequate nutrition
- exercises to maintain or improve muscle tone and function
- signs and symptoms of complications
- the importance of follow-up care
- the benefit of utilizing available community support groups such as the local chapter of the National Reye's Syndrome Foundation.

- Administer ordered I.V. fluids and medications as directed. Monitor the child for the desired effect. As ordered, give mannitol (Osmitrol) I.V., thiopental (Sodium Pentothal) I.V., or glycerol by nasogastric tube to control ICP.
- Maintain seizure precautions during the acute stage; seizures may occur at any time.
- Provide good skin care and perform range-of-motion exercises.
- Provide appropriate education to the child and his parents befoe discharge. (See *Teaching the patient with Reye's syndrome*.)

SKULL FRACTURE

A skull fracture is a break in the integrity of the skull bone. The first concern in a skull fracture is possible damage to the brain rather than the fracture itself; therefore, the injury is considered a neurologic emergency. Signs and symptoms reflect the severity and extent of the head injury.

A skull fracture may be simple (closed) or compound (open). It may also displace bone fragments. It may be linear (common hairline break, without displacement of structures), comminuted (splintering or crushing the bone into several fragments), or depressed (a fracture that pushes the bone toward the brain. It's classified according to location, such as cranial vault fracture and basilar fracture. A basilar skull fracture ocurrs at the base of the skull and involves the cribriform plate and frontal sinuses.

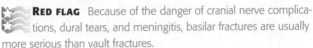 **RED FLAG** Because of the danger of cranial nerve complications, dural tears, and meningitis, basilar fractures are usually more serious than vault fractures.

Like concussions and cerebral contusions or lacerations, skull fractures invariably result from a traumatic blow to the head. Motor vehicle accidents, bad falls, and physical abuse or altercations (especially in children and elderly people) are among the most common causes of skull fracture.

A simple linear skull fracture is the most common type, especially in children younger than age 5.

Pathophysiology

With a skull fracture, trauma to the head causes a break at certain anatomic sites, such as:

- parietal bone
- squama of temporal bone
- foramen magnum
- petrous temporal ridge
- inner parts of the sphenoid wings at the skull base
- middle cranial fossa
- cribriform plate
- roof of orbits in the anterior cranial fossa
- bony areas between the mastoid and dural sinuses in the posterior cranial fossa. (See *Additional findings with skull fractures,* page 362.)

ADDITIONAL FINDINGS WITH SKULL FRACTURES

When jagged bone fragments pierce the dura mater of the cerebral cortex, skull fractures can cause subdural, epidural, or intracerebral hemorrhage or hematoma. Clinical findings caused by the resulting lesions may include hemiparesis, unequal pupils, dizziness, seizures, projectile vomiting, increased pulse and respiratory rates, and progressive unresponsiveness.

A sphenoidal fracture can damage the optic nerve, causing blindness. A temporal fracture may cause unilateral deafness or facial paralysis. A basilar skull fracture commonly produces hemorrhage from the nose, pharynx, or ears; blood under the periorbital skin (raccoon eyes) and under the conjunctiva; and Battle's sign (supermastoid ecchymosis), sometimes with bleeding behind the eardrum. Basilar skull fractures can cause cerebrospinal fluid or brain tissue to leak from the nose or ears.

Elderly patients may have cortical brain atrophy, which leaves more space for brain swelling under the cranium. Consequently, such patients may not show signs of increased intracranial pressure until the pressure is very high.

Complications
- Epilepsy
- Hydrocephalus
- Organic brain syndrome
- Headaches, giddiness, fatigability, neuroses, and behavior disorders
- Respiratory failure

Assessment findings
- History of head trauma
- Headache
- Loss of consciousness
- Decreased pulse and respirations
- Altered level of consciousness
- Scalp wound
- Bleeding in the periorbital area, nose, pharynx, ears, or under the conjunctivae

- Cerebrospinal fluid (CSF) leakage from the nose or ears; halo sign on pillowcase (a blood-tinged spot surrounded by a lighter ring)

Diagnostic test results
- Reagent strips turn blue if CSF is present.
- Computed tomography scan and magnetic resonance imaging show fracture, intracranial hemorrhage from ruptured blood vessels, and swelling.

Treatment
Treatment of a skull fracture is based on the type and severity of the fracture. Although a simple linear skull fracture can tear an underlying blood vessel or cause a CSF leak, most linear fractures require only supportive treatment. Such treatment includes mild analgesics (acetaminophen [Tylenol]) as well as cleaning, debriding, and suturing the wound after injection of a local anesthetic. Be sure to note the patient's coagulation time if he's taking anticoagulants at home. An increased International Normalized Ratio may necessitate treatment with fresh frozen plasma.

If the patient hasn't lost consciousness, he should be observed in the emergency department for at least 4 hours. After this time, a patient with stable vital signs can be discharged and observed at home.

More severe vault fractures, especially depressed fractures, usually require a craniotomy to elevate or remove fragments that have been driven into the brain and to extract foreign bodies and necrotic tissue. This reduces the risk of infection and further brain injury. Cranioplasty follows the use of tantalum mesh or acrylic plates to replace the removed skull section. The patient usually requires antibiotices, tetanus prophylaxis, and (with profound hemorrhage) blood transfusions. The patient may require a sedative, such as lorazepam (Ativan), to help reduce seizures, or an anticonvulsant may be required.

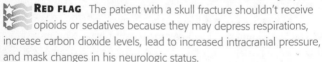

DISCHARGE TEACHING

TEACHING THE PATIENT WITH A SKULL FRACTURE

Before discharge, be sure to cover with the patient and his family:
● the disorder and its implications
● medication administration, dosage, and possible adverse effects, and when to notify the physician
● wound care
● activity restrictions
● signs and symptoms of complications
● the importance of follow-up care
● the benefit of available community support groups such as the local chapter of the Brain Injury Association of America.

A basilar fracture calls for immediate prophylactic antibiotics to prevent meningitis from CSF leaks. The patient also needs close observation for secondary hematomas and hemorrhages; surgery may be necessary. Also, a patient with either a basilar or a vault fracture requires I.V. dexamethasone (Decadron) to reduce cerebral edema and minimize brain injury.

RED FLAG The patient with a skull fracture shouldn't receive opioids or sedatives because they may depress respirations, increase carbon dioxide levels, lead to increased intracranial pressure, and mask changes in his neurologic status.

Nursing interventions
■ Establish and maintain a patent airway.

RED FLAG Nasal airways are contraindicated in patients with possible basilar skull fractures. Intubation may be necessary.

■ Suction through the mouth, not the nose, to prevent the introduction of bacteria.
■ Position the patient with a head injury for proper secretion drainage. Elevate the head of the bed 30 degrees if intracerebral injury is suspected.
■ Apply appropriate dressings; control bleeding as necessary.

- Institute seizure precautions.
- Monitor the patient's vital signs, neurologic status, and comfort level.
- Provide appropriate education to the patient before discharge. (See *Teaching the patient with a skull fracture*.)

SPINAL CORD INJURY

Usually the result of trauma to the head or neck, spinal cord injuries (SCIs) include fractures, contusions, and compressions of the vertebral column. SCIs most commonly occur at T12, L1, or C5, C6, or C7.

The prognosis for a patient with an SCI depends on the degree and location of injury, although many patients eventually regain some degree of independence. Morbidity most commonly results from pulmonary or renal complications such as infection.

Most serious SCIs are caused by motor vehicle accidents, falls, diving into shallow water, and gunshot wounds. Less serious injuries result from lifting heavy objects and minor falls. SCIs may also result from hyperparathyroidism and neoplastic lesions.

Approximately 10,000 people suffer SCIs each year; most are males ages 18 to 25.

Pathophysiology

SCI occurs from acceleration, deceleration, or other deforming forces, usually applied from a distance. Mechanisms involved with SCI include:

- hyperextension from acceleration-deceleration forces and sudden reduction in the anteroposterior diameter of the spinal cord
- hyperflexion from sudden and excessive force, propelling the neck forward or causing an exaggerated movement to one side

- vertical compression from force applied from the top of the cranium along the vertical axis through the vertebra
- rotational forces from twisting, which adds shearing forces.

The spinal cord is an important neurologic structure that plays a major role in nerve impulse transmission. Depending on the severity and location of the injury, effects can be widespread.

SCI causes microscopic hemorrhages in the gray matter and pia arachnoid. The hemorrhages gradually enlarge until the gray matter is completely filled with blood, which causes necrosis. From the gray matter, the blood enters the white matter, where it impedes the circulation within the spinal cord. Ensuing edema causes compression and decreases the blood supply; thus, the spinal cord loses perfusion and becomes ischemic. Edema and hemorrhage are greatest approximately two segments above and below the injury. Edema temporarily adds to the patient's dysfunction by also increasing pressure and compressing the nerves.

While edema builds up in the white matter, an inflammatory reaction prevents restoration of circulation in the gray matter. Phagocytes appear at the injury site within 36 to 48 hours after the injury, macrophages engulf degenerating axons, and collagen replaces normal tissue. Scarring and meningeal thickening leave the nerves in the area blocked or tangled.

Complications
- Paralysis
- Death
- Autonomic dysreflexia, spinal shock, and neurogenic shock (see *Spinal shock, neurogenic shock, and autonomic dysreflexia*)

Assessment findings
Assessment findings vary depending on the type, location, and degree of injury. (See *Types of spinal cord injury*, pages 368 to 371.)

SPINAL SHOCK, NEUROGENIC SHOCK, AND AUTONOMIC DYSREFLEXIA

Spinal shock

Spinal shock is the loss of autonomic, reflex, motor, and sensory activity below the level of the cord lesion. Signs include flaccid paralysis, loss of deep tendon and perianal reflexes, and loss of motor and sensory function. Until resolution (1 to 6 weeks after the injury is sustained), the extent of cord damage can't be assessed. The return of reflex activity heralds the resolution of spinal shock.

Neurogenic shock

Neurogenic shock is the loss of autonomic function below the level of injury, producing orthostatic hypotension, bradycardia, and loss of the ability to sweat below the level of the lesion. This abnormal vasomotor response occurs secondary to the disruption of sympathetic impulses from the brain stem to the thoracolumbar area. It's most commonly seen in cervical cord injury.

Autonomic dysreflexia

Autonomic dysreflexia, also known as *autonomic hyperreflexia,* is a serious condition that occurs after spinal shock with lesions at T5 or above. Symptoms include cold or goose-fleshed skin below the lesion level, bradycardia, hypertension, and severe pounding headache. The cause may be a noxious stimulus, such as a distended bladder or skin lesion. Rapid identification and removal of the stimulus may eliminate the need for pharmacologic treatment for headache and hypertension.

- History of trauma, a neoplastic lesion, an infection that could produce a spinal abscess, or an endocrine disorder
- Muscle spasm and back or neck pain that worsens with movement; in cervical fractures, pain that causes point tenderness; in dorsal and lumbar fractures, pain that may radiate to other areas such as the legs
- Mild paresthesia to tetraplegia and shock; in milder injury, symptoms that may be delayed several days or weeks
- Surface wounds that occurred with the spinal injury
- Pain
- Loss of sensation

(Text continues on page 370.)

TYPES OF SPINAL CORD INJURY

Injury to the spinal cord can be classified as complete or incomplete. An incomplete spinal injury may be a central cord syndrome, an anterior cord syndrome, or Brown-Séquard syndrome, depending on the area of the cord affected. This chart highlights the characteristic signs and symptoms of each.

TYPE

COMPLETE TRANSSECTION

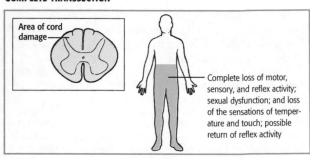

Area of cord damage

Complete loss of motor, sensory, and reflex activity; sexual dysfunction; and loss of the sensations of temperature and touch; possible return of reflex activity

INCOMPLETE TRANSSECTION: CENTRAL CORD SYNDROME

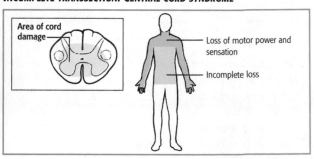

Area of cord damage

Loss of motor power and sensation

Incomplete loss

DESCRIPTION	SIGNS AND SYMPTOMS
● All tracts of the spinal cord completely disrupted ● All functions involving the spinal cord below the level of transsection lost ● Complete and permanent loss	● Loss of motor function (quadriplegia) with cervical cord transsection; paraplegia with thoracic cord transsection ● Muscle flaccidity ● Loss of all reflexes and sensory function below the level of the injury ● Bladder and bowel atony ● Paralytic ileus ● Loss of vasomotor tone in lower body parts with low and unstable blood pressure ● Loss of perspiration below the level of the injury ● Dry, pale skin ● Respiratory impairment
● Center portion of cord affected ● Typically from hyperextension injury	● Motor deficits greater in upper than lower extremities ● Variable degree of bladder dysfunction

TYPES OF SPINAL CORD INJURY *(continued)*

TYPE

INCOMPLETE TRANSSECTION: ANTERIOR CORD SYNDROME

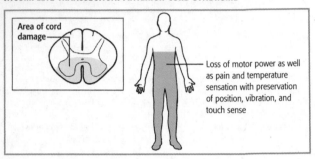

Area of cord damage

Loss of motor power as well as pain and temperature sensation with preservation of position, vibration, and touch sense

INCOMPLETE TRANSSECTION: BROWN-SÉQUARD SYNDROME

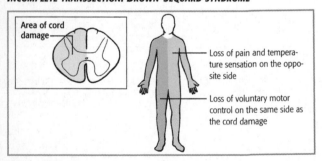

Area of cord damage

Loss of pain and temperature sensation on the opposite side

Loss of voluntary motor control on the same side as the cord damage

Diagnostic test results

■ Spinal X-rays, the most important diagnostic measure, detect the fracture.

■ Myelography, magnetic resonance imaging (MRI), and computed tomography (CT) scans locate the fracture and site of the compression. MRI or CT scans also reveal spinal cord edema and may reveal a spinal mass.

DESCRIPTION	SIGNS AND SYMPTOMS
● Occlusion of anterior spinal artery ● Occlusion from pressure of bone fragments	● Loss of motor function below the level of the injury ● Loss of pain and temperature sensations below the level of the injury ● Intact touch, pressure, position, and vibration senses
● Hemisection of cord affected ● Most common in stabbing and gunshot wounds ● Damage to cord on only one side	● Ipsilateral paralysis or paresis below the level of the injury ● Ipsilateral loss of touch, pressure, vibration, and position sense below the level of the injury ● Contralateral loss of pain and temperature sensations below the level of the injury

Adapted with permission from Hickey, J.V. *The Clinical Practice of Neurological and Neurosurgical Nursing,* 5th ed. Philadelphia: Lippincott Williams & Wilkins, 2003.

- Neurologic evaluation locates the level of injury and detects cord damage.
- Lumbar puncture may show increased cerebrospinal fluid pressure from a lesion or trauma in spinal compression.

Treatment

Initial treatment involves ensuring the patient's airway, breathing, and circulation and immobilizing him to stabilize his spine and prevent spinal cord damage.

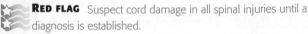 **RED FLAG** If the patient isn't intubated when admitted to the emergency department, hemorrhage and edema at the injury site can increase cord damage and lead to a higher level of dysfunction and altered respiratory function, necessitating mechanical ventilation. If the patient requires intubation and a cervical spine injury hasn't been ruled out, hyperextension of his neck is contraindicated. Perform nasal intubation or orotracheal intubation with the cervical spine immobilized manually.

Cervical injuries require immobilization using a hard cervical collar, skeletal traction with skull tongs, or a halo device. An unstable dorsal or lumbar fracture may be treated with a plaster cast, a turning frame and, in severe fracture, laminectomy and spinal fusion.

Surgery may be necessary to relieve pressure causing compression of the spinal column. Chemotherapy and radiation may be needed if spinal compression is caused by a neoplastic lesion. Methylprednisolone (Solu-Medrol) is administered to reduce inflammation. Assistive devices may be needed based on residual deficits.

Nursing interventions

■ Monitor the patient's vital signs and neurologic status. Maintain cervical immobility until cleared by a physician.

RED FLAG Suspect cord damage in all spinal injuries until a diagnosis is established.

■ Administer I.V. methylprednisolone to reduce inflammation. (Doses given in the first 3 hours appear to be most effective.)

■ Provide wound care and tetanus prophylaxis unless the patient has recently been immunized for surface wounds that may accompany the SCI.

- Perform a neurologic assessment to establish a baseline, including level of consciousness (LOC) and motor and sensory function. Continually assess the patient's LOC for changes, such as increasing restlessness or anxiety.
- Frequently assess the patient's respiratory status—at least every hour, initially. Establish baseline parameters for tidal volume, vital capacity, negative inspiratory forces, and minute volume. Auscultate lung sounds and monitor oxygen saturation levels.
- Assess cardiac function at least every hour, initially, including continuous cardiac, blood pressure, and hemodynamic monitoring, if indicated.

RED FLAG Loss of vascular motor control below the level of the SCI leads to hypotension, causing vasodilation and relative hypovolemia. Orthostatic hypotension may occur in a patient with an SCI to the cervical or high thoracic area. This sudden drop in blood pressure could lead to cerebral hypoxia and loss of consciousness. To prevent orthostatic hypotension, change the patient's position slowly and perform range-of-motion (ROM) exercises every 2 hours.

- Assess GI functioning for indications of ulceration, bleeding, abdominal distention, or decreased peristalsis. Paralytic ileus is a common problem for patients with SCI, usually occurring within the first 72 hours after the injury.
- Assess urinary output hourly during the initial period, reporting urine output less than 0.5 ml/kg/hour for 2 consecutive hours.
- Assess the patient frequently for signs and symptoms of autonomic dysreflexia. Be alert for throbbing headache, cutaneous vasodilation, and sweating above the level of the injury; sudden severe elevation in blood pressure; and piloerection, pallor, chills, and vasoconstriction below the level of injury.

RED FLAG If the patient develops signs and symptoms of autonomic dysreflexia, immediately elevate the head of the bed, monitor his blood pressure and heart rate every 3 to 5 minutes, and determine the underlying stimulus for the event (for example, a

DISCHARGE TEACHING

TEACHING THE PATIENT WITH A SPINAL CORD INJURY

Before discharge, be sure to cover with the patient and his family:
- the injury and its implications
- medication administration, dosage, and possible adverse effects, and when to notify the physician
- when to report changes in mental status, level of consciousness, or motor ability
- types of therapy that may be beneficial, such as physical therapy, occupational therapy, or counseling
- the importance of maintaining adequate nutrition
- exercises to maintain or improve muscle tone and function
- signs and symptoms of complications
- the importance of follow-up care
- the benefit of utilizing available community support groups such as the local chapter of the National Spinal Cord Injury Association.

blocked catheter, fecal impaction, or urinary tract infection) and re-move or correct it. Administer antihypertensive agents.

- Provide good skin care and perform ROM exercises; initiate rehabilitation measures as soon as possible.
- Provide appropriate education to the patient and his family before discharge. (See *Teaching the patient with a spinal cord injury.*)

SPINAL NEOPLASMS

Spinal neoplasms are similar to intracranial tumors but involve the spinal cord or its roots. Untreated spinal neoplasms can eventually cause paralysis. As primary tumors, they originate in the meningeal coverings, the parenchyma of the cord or its roots, the intraspinal vasculature, or the vertebrae. They can also occur as metastatic foci from primary tumors.

Little is known about the cause of spinal tumors. They have been associated with central von Recklinghausen's disease.

Spinal cord tumors are rare compared with intracranial tumors (ratio of 1:4). They occur with equal frequency in males and females, except for meningiomas, which are more common in females. Spinal cord tumors can grow anywhere along the cord or its roots. The prognosis depends on tumor control and the extent of residual neurologic deficit.

Pathophysiology

Primary tumors of the spinal cord may be extramedullary (occurring outside the spinal cord) or intramedullary (occurring within the cord itself). Extramedullary tumors may be intradural (meningiomas and schwannomas), which account for 60% of all primary malignant spinal cord neoplasms, or extradural (metastatic tumors from breasts, lungs, prostate, leukemia, or lymphomas), which account for 25% of these malignant neoplasms.

Intramedullary tumors, or gliomas (astrocytomas or ependymomas), are comparatively rare, accounting for only about 10%. In children, they're low-grade astrocytomas.

Complications

- Motor and sensory deficits
- Loss of sphincter control
- Bowel and bladder dysfunction
- Complications of immobility

Assessment findings

- Pain over the tumor site and radiating around the trunk or down the limb on the affected side
- Constipation
- Difficulty emptying the bladder or changes in the urinary stream
- Urine retention
- Symmetrical spastic weakness
- Decreased muscle tone
- Exaggerated reflexes
- Positive Babinski's sign

- Muscle wasting
- Contralateral loss of sensation to pain, temperature, and touch (Brown-Sequard syndrome)
- Paresthesia in the nerve pathway of the involved roots

Diagnostic test results

- Lumbar puncture reveals clear yellow cerebrospinal fluid (CSF) from increased protein levels if the flow is completely blocked.
- Papanicolaou test of CSF may show malignant cells of metastatic carcinoma.
- X-rays show distortion of the intervertebral foramina, changes in the vertebrae or collapsed areas in the vertebral body, and localized enlargement of the spinal canal.
- Myelography identifies the lesion's level and anatomic relation to the cord and dura.
- Radioisotope bone scan demonstrates metastatic invasion of the vertebrae.
- Computed tomography scanning and magnetic resonance imaging show cord compression and tumor location.
- Biopsy identifies tissue type.

Treatment

Spinal cord tumors are treated with decompression or radiation. Not usually indicated for metastatic tumors, laminectomy may be done for primary tumors that produce spinal cord or cauda equina compression. If the tumor progresses slowly or if it's treated before the cord degenerates from compression, signs and symptoms are likely to subside and function may be restored.

In a patient with metastatic carcinoma or lymphoma who suddenly experiences complete transverse myelitis with spinal shock, functional improvement is unlikely, even with treatment. The prognosis is poor.

If the patient has partial paraplegia of rapid onset, emergency surgical decompression may save cord function. Steroid therapy may minimize cord edema until the patient has surgery.

Partial removal of intramedullary gliomas, followed by radiation therapy, may temporarily ease signs and symptoms. Metastatic extradural tumors can be controlled with radiation therapy, analgesics and, in hormone-mediated tumors (breast and prostate), appropriate hormone therapy.

Transcutaneous electrical nerve stimulation may relieve radicular pain from spinal cord tumors and is a useful alternative to opioid analgesics.

Nursing interventions

- Perform a neurologic assessment to establish a baseline, including level of consciousness (LOC) and motor and sensory function. Continually assess the patient's LOC for changes, such as increasing restlessness or anxiety.
- Monitor the patient's respiratory status, especially if the spinal lesion involves the upper vertebrae.
- Monitor intake and output. Insert a urinary catheter if urine retention occurs.
- Monitor vital signs and pulse oximetry.
- Take steps to protect the patient's safety.
- Give prescribed drugs and note any adverse reactions.
- Monitor for changes in the patient's neurologic status and observe for signs of increased intracranial pressure.
- Monitor dressings if surgery was performed, and provide wound care.
- Assist with active and passive range-of-motion exercises.
- Reposition the patient every 2 hours and provide skin care.
- Consult with occupational, speech, and physical therapists.
- Assist with the application of a back brace, if ordered.
- Provide emotional support to the patient and his family. Encourage them to talk about their concerns. Listen carefully and answer their questions honestly and completely.

DISCHARGE TEACHING

TEACHING THE PATIENT WITH A SPINAL NEOPLASM

Before discharge, be sure to cover with the patient and his family:
- the disorder and its implications
- medication administration, dosage and possible adverse effects, and when to notify the physician
- the importance of good nutrition
- signs of infection or bleeding that may result from chemotherapy
- adverse effects of chemotherapy and other treatments and actions that may alleviate them
- physical limitations that may occur
- proper application and use of a back brace, if ordered
- how to prevent complications from immobility
- early signs of tumor recurrence
- wound and skin care
- types of therapy that would be beneficial, such as physical therapy, speech therapy, and occupational therapy
- signs and symptoms of complications, espically respiratory failure and infection
- information regarding end-of-life care, such as advance directives and hospice
- the importance of follow-up care
- the benefit of available community support groups such as the local chapter of the American Cancer Society.

■ Provide appropriate education to the patient and his family before discharge. (See *Teaching the patient with a spinal neoplasm.*)

TRAUMATIC BRAIN INJURY

A traumatic brain injury is an insult to the brain resulting in physical, cognitive, or vocational impairment. Children ages 6 months to 2 years, those ages 15 to 24, and elderly people are at highest risk for traumatic brain injury. Men are twice as likely as women to experience traumatic brain injury.

Traumatic brain injury commonly results from:

- transportation or motor vehicle accidents (most common cause)
- falls
- sports-related accidents
- assault.

Pathophysiology

Traumatic brain injuries are classified as closed or open, depending on whether the cranial vault—the protective structure consisting of hair, skin, bone, meninges, and cerebrospinal fluid (CSF)—is breached. Closed trauma, the most common type of brain injury, typically results from acceleration-deceleration (also called *coup-contrecoup*). Forceful impact between the head and a stationary object causes the brain to strike the skull, injuring cranial tissues near the point of contact (coup). Residual force then causes the brain to rebound, driving it against the opposite side of the skull (contrecoup). Although the brain isn't exposed in closed trauma injuries, contusions and lacerations may occur as brain tissues slide over the rough bone of the cranial cavity. Diffuse axonal injury (or shearing) also occurs, damaging and severing connections between neurons.

In open trauma injuries, the cranial vault and dura are breached and brain tissues are exposed. Open trauma may result from impact (for example, in a fall or motor vehicle accident) or penetration (for example, by a knife or bullet). Open brain injuries are typically associated with skull fractures; bone fragments commonly cause hematomas and meningeal tears with consequent loss of CSF. The patient with an open trauma brain injury is also at high risk for infection.

 RED FLAG All patients with head injuries must be presumed to have spine injury until X-rays have shown otherwise.

Complications

- Intracranial hemorrhage or hematoma
- Tentorial herniation
- Residual headache

- Cerebral edema
- Infection
- Impaired physical or mental function
- Depression
- Complications from immobility
- Death

Assessment findings

Assessment findings vary, depending on the type and location of the head injury. Types of head injury include concussion, epidural hematoma, subdural hematoma, intracerebral hematoma, and skull fractures. (See *Types of brain injury,* pages 382 to 387.)

- History of traumatic injury (obtained from the patient, his family, eyewitnesses, or emergency personnel) to the head, possibly followed by a period of unconsciousness
- Altered level of consciousness (LOC) ranging from drowsy or easily disturbed by any form of stimulation (such as noise or light) to unconsciousness

Diagnostic test results

- Skull X-rays locate a fracture, if present, unless the fracture occurs in the cranial vault. (These fractures aren't visible or palpable.)
- Cerebral angiography locates vascular disruptions from internal pressure or injuries due to cerebral contusion or skull fracture.
- Computed tomography scan reveals intracranial hemorrhage from ruptured blood vessels, ischemic or necrotic tissue, cerebral edema, areas of petechial hemorrhage, a shift in brain tissue, and subdural, epidural, and intracerebral hematomas.
- Magnetic resonance imaging and a radioisotope scan may also show intracranial hemorrhage from ruptured blood vessels in a patient with a skull fracture.

Treatment

Immediate treatment may include establishing a patent airway and, if necessary, endotracheal (ET) intubation. Treatment may also consist of careful administration of I.V. fluids (lactated Ringer's or normal saline solution), I.V. mannitol (Osmitrol) to reduce intracranial pressure (ICP), and restricted fluid intake to decrease intracerebral edema. Dexamethasone (Decadron) may be given I.M. or I.V. for several days to control cerebral edema.

Serial arterial blood gas studies allow monitoring of oxygenation and carbon dioxide levels to adjust ventilator settings appropriately.

Surgical treatment of traumatic brain injury may include evacuation of the hematoma or a craniotomy to elevate or remove fragments that have been driven into the brain and to extract foreign bodies and necrotic tissue, thereby reducing the risk of infection and further brain damage from fractures.

Physical therapy, occupational therapy, and social services may be necessary if the patient has physical or cognitive deficits from the injury and requires assistance with activities of daily living.

AGE AWARE A child with a head injury may be referred to a child life therapist for care to facilitate normal growth and development through the use of play and self-expression therapy. In cases of severe injury, the family may require spiritual support and help in considering whether the patient may be a candidate for organ donation.

Nursing interventions

- Observe the patient closely to detect changes in neurologic status, including LOC and pupil size, which suggest further damage or expanding hematoma.
- Clean and debride wounds associated with skull fractures.
- Administer medications, as ordered, including diuretics (such as mannitol) and corticosteroids (such as dexametha-

(*Text continues on page 386.*)

TYPES OF BRAIN INJURY

TYPE	DESCRIPTION
Concussion (closed head injury)	● A blow to the head hard enough to make the brain hit the skull, but not hard enough to cause a cerebral contusion; causes temporary neural dysfunction. ● Recovery is usually complete within 24 to 48 hours. ● Repeated injuries exact a cumulative toll on the brain.
Epidural hematoma	● Acceleration-deceleration injuries disrupt normal nerve functions in bruised area. ● Injury is directly beneath the site of impact when the brain rebounds against the skull from the force of a blow (for example, a beating with a blunt instrument), when the force of the blow drives the brain against the opposite side of the skull, or when the head is hurled forward and stopped abruptly (for example, in an automobile accident when a driver's head strikes the windshield). ■ Brain continues moving and slaps against the skull (acceleration), and then rebounds (deceleration). Brain may strike bony prominences inside the skull (especially the sphenoidal ridges), causing intracranial hemorrhage or hematoma that may result in tentorial herniation.

SIGNS AND SYMPTOMS

- Short-term loss of consciousness secondary to disruption of reticular activating system (RAS), possibly due to abrupt pressure changes in the areas responsible for consciousness, changes in polarity of the neurons, ischemia, or structural distortion of neurons
- Vomiting from localized injury and compression
- Anterograde and retrograde amnesia (patient can't recall events immediately after the injury or events that led up to the traumatic incident) correlating with severity of injury; all related to disruption of RAS
- Irritability or lethargy from localized injury and compression
- Behavior out of character due to focal injury
- Complaints of dizziness, nausea, or severe headache due to focal injury and compression

- Brief period of unconsciousness after injury reflecting the concussive effects of head trauma, followed by a lucid interval varying from 10 to 15 minutes to hours or, rarely, days
- Severe headache
- Progressive loss of consciousness and deterioration in neurologic signs resulting from expanding lesion and extrusion of medial portion of temporal lobe through tentorial opening
- Compression of brain stem by temporal lobe causing clinical manifestations of intracranial hypertension
- Deterioration in level of consciousness resulting from compression of brainstem reticular formation as temporal lobe herniates on its upper portion
- Respirations, initially deep and labored, becoming shallow and irregular as brain stem is impacted

DIAGNOSTIC TEST RESULTS

- Computed tomography (CT) scan reveals no sign of fracture, bleeding, or other nervous system lesion.

- CT scan or magnetic resonance imaging (MRI) identifies abnormal masses or structural shifts within the cranium.

(continued)

TYPES OF BRAIN INJURY *(continued)*

TYPE	DESCRIPTION
Epidural hematoma *(continued)*	
Intracerebral hematoma	● Subacute hematomas have better prognosis because venous bleeding tends to be slower. ● Traumatic or spontaneous disruption of cerebral vessels in brain parenchyma cause neurologic deficits, depending on site and amount of bleeding. ● Shear forces from brain movement frequently cause vessel laceration and hemorrhage into the parenchyma. ● Frontal and temporal lobes are common sites of injury. Trauma is associated with few intracerebral hematomas; most result from hypertension.
Skull fracture	● There are four types of skull fractures: linear, comminuted, depressed, and basilar. ● Fractures of the anterior and middle fossae are associated with severe head trauma and are more common than those of the posterior fossa. ● Blow to the head causes one or more of the types. May not be problematic unless brain is exposed or bone fragments are driven into neural tissue.

SIGNS AND SYMPTOMS

DIAGNOSTIC TEST RESULTS

● Contralateral motor deficits reflecting compression of corticospinal tracts that pass through the brain stem
● Ipsilateral pupillary dilation due to compression of cranial nerve (CN) III
● Seizures possible from increased intracranial pressure (ICP)
● Continued bleeding leading to progressive neurologic degeneration, evidenced by bilateral pupillary dilation, bilateral decerebrate response, increased systemic blood pressure, decreased pulse, and profound coma with irregular respiratory patterns

---

● Unresponsive immediately or experiencing a lucid period before lapsing into a coma from increasing ICP and mass effect of hemorrhage
● Possible motor deficits and decorticate or decerebrate responses from compression of corticospinal tracts and brain stem

● CT scan or cerebral arteriography identifies bleeding site. CSF pressure is elevated; fluid may appear bloody or xanthochromic (yellow or straw-colored) from hemoglobin breakdown.

● Possibly asymptomatic, depending on underlying brain trauma
● Discontinuity and displacement of bone structure with severe fracture
● Motor sensory and cranial nerve dysfunction with associated facial fractures
● CSF rhinorrhea (leakage through nose), CSF otorrhea (leakage from the ear), and hemotympanum (blood accumulation at eardrum)
● With anterior fossa basilar skull fractures, possible periorbital ecchymosis ("raccoon eyes"), anosmia (loss of smell due to CN I involvement), and pupil abnormalities (CN II and III involvement)

● CT scan and MRI reveal intracranial hemorrhage from ruptured blood vessels and swelling.
● Skull X-ray may reveal fracture.
● Lumbar puncture is contraindicated if there's evidence of expanding lesions.

(continued)

TYPES OF BRAIN INJURY *(continued)*

TYPE	DESCRIPTION
Skull fracture *(continued)*	
Subdural hematoma	● Meningeal hemorrhages, resulting from accumulation of blood in subdural space (between dura mater and arachnoid) are most common.
	● It may be acute, subacute, and chronic and unilateral or bilateral.
	● It's usually associated with torn connecting veins in cerebral cortex and rarely from arteries.
	● Acute hematomas are a surgical emergency.

sone) to reduce cerebral edema, analgesics (such as acetaminophen [Tylenol]) to relieve complaints of headache, anticonvulsants (such as phenytoin [Dilantin]) to prevent and treat seizures, and prophylactic antibiotics to prevent the onset of meningitis from CSF leakage.

■ Provide respiratory support, as indicated, including ET intubation and mechanical ventilation, to prevent respiratory failure from brain stem involvement.

■ Assess for cardiopulmonary changes.

RED FLAG Abnormal respirations could indicate a breakdown in the brain's respiratory center and, possibly, impending tentorial herniation—a neurologic emergency. Elderly patients require close monitoring because brain atrophy caused by aging leads to greater space for cerebral edema, and ICP may increase despite an absence of signs or symptoms.

■ Maintain a patent airway and monitor oxygen saturation levels; administer supplemental oxygen, as necessary.

■ Carefully observe for CSF leakage. Check sheets for a blood-tinged spot surrounded by a lighter ring (halo sign) or test fluid with a reagent strip for glucose.

SIGNS AND SYMPTOMS	DIAGNOSTIC TEST RESULTS
● With posterior fossa basilar skull fracture, signs of medullary dysfunction such as cardiovascular and respiratory failure	
● Similar to epidural hematoma but significantly slower in onset because bleeding typically originates in veins	● CT scan, X-rays, and arteriography reveal mass and altered blood flow in the area, confirming hematoma. ● CT scan or MRI reveals evidence of masses and tissue shifting. ● CSF is yellow and has relatively low protein (chronic subdural hematoma).

RED FLAG If the patient has CSF leakage or is unconscious, elevate the head of the bed to 30 degrees to reduce the risk of jugular compression, which can lead to increased ICP. Keep his head properly aligned.

- Assist with the insertion of the ICP monitoring system, and continuously monitor ICP waveforms and pressure, as appropriate.
- Determine cerebral perfusion pressure (CPP) by calculation or with a cerebral blood flow monitoring system.
- Assess hemodynamic parameters to help evaluate CPP.
- Administer medications, as ordered. If necessary, use continuous infusions of medications, such as midazolam, fentanyl (Actiq), morphine, or propofol (Diprivan) to help reduce metabolic demand and reduce the risk of increased ICP. If ICP increases, administer mannitol or furosemide (Lasix), as ordered.
- Monitor intake and output frequently to help maintain a normovolemic state.
- Institute safety and seizure precautions, if indicated.
- Prepare the patient for a craniotomy, as indicated.

TEACHING THE PATIENT WITH A BRAIN INJURY

Before discharge, be sure to cover with the patient and his family:
- the injury and its implications
- medication administration, dosage, and possible adverse effects, and when to notify the physician
- when to report changes in mental status, level of consciousness, or motor ability
- types of therapy that may be beneficial, such as physical therapy, occupational therapy, or counseling
- exercises to maintain or improve muscle tone and function
- signs and symptoms of complications
- the importance of follow-up care
- the benefit of utilizing available community support groups such as the local chapter of the Brain Injury Association of America.

- After the patient is stabilized, clean and dress superficial scalp wounds using strict sterile technique.
- Provide appropriate education to the patient and his family before discharge. (See *Teaching the patient with a brain injury.*)

Appendices
Selected references
Index

Selected signs and symptoms

───────────○───────────

This appendix supplements chapter 2—Assessment, which provides assessment guidelines for patients with neurologic disorders. The appendix provides the definition and common causes of less familiar, accessory, or nonspecific signs and symptoms. It may also more formally define some symptoms already mentioned throughout the text. For an elicited sign, such as Chaddock's sign, it also includes the technique for evoking the patient's response.

A

adipsia Abnormal absence of thirst. This symptom commonly occurs in hypothalamic injury or tumor, head injury, bronchial tumor, and cirrhosis.

agnosia Inability to recognize and interpret sensory stimuli, even though the principal sensation of the stimulus is known. Auditory agnosia refers to the inability to recognize familiar sounds. Astereognosis, or tactile agnosia, is the inability to recognize objects by touch or feel. Anosmia is the inability to recognize familiar smells; gustatory agnosia, the inability to recognize familiar tastes. Visual agnosia refers to the inability to recognize familiar objects by sight. Autotopagnosia is the inability to recognize body parts. Anosognosia refers to the denial or unawareness of a disease or defect (especially paralysis).

Agnosias stem from lesions that affect the association areas of the parietal sensory cortex. They're a common sequelae of stroke.

agraphia Inability to express thoughts in writing. Aphasic agraphia is associated with spelling and grammatical errors, whereas constructional agraphia refers to the reversal or incorrect ordering of correctly spelled words. Apraxic agraphia refers to the inability to form letters in the absence of significant motor impairment.

Agraphia commonly results from a stroke.

Amoss' sign A sparing maneuver to avoid pain upon flexion of the spine. To detect this sign, ask the patient to rise from a supine to a sitting position. If he supports himself by placing his hands far behind him on the examination table, you've observed this sign.

anesthesia Absence of cutaneous sensation of touch, temperature, and pain. This sensory loss may be partial or total, and unilateral or bilateral. To detect anesthesia, ask the patient to close his eyes. Then touch him and ask him to specify the location. If the patient's verbal skills are immature or poor, watch for movement or changes in facial expression in response to your touch.

anisocoria A difference of 0.5 to 2 mm in pupil size. Anisocoria occurs normally in about 2% of people, in whom the pupillary inequality remains constant over time and despite changes in light. However, if anisocoria results from fixed dilation or constriction of one pupil or from slowed or impaired constriction of one pupil in response to light, it may indicate neurologic disease. Determining whether the abnormal pupil is dilated or constricted aids diagnosis.

apathy Absence or suppression of emotion or interest in the external environment and personal affairs. This indifference can result from many disorders, chiefly neurologic, psychological, respiratory, and renal as well as from alcohol and drug use and abuse. It's associated with many chronic disorders that cause personality changes and depression. In fact, apathy may be an early indicator of a severe disorder, such as a brain tumor or schizophrenia.

aphonia Inability to produce speech sounds. This sign may result from overuse of the vocal cords, disorders of the larynx or laryngeal nerves, psychological disorders, or muscle spasm.

Argyll Robertson pupil A small, irregular pupil that constricts normally in accommodation for near vision but poorly or not at all in response to light. Response to mydriatics is also poor or absent. This condition may be unilateral or bilateral, or the degree of involvement in the eyes may be asymmetrical. Chronic syphilitic meningitis or other forms of late syphilis are the most common causes.

asthenocoria Slow dilation or constriction of the pupils in response to light changes. Photophobia may be present if constriction occurs slowly. Asthenocoria occurs in adrenal insufficiency. Also known as *Arroyo's sign.*

asynergy Impaired coordination of muscles or organs that normally function harmoniously. This extrapyramidal symptom stems from disorders of the basal ganglia and cerebellum.

atrophy Shrinkage or wasting away of a tissue or organ due to a reduction in the size or number of its cells. Its etiology may be physiologic, as in ovary, brain, and skin atrophy, or pathologic, such as atrophy commonly associated with neurologic disorders or spleen, liver, and thyroid abnormalities. This symptom is normally observed using inspection and palpation techniques.

attention span decrease Inability to focus selectively on a task while ignoring extraneous stimuli. Anxiety, emotional upset, and any dysfunction of the central nervous system may decrease the attention span.

B

Bárány's sign With warm water irrigation of the ear, rotary nystagmus toward the irrigated side; with cold water irrigation, rotary nystagmus away from the irrigated side. Absence of this symptom indicates labyrinthine dysfunction. Also called the *caloric test.*

Barré's pyramidal sign Inability to hold the lower legs still with the knees flexed. To detect this sign, help the patient into a prone position and flex his knees 90 degrees. Then ask him to hold his lower legs still. If he can't maintain this position, you've observed this sign of pyramidal tract or prefrontal brain disease.

Barré's sign Delayed contraction of the iris, seen in mental deterioration.

Beevor's sign Upward movement of the umbilicus upon contraction of the abdominal muscles. To detect this sign, help the patient into a supine position and then ask him to sit up. If the umbilicus moves upward, you've observed this sign—an indicator of paralysis of the lower rectus abdominis muscles associated with lesions at T10.

Bell's sign Reflexive upward and outward deviation of the eyes that occurs when the patient attempts to close his eyelid. It occurs on the affected side in Bell's palsy and indicates that the defect is supranuclear. Also known as *Bell's phenomenon.*

blepharoclonus Excessive blinking of the eyes. This extrapyramidal sign occurs in disorders of the basal ganglia and cerebellum.

Bonnet's sign Pain on adduction of the thigh, seen in sciatica.

bradykinesia Slowness of all voluntary movement and speech, believed to be due to a reduced level of dopamine in the neurons in the brain stem region. Bradykinesia can be a symptom of inhibited central nervous system functioning and is usually associated with parkinsonism or extrapyramidal or cerebellar disorders. It can also result from the use of certain drugs. Bradykinesia usually affects patients older than age 50, but it may also occur in children who have suffered hypoxic accidents. Associated findings include tremor and muscle rigidity.

C

Chaddock's sign Chaddock's toe sign: extension (dorsiflexion) of the great toe and fanning of the other toes. To elicit this sign, firmly stroke the side of the patient's foot just distal to the lateral malleolus. A positive sign indicates pyramidal tract disorders.

Chaddock's wrist sign: flexion of the wrist and extension of the fingers. To elicit this sign, stroke the ulnar surface of the patient's forearm near the wrist. A positive sign occurs on the affected side in hemiplegia. Although Chaddock's sign signals pathology in children and adults, it's a normal finding in infants up to age 7 months.

cherry-red spot The choroid appearing as a red circular area surrounded by an abnormal gray-white retina. It's viewed through the fovea centralis of the eye with an ophthalmoscope. A cherry-red spot appears in infantile cerebral sphingolipidosis; for example, this spot is detected in more than 90% of patients with Tay-Sachs disease.

circumstantiality Speech in which the main point is obscured by minute detail. Although the speaker may recognize his main point and return to it after many digressions, the listener may fail to recognize it. Circumstantiality commonly occurs in compulsive disorders, organic brain disorders, and schizophrenia.

clonus Abnormal response of a muscle to stretching. It's a sign of damage to nerve fibers that carry impulses to a particular muscle from the motor cortex. Usually, a muscle that's stretched responds by contracting once and then relaxing. In clonus, stretching sets off a series of muscle contractions in rapid succession. Clonuslike, or clonic, muscle contractions are also a feature of generalized tonic-clonic seizures.

cognitive dysfunction   Inability to perceive, organize, and interpret sensory stimuli and to think and solve problems. It may arise from various causes, including central nervous system disturbances, extrapyramidal conditions, systemic illness, endocrine diseases, and deficiency states, or from unknown causes, as in chronic fatigue syndrome.

complementary opposition sign   Increased effort in lifting a paretic leg, demonstrated in the opposite leg. To elicit this sign, help the patient into a supine position, and place your hand under the heel of the unaffected leg. Then ask the patient to lift the paretic leg. If his effort produces marked downward pressure on your hand, you've detected this sign. Also known as *Grasset-Gaussel-Hoover sign.*

confabulation   Fabrication of facts and experiences to cover gaps in memory. The fabrications are generally plausible and detailed. Confabulation is most commonly seen in alcoholism, Korsakoff's syndrome, dementia, lead poisoning, and head injuries.

crossed extensor reflex   Extension of one leg in response to stimulation of the opposite leg; a normal reflex in neonates. It's mediated at the spinal cord level and should disappear after age 6 months. To elicit this sign, place the infant in a supine position with his legs extended. Tap the medial aspect of the thigh just above the patella. The infant should respond by extending and adducting the opposite leg and fanning the toes of that foot. Persistence of this reflex beyond age 6 months indicates anoxic brain damage. Its appearance in a child signals a central nervous system lesion or injury.

D

delirium Acute confusion characterized by restlessness, agitation, incoherence, and often hallucinations. Typically, delirium develops suddenly and lasts for a short period. It's a common effect of drug and alcohol abuse, metabolic disorders, and high fever. Delirium may also follow head trauma or seizures.

disorientation Inaccurate perception of time, place, or identity. Disorientation may occur in organic brain disorders, cerebral anoxia, and drug and alcohol intoxication. It occurs occasionally after prolonged, severe stress.

dysdiadochokinesia Difficulty performing rapidly alternating movements. This extrapyramidal sign occurs in disorders of the basal ganglia and cerebellum.

dysphonia Hoarseness or difficulty producing voice sounds. This sign may reflect disorders of the larynx or laryngeal nerves, overuse or spasm of the vocal cords, or central nervous system disorders such as Parkinson's disease. Pubertal voice changes are termed *dysphonia puberum*.

E

echolalia In an adult: repetition of another's words or phrases with no comprehension of their meaning. This sign occurs in schizophrenia and frontal lobe disorders.

In a child: an imitation of sounds or words produced by others.

echopraxia Repetition of another's movements with no comprehension of their meaning. This sign may occur in catatonic schizophrenia and certain neurologic disorders.

ectropion Eversion of the eyelid. It may affect the lower eyelid or both lids, exposing the palpebral conjunctiva. If the lacrimal puncta are everted, the eye can't drain properly, and tearing occurs. Ectropion may occur gradually as part of aging, or it may result from injury or paralysis of the facial nerve.

entropion Inversion of the eyelid. It typically affects the lower lid but may also affect the upper lid. The eyelashes may touch and irritate the cornea. Usually associated with aging, entropion may also stem from chemical burns, mechanical injuries, spasm of the orbicularis muscle, pemphigoid, Stevens-Johnson syndrome, or trachoma.

extensor thrust reflex In neonates, extension of the leg upon stimulation of the sole. This normal reflex is mediated at the spinal cord level and should disappear after age 6 months.

To elicit the extensor thrust reflex, place the infant in a supine position with the leg flexed; then stimulate the sole. If the extensor thrust reflex is present, the leg will slowly extend. In premature neonates, this reflex may be weak. Its persistence beyond age 6 months indicates anoxic brain damage. Its recurrence in a child signals a central nervous system lesion or injury.

extinction In neurology: inability to perceive one of two stimuli presented simultaneously. To detect this sign, simultaneously stimulate two corresponding areas on opposite sides of the body. Extinction is present if the patient fails to perceive one sensation.

In neurophysiology: loss of excitability of a nerve, synapse, or nervous tissue in response to stimuli that were previously adequate.

In psychology: disappearance of a conditioned reflex resulting from lack of reinforcement.

extrapyramidal signs and symptoms Movement and posture disturbances characteristically resulting from disorders of the basal ganglia and cerebellum. These disturbances include asynergy, ataxia, athetosis, blepharoclonus, chorea, dysarthria, dysdiadochokinesia, dystonia, muscle rigidity and spasticity, myoclonus, spasmodic torticollis, and tremors.

F

Fajersztajn's crossed sciatic sign In sciatica, pain on the affected side caused by lifting the extended opposite leg. To elicit this sign, place the patient in a supine position and have him flex his unaffected hip, keeping his knee extended. Flexion at the hip will produce pain on the affected side due to stretching of the irritated sciatic nerve.

fan sign Spreading apart of the toes after the patient's foot is firmly stroked; a component of Babinski's reflex.

flexor withdrawal reflex In neonates, flexion of the knee upon stimulation of the sole. This normal reflex is mediated at the spinal cord level and should disappear after age 6 months. To elicit this reflex, place the infant in a supine position, extend his legs, and pinch the sole. Normally, an infant younger than age 6 months will respond with slow, uncontrolled flexion of the knee. This reflex may be weak in premature neonates. Its persistence beyond age 6 months may indicate anoxic brain damage. Its recurrence signals a central nervous system lesion or injury.

G

Galant's reflex Movement of the pelvis toward the stimulated side when the back is stroked laterally to the spinal column. Normally present at birth, this reflex disappears by age 2 months. To elicit this reflex, place the infant in a prone position on the examination table or on your hand. Then using a pin or your finger, stroke the back laterally to the midline. Normally, the infant responds by moving the pelvis toward the stimulated side, indicating integrity of the spinal cord from T1 to S1. The absence, irregularity, or asymmetry of this reflex may indicate a spinal cord lesion.

glabella tap reflex Persistent blinking in response to repeated light tapping on the forehead between the eyebrows. This reflex occurs in Parkinson's disease, pre-senile dementia, and diffuse tumors of the frontal lobes.

Goldthwait's sign Pain elicited by maneuvers of the leg, pelvis, and lower back to differentiate irritation of the sacroiliac joint from irritation of the lumbosacral or sacroiliac articulation. To elicit this sign, help the patient into a supine position and place one hand under the small of his back. With your other hand, raise the patient's leg. If the patient reports pain, suspect sacroiliac joint irritation. If he reports no pain, place your hand under his lower back and apply pressure. If the patient reports pain, suspect irritation of the lumbosacral or sacroiliac articulation.

Gowers' sign In an adult: irregular contraction of the iris when the eye is illuminated. This sign can be detected in certain stages of tabes dorsalis. In a child: the characteristic maneuver used to rise from the floor or a low sitting position to compensate for proximal muscle weakness in Duchenne's or Becker's muscular dystrophy.

grasp reflex In infants, flexion of the fingers when the palmar surface is touched, and of the toes when the plantar surface is touched. This normal reflex develops at 26 to 28 weeks' gestation but may be weak until term. The absence, weakness, or asymmetry of this reflex during the neonatal period may indicate paralysis, central nervous system depression, or injury. To elicit this reflex, place a finger in each of the infant's palms. His reflexive grasping should be symmetrical and strong enough at term to allow him to be lifted. Elicit flexion of the toes by gently touching the ball of the foot. The grasp reflex is an abnormal finding in adults, indicating a disorder of the premotor cortex.

Grasset's phenomenon Inability to raise both legs simultaneously, even though each can be raised separately; a normal
finding in infants until age 5 to 7 months. In adults, this phenomenon occurs in complete organic hemiplegia. To elicit it,
help the patient into a supine position, lift and support the affected leg, and then try to lift the opposite leg. In Grasset's
phenomenon, the unaffected leg will drop—the result of an
upper-motor-neuron lesion.

Guilland's sign Quick, energetic flexion of the hip and knee
in response to pinching of the contralateral quadriceps muscle.
This sign indicates meningeal irritation.

HI

---

hallucination A sensory perception without corresponding
external stimuli that occurs while awake. Hallucinations may
occur in depression, schizophrenia, bipolar disorder, organic
brain disorders, and drug-induced and toxic conditions.

 An auditory hallucination refers to the perception of non-
existent sounds—typically voices but occasionally music or
other sounds. Occurring in schizophrenia, this is the most
common type of hallucination.

 An olfactory hallucination—a perception of nonexistent
odors from the patient's own body or from some other person
or object—is typically associated with somatic delusions. It occurs most commonly in temporal lobe lesions and sometimes
in schizophrenia.

 A tactile hallucination refers to the perception of nonexistent tactile stimuli, generally described as something crawling
on or under the skin. It occurs mainly in toxic conditions and
addiction to certain drugs. Formication—the sensation of in-
sects crawling on the skin—usually occurs in alcohol withdrawal syndrome and cocaine abuse.

 A visual hallucination is a perception of images of nonexistent people, flashes of light, or other scenes. It usually occurs

in acute, reversible organic brain disorders but may also occur in drug and alcohol intoxication, schizophrenia, febrile illness, and encephalopathy.

A gustatory hallucination refers to the perception of non-existent, usually unpleasant tastes.

Hoffmann's sign Flexion of the terminal phalanx of the thumb and the second and third phalanges of another finger when the nail of the index, middle, or ring finger is snapped or flicked. A bilateral or strongly unilateral response suggests a pyramidal tract disorder such as spastic hemiparesis. To elicit this sign, dorsiflex the patient's wrist, have him flex his fingers, and then snap the nail of his index, middle, or ring finger.

Hoffmann's sign also refers to increased sensitivity of sensory nerves to electrical stimulation, as in tetany.

hyperesthesia Increased or altered cutaneous sensitivity to touch, temperature, or pain.

hypoesthesia Decreased cutaneous sensitivity to touch, temperature, or pain.

J

Joffroy's sign Immobility of the facial muscles with upward rotation of the eyes; associated with exophthalmos in Graves' disease. To detect this sign, observe the patient's forehead as he quickly rotates his eyes upward.

Joffroy's sign also refers to the inability to perform simple mathematics, a possible early sign of organic brain disorder.

K

Kleist's sign Flexion, or hooking, of the fingers when passively raised; associated with frontal lobe and thalamic lesions. To elicit this sign, have the patient turn his palms down; then gently raise his fingers. If his fingers hook onto yours, you've detected Kleist's sign.

Kussmaul's sign Distention of the jugular veins on inspiration, occurring in constrictive pericarditis and mediastinal tumor. Kussmaul's sign also refers to a paradoxical pulse and to seizures and coma that result from absorption of toxins.

L

Lasègue's sign Pain upon passive movement of the leg, distinguishing hip joint disease from sciatica. To elicit this sign, help the patient into a supine position, raise one of his legs, and bend the knee to flex the hip joint. Pain with this movement indicates hip joint disease. With the hip still flexed, slowly extend the knee. Pain with this movement results from stretching an irritated sciatic nerve, indicating sciatica.

lead-pipe rigidity Diffuse muscle stiffness occurring, for example, in Parkinson's disease.

Leichtenstern's sign Pain upon gentle tapping of the bones of an extremity. This sign occurs in cerebrospinal meningitis. The patient may wince, draw back suddenly, or cry out loudly.

Lhermitte's sign Sensations of sudden, transient, electric-like shocks spreading down the back and into the extremities, precipitated by forward flexion of the head. This sign occurs in multiple sclerosis, spinal cord degeneration, and cervical spinal cord injury.

Lichtheim's sign An inability to speak that's associated with subcortical aphasia. However, the patient can indicate with his fingers the number of syllables in the word he wants to say.

Linder's sign Pain upon neck flexion, indicating sciatica. To elicit this sign, help the patient into a supine or sitting position with his legs fully extended. Then passively flex his neck, noting whether he experiences pain in the lower back or the affected leg from stretching of the irritated sciatic nerve.

lumbosacral hair tuft Abnormal growth of hair over the lower spine, possibly accompanied by skin depression or discoloration. This may mark the site of spina bifida occulta or spina bifida cystica.

M

Macewen's sign A "cracked pot" sound heard on light percussion with one finger over an infant's or young child's anterior fontanel. An early indicator of hydrocephalus, this sign may also occur in cerebral abscess.

malaise Listlessness, weariness, or absence of the sense of well-being. This nonspecific symptom may begin suddenly or gradually and may precede characteristic signs of an illness by several days or weeks. Malaise may reflect the metabolic alterations that precede or accompany infectious, endocrine, or neurologic disorders.

Moro's reflex An infant's generalized response to a loud noise or sudden movement. Usually, this reflex disappears by about age 3 months. Its persistence after age 6 months may indicate brain damage. To elicit this reflex, make a sudden loud noise near the infant, or carefully hold his body with one hand while allowing his head to drop a few centimeters with the other hand. In a complete response, the infant's arms extend and abduct, and his fingers open; then his arms adduct and flex over his chest in a grasping motion. The infant may also extend his hips and legs and cry briefly. A bilaterally equal response is normal; an asymmetrical response may indicate a fractured clavicle or brachial nerve damage. The absence of a response may indicate hearing loss or severe central nervous system depression. Also called the *startle reflex*.

muscle rigidity Muscle tension, stiffness, and resistance to passive movement. This extrapyramidal symptom occurs in disorders affecting the basal ganglia and cerebellum, such as Parkinson's disease, Wilson's disease, Hallervorden-Spatz disease in adults, and kernicterus in infants.

myalgia Diffuse muscle pain, usually accompanied by malaise, occurring in many infectious diseases. These diseases include brucellosis, dengue, influenza, leptospirosis, measles, and poliomyelitis. Myalgia also occurs in arteriosclerosis obliterans, fibrositis, fibromyositis, Guillain-Barré syndrome, hyperparathyroidism, hypoglycemia, hypothyroidism, muscle tumor, myoglobinuria, myositis, and renal tubular acidosis. In addition, various drugs may cause myalgia, including amphotericin B, chloroquine, clofibrate, and corticosteroids.

N

neologism A new word or condensation of several words with special meaning for the patient but not readily understood by others. This coining occurs in schizophrenia and organic brain disorders.

neuralgia Severe, paroxysmal pain over an area innervated by specific nerve fibers. Neuralgia may be precipitated by pressure, cold, movement, or stimulation of a trigger zone; however, in many cases, the cause is unknown. Usually brief, neuralgia may be accompanied by vasomotor symptoms, such as sweating or tearing.

O

orbicularis sign Inability to close one eye at a time, occurring in hemiplegia.

orthotonos A form of tetanic spasm producing a rigid, straight line of the neck, limbs, and body.

PQ

peroneal sign Dorsiflexion and abduction of the foot upon tapping over the common peroneal nerve. To elicit this sign of latent tetany, tap over the lateral neck of the fibula with the patient's knee relaxed and slightly flexed.

Piotrowski's sign Dorsiflexion and supination of the foot on percussion of the anterior tibial muscle. Excessive flexion may indicate a central nervous system disorder.

Prévost's sign Conjugate deviation of the head and eyes in hemiplegia. Typically, the eyes gaze toward the affected hemisphere.

R

Rosenbach's sign Absence of the abdominal skin reflex, associated with intestinal inflammation and hemiplegia. This sign also refers to the fine, rapid tremor of gently closed eyelids in Graves' disease and to the inability to close the eyes immediately on command, as occurs in neurasthenia.

S

Seeligmüller's sign In facial neuralgia, pupillary dilation on the affected side.

Simon's sign Incoordination of the movements of the diaphragm and thorax, occurring early in meningitis. This sign also refers to retraction or fixation of the umbilicus during inspiration.

Soto-Hall sign Pain in the area of a lesion, occurring on passive flexion of the spine. To elicit this sign, help the patient into a supine position and progressively flex his spine from the neck downward. The patient will complain of pain in the area of the lesion.

spasmodic torticollis Intermittent or continuous spasms of the shoulder and neck muscles that turn the head to one side. Typically transient and idiopathic, this sign can occur in patients with extrapyramidal disorders or shortened neck muscles.

stepping reflex In neonates, spontaneous stepping movements that simulate walking. This reciprocal flexion and extension of the legs disappears after about age 4 weeks. To elicit this sign, hold the infant erect with the soles touching a hard surface. Although the stepping reflex is normal, scissoring movements with persistent extension and crossing of the legs or asymmetrical stepping is abnormal, possibly indicating central nervous system damage.

sucking reflex Involuntary circumoral sucking movements in response to stimulation. Present at about 26 weeks' gestation, this reflex is initially weak and isn't synchronized with swallowing. It persists through infancy, becoming more discriminating during the first few months and disappearing by age 1. To elicit this response, place your finger in the infant's mouth. Rhythmic sucking movements are normal. Weak or absent sucking movements may indicate elevated intracranial pressure.

TUVWX

tangentiality Speech characterized by tedious detail that never gets to the point. This occurs in schizophrenia and organic brain disorders.

tibialis sign Involuntary dorsiflexion and inversion of the foot upon brisk, voluntary flexion of the patient's knee and hip, occurring in spastic paralysis of the lower limb. Also known as *Strümpell's sign*.

To detect this sign, help the patient into a supine position and have him flex his leg at the hip and knee so that the thigh touches the abdomen. Or, help the patient into a prone position, and have him flex his leg at the knee so that the calf touches the thigh. If this sign is present, you may observe dorsiflexion of the great toe, or of all the toes, as the foot dorsiflexes and inverts. Normally, plantar flexion of the foot occurs with this action.

tonic neck reflex Extension of the limbs on the side to which the head is turned and flexion of the opposite limbs. In the neonate, this normal reflex appears between 28 and 32 weeks' gestation, diminishes as voluntary muscle control increases, and disappears by age 3 to 4 months. The absence or persistence of this reflex may indicate central nervous system damage. To elicit this response, place the infant in a supine position, and then turn his head to one side.

twitching Nonspecific intermittent contraction of muscles or muscle bundles.

YZ

---

yawning, excessive Persistent involuntary opening of the mouth, accompanied by attempted deep inspiration. In the absence of sleepiness, excessive yawning may indicate cerebral hypoxia.

Rare neurologic disorders

————————◯————————

This table provides information on additional neurologic disorders, or complications of neurologic disorders, along with their description, cause, signs and symptoms, and treatment.

DISORDERS	DESCRIPTION	CAUSES
Alpers' disease	Progressive degeneration of the grey matter of the cerebrum	● Genetic metabolic defect (possible)
Brown-Sequard syndrome	Rare neurologic condition that occurs from spinal cord dysfunction	● Spinal cord lesion or tumor ● Trauma to spinal cord ● Ischemia of spinal cord ● Infectious or inflammatory disease
Cavernous malformation	Rare disorder of the capillaries and small veins in one part of the brain	● Hemangioma formation that affects small capillaries of the brain
Dandy-Walker syndrome	Congential malformation of the cerebellum and the fourth ventricle	● Congenital brain malformation
Empty sella syndrome	Disorder that affects the bony protective covering of the pituitary gland (sella tunica)	● Anatomical defect above the pituitary gland causes it to flatten (primary) ● Surgery, injury, or radiation that causes the pituitary gland to regress within the cavity (secondary)
Farber's disease	Metabolic disorder that causes buildup of lipids in joints, tissues, and central nervous system	● Inherited metabolic disorder

SIGNS AND SYMPTOMS	TREATMENT
• Convulsions • Developmental delay • Mental retardation • Hypotonia and muscle spasticity	• Symptomatic and supportive • Anticonvulsants • Physical therapy
• Loss of pain, temperature, and touch sensation on one side of the body with weakness or paralysis on the other side	• Treatment of underlying cause • Steroids • Symptomatic, supportive care
• Headaches • Seizures	• Symptomatic and supportive • Surgery if hemangioma accessible or bleeding
• Slow motor development • Progressive enlargement of the skull • Signs and symptoms of increased intracranial pressure	• Ventricular-peritoneal shunt
• Obesity and hypertension in women (primary) • Amenorrhea, infertility, fatigue, intolerance to stress (secondary) • Early onset puberty, growth hormone deficiency, pituitary tumors or dysfunction (in children)	• Treatment for pituitary malfunction
• Impaired motor and metal ability • Difficulty swallowing	• Corticosteroids • Bone marrow transplant • Surgical removal of nodes

DISORDERS	DESCRIPTION	CAUSES
Gerstmann's syndrome	Neurologic disorder that occurs after damage to the parietal lobe	• Stroke • Injury to parietal lobe
Hallervorden-Spatz disease	Neurologic movement disorder that results in progressive degeneration of the nervous system, characterized by iron deposition in the brain	• Inherited
Issac's syndrome	Neuromuscular disorder of continuous muscle fiber activity	• Inherited • Toxins (mercury or gold) • Tumor (lung or thymus) • Autoimmune condition
Joubert syndrome	Underdevelopment of the cerebellar vermis of the brain	• Inherited
Kennedy's disease	Motor neuron disease; affects males (onset between ages 20 and 40)	• Inherited: X-linked recessive gene
Landau-Kleffner syndrome	Rare childhood neurologic disorder that affects the part of the brain that controls comprehension and speech	• Unknown
Machado-Joseph disease	Neuromuscular disorder	• Inherited
Neuroacanthocytosis	Neuromuscular disorder that causes degeneration of the basal ganglia and neuron loss in the brain and spinal cord	• Inherited autosomal recessive disorder

SIGNS AND SYMPTOMS	TREATMENT
• Writing disability • Inability to do calculations • Inability to distinguish left from right or identify fingers • Aphasia	• Symptomatic and supportive • Occupational and speech therapy
• Dystonia • Tremor • Rigid extremities • Slow movement • Speech disturbances	• Symptomatic and supportive • Occupational and physical therapy • Dopaminergic agents
• Continuous twitching muscles • Progressive muscle stiffness • Muscle cramping • Increased sweating	• Symptomatic and supportive • Immunosuppressives • Anticonvulsants • Plasma exchange
• Tongue protrusion • Abnormal eye movements • Hypotonia, ataxia • Developmental delay • Hypernea	• Symptomatic and supportive • Physical, occupational, and speech therapy
• Hand tremors • Fasciculations • Limb weakness • Dysphagia • Dysarthria	• Symptomatic and supportive • Physical, occupational, and speech therapy
• Aphasia • Loss of language skills • Seizures	• Corticosteroids • Anticonvulsants • Speech therapy
• Ataxia • Muscle spasticity • Lurching gait • Dystonia	• Levodopa therapy • Antispasmodics • Physical and speech therapy
• Progressive muscle weakness • Muscle atrophy • Chorea • Loss of cognitive function	• Symptomatic and supportive • Antipsychotics • Sedatives • Anticonvulsants • Antidepressants • Physical and speech therapy

DISORDERS	DESCRIPTION	CAUSES
Ohtahara syndrome	Type of seizure disorder	● Unknown
Pelizaeus-Merzbacher disease	Central nervous system disorder that affects the growth of the myelin sheath (leukodystrophy); affects males	● Inherited: X-linked recessive trait
Ramsay-Hunt–type II syndrome	Degenerative neuromuscular disorder	● Mitochondrial defect; possible autosomal recessive trait
Syringomyelia	Cyst formation in the spinal cord that progressively destroys the center of the spinal cord	● Related to congenital abnormality of the brain (Chiari I malformation) ● Trauma ● Meningitis ● Hemorrhage, tumor
Tarlov cysts	Cerebral spinal fluid filled sacs that contain spinal root fibers within the cyst wall or the cyst cavity	● Possible congenital defect
Von Recklinghausen's disease	Neurofibromatosis: tumor growth on nerves	● Genetic disorder
Wernicke-Korsakoff syndrome	Encephalopathy resulting from thiamine deficiency	● Alcoholism ● Dietary deficiency ● Prolonged vomiting, as with eating disorders ● Chemotherapy

SIGNS AND SYMPTOMS	TREATMENT
● Seizures, beginning within the first 10 days to 3 months of birth	● Symptomatic and supportive ● Anticonvulsants ● Corticosteroids
● Nystagmus ● Spastic paraparesis ● Ataxia ● Speech and mental function deterioration	● Symptomatic and supportive ● Anticonvulsants ● Antispasmodics ● Physical and speech therapy
● Tremors ● Seizures ● Muscle incoordination ● Cognitive impairment	● Symptomatic and supportive ● Anticonvulsants
● Progressive weakness of the arms and legs ● Chronic, severe pain ● Loss of hand sensation	● Surgical repair
● Lower back pain ● Sciatica ● Urinary or sexual dysfunction	● Corticosteroid injections ● Surgical drainage or removal ● Fibrin glue injection
● Café-au-lait spots on skin ● Tumors under the skin ● Tumor on the optic nerve ● Small clumps of pigment in the iris ● Bone defects such as bowing of the legs	● Symptomatic ● Surgical removal of tumors
● Altered mental status ● Decreased level of consciousness ● Memory loss ● Vision defects	● Thiamine replacement ● Nutritional therapy and hydration

Resources

———————O———————

This appendix provides contact information for organizations associated with neurologic disorders.

ALS Association
National Office
27001 Agoura Road, Suite 150
Calabasas Hills, CA 91301-5104
Phone: (818) 880-9007
Fax: (818) 880-9006
www.alsa.org

Alzheimer's Association
National Office
225 N. Michigan Ave., Fl. 17
Chicago, IL 60601-7633
Toll free: 1-800-272-3900
TDD: (312) 335-8700
Fax: 1-866-699-1246
www.alz.org

American Cancer Society
P.O. Box 22718
Oklahoma City, OK 73123
Toll free: 1-800-ACS-2345
www.cancer.org

American Stroke Association
National Center
7272 Greenville Avenue
Dallas, TX 75231
Toll free: 1-888-478-7653
www.strokeassociation.org

Bell's Palsy Research Foundation
9713 Lookout Place
Montgomery Village, MD 20886
Phone: (301) 330-FACE (3223)
Fax: (301) 216-2477
www.bellspalsy.com

Brain and Spine Foundation
7 Winchester House
Cranmer Road
Kennington Park
London
SW9 6EJ
Phone: 020 7793 5900
Fax: 020 7793 5939
www.brainandspine.org.uk

Brain Aneurysm Foundation
612 East Broadway
South Boston, MA 02127
Phone: (617) 269-3870
www.bafound.org

Brain Injury Association of America
8201 Greensboro Drive, Suite 611
McLean, VA 22102
Phone: (703) 761-0750
www.biausa.org

Creutzfeldt-Jakob Disease Foundation, Inc.
843 N. Cleveland-Massillon Road, Suite 7A
Akron, OH 44333
Toll free: 1-800-659-1991
www.cjdfoundation.org

Epilepsy Foundation
8301 Professional Place
Landover, MD 20785-7223
Toll free: 1-800-332-1000
www.epilepsyfoundation.org

Guillain-Barré Syndrome Foundation International
GBS/CIDP Foundation International
The Holly Building
104 1/2 Forrest Avenue
Narberth, PA 19072
Phone: (610) 667-0131
Fax: (610) 667-7036
www.gbsfi.com

Huntington's Disease Society of America
505 Eighth Avenue, Suite 902
New York, NY 10018
Phone: (212) 242-1968
Toll free: 1-800-345-HDSA (4372)
Fax: (212) 239-3430
www.hdsa.org

Hydrocephalus Association
870 Market Street, Suite 705
San Francisco, CA 94102.
Toll free: 1-888-598-3789.
Fax: (415) 732-7044
www.hydroassoc.org

Muscular Dystrophy Association
National Headquarters
3300 E. Sunrise Drive
Tucson, AZ 85718
Toll free: 1-800-FIGHT-MD (344-4863)
www.mda.org

Myasthenia Gravis Foundation of America
1821 University Ave. W., Suite S256
St. Paul, MN 55104
Phone: (651) 917-6256
Toll free: 1-800-541-5454
Fax: (651) 917-1835
www.myasthenia.org

National Brain Tumor Foundation
22 Battery St., Suite 612
San Francisco, CA 94111
Toll free: 1-800-934-CURE
www.braintumor.org

National Headache Foundation
820 N. Orleans, Suite 217
Chicago, IL 60610
Toll free: 1-888-NHF-5552
www.headaches.org

National Hydrocephalus Foundation.
12413 Centralia Road
Lakewood, CA 90715-1623
Phone: (562) 402-3523
Toll free: 1-888-857-3434
Fax: (562) 924-6666
www.nhfonline.org

National Institute of Neurological Disorders and Stroke
NIH Neurological Institute
P.O. Box 5801
Bethesda, MD 20824
Phone: (301) 496-5751
Toll free: 1-800-352-9424
TTY (for people using adaptive equipment): (301) 468-5981
www.ninds.nih.gov

National Meningitis Association
738 Robinson Farms Drive
Marietta, GA 30068
Phone: 1-866-366-3662 (1-866-FONE-NMA)
Fax: (877) 703-6096
www.nmaus.org

National Multiple Sclerosis Society
733 Third Avenue
New York, NY 10017
Toll free: 1-800-344-4867
www.nmss.org

National Parkinson Foundation
1501 N.W. 9th Avenue/Bob Hope Road
Miami, FL 33136-1494
Phone: (305) 243-6666
Toll free: 1-800-327-4545
Fax: (305) 243-5595
www.parkinson.org

National Reye's Syndrome Foundation
426 North Lewis Street
Bryan, OH 43506
Phone: (419) 636-2679
Toll free: 1-800-233-7393 (U.S. only)
Fax: (419) 636-9897
www.reyessyndrome.org

National Spinal Cord Injury Association
6701 Democracy Blvd., Suite 300-9
Bethesda, MD 20817
Toll free: 1-800-962-9629
Fax: (301) 990-0445
www.spinalcord.org

National Stroke Association
9707 E. Easter Lane
Centennial, CO 80112
Toll free: 1-800-787-6537
www.stroke.org

Neuropathy Association
60 E 42nd St., Suite 942
New York, NY 10165-0930
Phone: (212) 692-0662
www.neuropathy.org

Reflex Sympathetic Dystrophy Syndrome Association
P.O. Box 502
Milford, CT 06460
Phone: (203) 877-3790
Toll free: 1-877-662-7737
Fax: (203) 882-8362
www.rsds.org

Spina Bifida Association of America.
4590 MacArthur Blvd., NW, Suite 250
Washington, DC 20007 4226
Phone: (202) 944-3285
Toll free: 1-800-621-3141
Fax: (202) 944-3295
www.sbaa.org

Transverse Myelitis Association
1787 Sutter Parkway
Powell, OH 43065-8806
Phone: (614) 766-1806
www.myelitis.org

United Cerebral Palsy Association
1660 L Street, NW, Suite 700
Washington, DC 20036
Phone: (202) 776-0406
Toll free: 1-800-872-5827
Fax: (202) 776-0414
www.ucpa.org

Selected references

———————————○———————————

Barnes, L.L., et al. "Memory Complaints are Related to Alzheimer Disease Pathology in Older Persons," *Neurology* 67(9):1581-85, November 2006.

Bickley, L., and Szilagyi, P. *Bates' Guide to Physical Examination and History Taking,* 9th ed. Philadelphia: Lippincott Williams & Wilkins, 2005.

Cook, R., et al. "Mild Traumatic Brain Injury in Children: Just Another Bump on the Head?" *Journal of Trauma Nursing* 13(2):58-65, April-June 2006.

Coulthard, E., et al. "Treatment of Attention Deficits in Neurological Disorders," *Current Opinion in Neurology* 19(6):613-18, December 2006.

Durand, M.C., et al. "Clinical and Electrophysiological Predictors of Respiratory Failure in Guillain-Barré Syndrome: A Prospective Study," *Lancet Neurology* 5(12):1021-28, December 2006.

Haldemena, D., and Zulkosky, K. "Treatment and Nursing Care for a Patient with Guillain-Barré Syndrome," *Dimensions of Critical Care Nursing* 24(6):267-72, November-December 2005.

Handbook of Pathophysiology. Philadelphia: Lippincott Williams & Wilkins, 2006.

Hayes, J.S., and Arriola, T. "Pediatric Spinal Injuries," *Pediatric Nursing* 31(6):464-67, November-December 2005.

Jankovic, J., and Tolosa, E. *Parkinson's Disease and Movement Disorders,* 5th ed. Philadelphia: Lippincott Williams & Wilkins, 2006.

Lew, H., et al. "Prognostic Value of Evoked and Event-related Potentials in Moderate to Severe Brain Injury," *Journal of Head Trauma Rehabilitation* 21(4):350-60, July-August 2006.

Powe, C. "Cervical Spine Clearance in the Blunt Trauma Patient: A Review of Current Management Strategies," *Journal of Trauma Nursing* 13(2):80-84, April-June 2006.

Professional Guide to Diagnostic Tests. Philadelphia: Lippincott Williams & Wilkins, 2004.

Riazi, A. "Patient-reported Outcome Measures in Multiple Sclerosis," *International MS Journal* 13(3):92-99, November 2006.

Richardson, J., et al. "Successful Implementation of the National Institutes of Health Stroke Scale on a Stroke/Neurovascular Unit," *The Journal of Neuroscience Nursing* 38(4 Supp):309-15, September 2006.

Saburi, G., et al. "Perceived Family Reactions and Quality of Life of Adults with Epilepsy," *The Journal of Neuroscience Nursing* 38(3):156-65, June 2006.

Valvano, J., and Rapport, M.J. "Activity-focused Motor Interventions for Infants and Young Children with Neurological Conditions," *Infants & Young Children* 19(4):292-307, October-December 2006.

Wagner, M., and Stenger, K. "Unruptured Intracranial Aneurysms; Using Evidence and Outcomes to Guide Patient Teaching," *Critical Care Nursing Quarterly* 28(4):341-54, October-December 2005.

Weaver, F.M., et al. "Deep-brain Stimulation in Parkinson's Disease," *Lancet Neurology* 5(11):900-901, November 2006.

Whitnall, M., and Richardson, D.R. "Iron: A New Target for Pharmacological Intervention in Neurodegenerative Diseases," *Seminars in Pediatric Neurology* 13(3):186-97, September 2006.

Zeisel, J. "Environment, Neuroscience, and Alzheimer's Disease," *Alzheimer's Care Quarterly* 6(4):273-79, October-December 2005.

Index

---

i refers to an illustration; t refers to a table.

---

i refers to an illustration; t refers to a table.

---

i refers to an illustration; t refers to a table.

---

i refers to an illustration; t refers to a table.

---

i refers to an illustration; t refers to a table.

---

i refers to an illustration; t refers to a table.

---

i refers to an illustration; t refers to a table.

i refers to an illustration; t refers to a table.

i refers to an illustration; t refers to a table.

---

i refers to an illustration; t refers to a table.

---

i refers to an illustration; t refers to a table.

i refers to an illustration; t refers to a table.

---

i refers to an illustration; t refers to a table.